# INFUSION SYSTEMS IN MEDICINE


*edited by*

## William D. Ensminger, M.D., Ph.D.

Professor, Internal Medicine and Pharmacology
Upjohn Center for Clinical Pharmacology
University of Michigan Medical School
Ann Arbor, Michigan

*and*

## Jean-Louis Selam, M.D.

Associate Professor of Medicine
Director of Clinical Research
University of California, Irvine
UCI/AMI Diabetes Center
Garden Grove, California


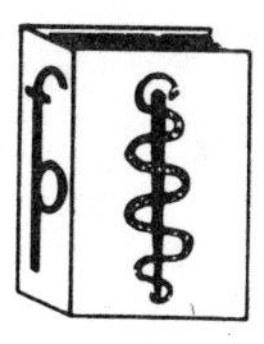


Futura Publishing Company
Mount Kisco, New York
1987

**Library of Congress Cataloging-in-Publication Data**

Infusion systems in medicine.

Proceedings of the Drug Delivery System Symposium, held June
19—21, 1986 in Monaco.
Includes bibliographies and index.
1. Drug infusion pumps—Congresses. 2. Infusion therapy—Con-
gresses. I. Ensminger, William D. II. Selam, Jean-Louis. III. Drug
Delivery System Symposium (1986 : Monaco, Monaco) [DNLM: 1.
Infusion Pumps—congresses. WB 354 I428 1986]
RM170.5.U54   1987                    615'.6              87—23607
ISBN 0—87993—312—7

# Contributors

**P. Abel**
Karlsburg, Germany

**H. Achterberg**
Mainz, West Germany

**Robert C. Arzbaecher**
Chicago, Illinois

**N. Avetyan**
Paris, France

**Anthony Bailey**
Norwood, Massachusetts

**Jurgen Beyer**
Mainz, West Germany

**Perry J. Blackshear**
Durham, North Carolina

**Arthur Boddie**
Houston, Texas

**Jeffrey Brown**
Chicago, Illinois

**Thomas E. Bump**
Chicago, Illinois

**C.W. Burger**
Amsterdam, The Netherlands

**Paul Burke**
Norwood, Massachusetts

**M. Castot**
Paris, France

**William F. Chandler**
Ann Arbor, Michigan

**Laura Claghorn**
Houston, Texas

**Jerry M. Collins**
Bethesda, Maryland

**S. Crepin**
Paris, France

**S. Crespy**
Montpellier, France

**J.C. Daubresse**
Charleroi, Belgium

**Kenneth Davenport**
Chicago, Illinois

**Richard F. Diaz**
Ann Arbor, Michigan

**A. El Harfi**
Montpellier, France

**William D. Ensminger**
Ann Arbor, Michigan

**Uwe Fischer**
Karlsburg, Germany

**F. Fraioli**
Paris, France

**J.P. Fraioli**
Paris, France

**Stephen S. Gebarski**
Ann Arbor, Michigan

**Ulrich Grau**
Frankfurt, Germany

**Harry S. Greenberg**
Ann Arbor, Michigan

**D. Gregonis**
Salt Lake City, Utah

**Alain Guezennec**
Chicago, Illinois

**Franz Halberg**
Minneapolis, Minnesota

**B.K. Hanover**
Salt Lake City, Utah

**P. Henrivaux**
Liège, Belgium

**K.D. Hepp**
Munich, West Germany

**F. Hohleweg**
Mainz, West Germany

**David L. Holmberg**
Salt Lake City, Utah

**Terry W. Wood**
Ann Arbor, Michigan

**William J.M. Hrushesky**
Minneapolis, Minnesota

**Karl Irsigler**
Vienna, Austria

**M.Y. Jaffrin**
Compiègne, France

**Seo Young Jeong**
Salt Lake City, Utah

**Larry Junck**
Ann Arbor, Michigan

**Sung Wan Kim**
Salt Lake City, Utah

**G. Klausmann**
Mainz, West Germany

**Kirsi-Marja Lähteenoja**
Helsinki, Finland

**C.B. Lambalk**
Amsterdam, The Netherlands

**Yves Lazorthes**
Toulous, France

**Pierre J. Lefebvre**
Liège, Belgium

**Allen S. Lichter**
Ann Arbor, Michigan

**Eeva-Liisa Maunuksela**
Helsinki, Finland

**Jacques Mirouze**
Montpellier, France

**André Orsetti**
Montpellier, France

**Geraldine M. O'Shea**
Willowdale, Ontario, Canada

**Michaelyn A. Page**
Ann Arbor, Michigan

**G. Paleirac**
Montpellier, France

**Yehuda Z. Patt**
Houston, Texas

**Clayton R. Perry**
St. Louis, Missouri

**Klaus Piwernetz**
Munich, West Germany

**Jeffrey T. Rabatin**
Minneapolis, Minnesota

**Jukka Rajantie**
Helsinki, Finland

**Gerard Reach**
Compiègne, France

**R. Renner**
Munich, West Germany

**A.M. Rinaldi**
Liège, Belgium

**Reinhard V. Roemeling**
Minneapolis, Minnesota

**A.J. Scheen**
Liège, Belgium

**J. Schoemaker**
Amsterdam, The Netherlands

**J. Schrezenmeir**
Mainz, West Germany

**F. Schue**
Montpellier, France

**G. Schulz**
Mainz, West Germany

**L. Schwartzenberg**
Villejuif, France

**Jean-Louis Selam**
Irvine, California

**Martti A. Siimes**
Helsinki, Finland

**J. Sledz**
Montepellier, France

**Jim Sluetz**
Norwood, Massachusetts

**Marilyn Soski**
Houston, Texas

**Robert L. Stephen**
Salt Lake City, Utah

**Philip L. Stetson**
Ann Arbor, Michigan

**T. Strack**
Mainz, West Germany

**Anthony M. Sun**
Willowdale, Ontario, Canada

**Mark K. Vossen**
St. Louis, Missouri

**D.F. Williams**
Liverpool, United Kingdom

**Dana E. Wilson**
Salt Lake City, Utah

**Charles Yurkonis**
Chicago, Illinois

# Preface

In 1978, Dr. Jacques Mugica (St. Cloud, France) created Cardiostim, soon to become a world famous biennial international congress devoted to cardiostimulation. In 1984, he attached to the congress several satellite congresses, all related to medical bioengineering, such as sensors, biostimulation, and drug delivery systems.

In 1984, the Drug Delivery Symposium was only a one-day meeting. The 1986 symposium, chaired by J. Mirouze and W. Ensminger, and organized by A. Ripart and J.L. Selam, was a very successful three-day symposium.

This book reports the major presentations of the 1986 Drug Delivery System Symposium and, in addition, includes several invited articles from leaders in the field. The articles have been reorganized so that the chapters will roughly cover successively basic concepts/historical background, design and biocompatibility, and clinical applications of drug delivery systems. The Drug Delivery Systems Symposia should continue to grow as more devices become available and clinical applications expand. As a consequence, *Infusion Systems in Medicine* will also appear on a biennial basis with an emphasis in successive years on increasing rapidity of publication.

We hope the vintage 1987 will be a good reflection of the interest and optimism which participants expressed at the 1986 conference.

J. L. Selam, M.D.
University of California at Irvine

W.D. Ensminger, M.D.
University of Michigan

# Contents

IV.  Applications in Oncology

## V. Other Applications

# Conceptual and Historical Background

# Chapter 1

# Pharmacology and Drug Delivery Systems

Jerry M. Collins

## Introduction

Most of our ingrained patterns of drug delivery are a compromise among issues such as convenience for the physician or hospital staff, convenience for the patient, and currently available technology, as well as technical limitations that existed at the time that these patterns became established. Although there have been many unfulfilled promises in the past, there are a wide variety of dependable delivery systems now available that make practical certain types of therapy, which could not be considered in the past. The existence of these new delivery systems dictates that some of our ingrained patterns must be challenged and, ultimately, revised.

As a result of these advances, infusional therapy (also known as controlled-rate delivery) has been broadly applied. Table 1 lists many medical subspecialties[1-10] for which fruitful use has been accomplished. In addition, the conceptual framework, hardware, and technical expertise are now available for many modes of regional drug delivery.[11]

The mere existence of fancy new technology can also provide an inappropriate stimulus toward drug delivery. Every sophisticated patient wants access to the most up-to-date therapy available. Also,

*From:* Ensminger WD, Selam JL (eds): *Infusion Systems in Medicine.* Mount Kisco, NY, Futura Publishing Co., Inc.,©1987.

---

**Table 1**
**Applications of Infusional Therapy**

---

*(Reference Numbers in Brackets)*
Cardiovascular [1,2]
Analgesic [3]
Anesthetic [4]
Endocrine [5]
Psychoactive [6]
Antiasthmatic [7]
Ocular therapy [8]
Anticancer [9]
Infectious diseases [10]

---

some physicians and institutions find prestige in the acquisition and use of the latest gadgetry available. Once an individual or institution has invested in the training, staff, and hardware necessary for a sophisticated approach to drug delivery, it may be very difficult to admit that most situations can be readily handled with a prescription as simple as a monthly injection.

One approach to rethinking therapeutic patterns is to imagine that there are no limitations on the technical ability to produce any desired drug delivery pattern and no economic constraints. What would be the truly ideal delivery pattern in this case? Although it is convenient to blame technical difficulties or cost factors, there are many clinical circumstances for which the optimal solution has not been established.

The role of pharmacology should be to suggest the most desirable delivery pattern and to make a realistic assessment of the relative advantages and disadvantages of various proposed approaches. In some cases, there are sound pharmacologic rationales for the investigation and use of infusional and regional drug delivery systems. Failure to consider the role of delivery pattern should not be a major contributing factor to suboptimal attempts at therapy. Of course, the final selection of hardware, etc. encompasses more than pharmacologic considerations.

To summarize, pharmacology provides the scientific rationale for ideal drug delivery, while economic and technical factors exert a moderating influence. In the final analysis, the clinical utility of these approaches must be demonstrated by clinical trials that are designed and implemented in a definitive fashion.

## Interplay Between Hardware and
## Delivery Schedules

Totally implantable delivery systems are especially useful for situations in which long-term therapy (e.g., more than a few months) is expected. The principal drawbacks of this approach are the expense (and surgical risk) of the device and implantation procedure as well as the pharmaceutical constraints upon the types of drugs that can be delivered with this technology. These constraints include: stability at body temperature, compatibility with other drugs in the same reservoir (if any), and sufficient solubility in order that the desired infusion rate can be delivered within the limits of volumetric output of the device.

External devices are more cumbersome in day-to-day living, and probably subject the patient to a considerably higher risk of infection or catheter-related problems than an internal pump. However, external pumps provide viable solutions to solubility problems, and can be creatively managed to overcome stability and compatibility issues. Further, for short-term therapy, external devices are most frequently used with semipermanent venous access devices which are implanted at lower cost and with a lower risk of morbidity than permanent access devices.

There are some patterns of drug delivery that can only be tested effectively in the clinic. The role of preclinical studies is to orient initial clinical trials in the right direction. Specifically, preclinical studies can guide the choice between brief, intensive periods of therapy versus prolonged therapy. But how long should therapy be continued? The time scale for *continuous* delivery depends upon the nature of the response of the disease as well as the pharmacokinetic properties of the drug.

In some clinical settings, such as oral digoxin therapy, once per day for the lifetime of the patient constitutes effective continuous therapy. When intravenous delivery is required, technical considerations often dominate the decisions regarding length of therapy. Some studies might choose 48 hours, not only because of considerations of the target response, but also because that is the maximum length of time that most institutions use for an ordinary peripheral intravenous infusion set. Five to seven days is another common limit for many types of continuous therapy, as well as a common limit for centrally-placed infusion catheters. In most oncology protocols, it is then accepted practice to wait three to four weeks before starting another cycle of therapy. At our institution, we have used peripheral catheters for 24-hour infusions of carboplatin[12] and dihydroazacytidine,[13] and central lines for five-day infusions of tiazofurin.[14]

The advent of permanent indwelling catheters and pumps that work on 14-day cycles has coincided with several promising trials for the treatment of hepatic metastases from colorectal cancer.[15,16] A new time scale of 14 days on-therapy, 14 days off-therapy has been created. Thousands of patients have been treated on this schedule, most likely with improved response compared with the five-day treatment schedule (randomized comparisons are still in progress). At our institution, we have adopted the 14-day alternating cycle for infusions of bromodeoxyuridine[17] and iododeoxyuridine.[18]

These promising results should not lure us into thinking that we have finally optimized scheduling. Indeed, infusions of 28 to 300 days have been reported[19,20] with considerable apparent benefit.

Sorting out these issues has been complicated by substantial differences in patient populations as well as the drugs under study. Clearly, they serve both to encourage further work on scheduling and also to keep us humble about the actual limitations of our current understanding.

In the discussion of clinical use of drug delivery systems, there was an emphasis on the key role of currently-available technology in defining the types of trials that are undertaken. A similar set of circumstances now exists at the preclinical level.

Despite an increased emphasis upon in vitro screening, all new drugs must undergo safety evaluation in animals in vivo before entering human testing. Exact requirements vary with the class of drug (benefit:risk ratio) and the regulatory climate in each country. Beyond the formality of meeting statutory requirements, there is a wealth of data to be obtained from in vivo testing at the preclinical stage.

Mice are the most commonly used animal species. The implantable osmotic infusion pumps that are usable in mice may not be as fancy as implantable human pumps, but their existence has already changed the way some research is carried out and is beginning to influence the development process for new drugs. Over 1,500 papers have been published that utilized these devices (ALZET Corporation bibliography).

After extensive screening in rodents, many drugs receive final testing in dogs before entry into the clinic. One recent project clearly demonstrated the utility of bringing infusional technology to preclinical testing. Hexamethylene bisacetamide, an investigational anticancer agent, was given by five-day continous infusion to dogs in the final preclinical toxicology testing. A harness was used to place ambulatory infusion pumps on the backs of the dogs. For a variety of reasons, it had been decided that initial clinical testing of this agent would only occur via continuous infusion. Thus, the design of these toxicology studies permitted a close mimicry of expected clinical conditions. Indeed, the starting dose information generated from these studies, as well as the pattern of toxic reactions, facilitated a safe and rapid phase I evaluation of this compound in humans.[21,22]

In summary, the revolution in drug delivery, which has had a major impact upon clinical drug use, is now penetrating preclinical studies and influencing drug development. Presumably, one of the most important rewards will be a more logical selection of those candidates for infusional and/or regional delivery, as well as an opportunity to bring forward candidates with short half-lives, who would have been selected against by traditional screening methods.

## Schedule Selection:
## The Decision-making Process

If the biological effect of a drug depends upon the rate of its delivery, the drug is said to be "schedule-dependent." Both the tolerance of normal host tissues and the target response may be schedule-dependent. The general motivation for the study of schedule-dependence is to improve the therapeutic index for a drug, i.e., to maximize the ratio of therapeutic effects to toxic effects.

The first inclination is to think about schedule-selection for established drugs. While this is an important area in itself, attention must also be focused on the roles of schedule-selection in the process of new drug development. In the context of new drug development, there are several areas of concern that relate to schedule-dependence: (1) Is there an attempt to match exposure conditions between the clinical and preclinical settings? (2) Is the maximal clinical activity of a new drug missed due to initial testing on inappropriate schedules? (3) During preclinical development, is there a failure to discover potentially useful drugs due to testing on inappropriate schedules?

A careful matching of exposure conditions in preclinical and early clinical testing is essential in order to avoid underestimation of the potential of a new drug. Once a drug enters widespread clinical use, it might be argued that empirical testing will eventually optimize its schedule. However, the decision to invest enormous resources for full-scale clinical testing is not made lightly. If preliminary clinical tests do not show promise, there is considerable reluctance for further investment. Thus, there is a burden on even the earliest clinical trials to use the best estimate of an optimal schedule.

Of course, the most promising drugs may never make it to the clinic due to inappropriate testing schedules. If an inappropriate schedule fails to produce the full potential of a drug, its chances for subsequent optimization in the clinic are vanishingly small. It would be an interesting (though ethically difficult) experiment to clinically evaluate compounds that are negative in preclinical screening. In practice, false-negative results are safely buried from further scrutiny.

Although we must be humble about the ability to specify the optimal schedule for drug delivery, it is possible to develop a systematic approach. Some of the factors that can be used as a guide in decision-making are listed in Table 2. For each element, selectivity is the principal concern. Even though the target response might best be achieved via continous exposure to some effective concentration of drug, undesirable drug effects on host tissue must be balanced against the therapeutic goals.

If the mechanism of drug action is known, it can provide some indications about scheduling. For example, if a drug is an irreversible enzyme inhibitor, then the frequency of administration might be matched to the rate of synthesis of new enzyme. Thus, daily administration might be appropriate. On the other hand, if the drug acts as a reversible inhibitor of its target enzyme, then the most important consideration is to keep the drug concentration continuously above some threshold for the desired level of enzyme inhibition.

Early in drug development, the mechanism of action of a new

---

**Table 2**
**Elements of Decision-Making for Schedule-Selection**

Mechanism of action (e.g., reversible or irreversible)
In vitro exposure conditions
Animal models of target response
Animal tolerance
Pilot clinical studies

---

compound may not be known. Empirically, schedule-dependency can be tested in vitro by exposure of cells to the test compound for varying periods of time. The essence of schedule-dependence is variation in effects with time, which is readily tested in cell culture. One common difficulty with this approach is a failure to ensure that the drug is stable for the entire length of incubation.

Testing in vivo is usually performed separately on normal animals and on animals serving as models for the target disease (e.g., a hypertensive strain of rats, or tumor-bearing mice). For some diseases, in vivo models of target response are not available. In these cases, the reliance upon in vitro results will be even greater.

Even when animal models of disease are available, they are usually more expensive and more difficult to manage than normal animals. Therefore, it is more logical to define the set of tolerable conditions in normal animals, and then the set of experiments in the disease model will be reduced. The testing in normal animals provides the physiological constraints that do not exist during studies in vitro.

Thus, there should be an emphasis on tolerance as a function of schedule. Tolerance studies should address: (a) moderation of acute toxicity (peak concentration effects, discussed in the next section); (b) threshold effects; and (c) time-dependence of effects. As noted in the previous section, the technology for addressing these issues is now available.

In addition to acute toxicities, the cumulative effect of repetitive bolus doses may produce undesirable side effects such as cardiotoxicity[23] and pulmonary toxicity.[24]

Pilot clinical studies may considerably modify the impression gained from preclinical studies. For example, the half-life of the drug may be substantially different in humans than in animals. An example occurred in recent studies of a potential anticancer agent, trimetrexate. The half-life in mice was short, 50 minutes,[25] which combined with some indication of improved efficacy in the mouse via continous infusion, led to trials of continuous infusion in man. However, the half-life of 16 hours in humans[26] certainly dampens the basis for infusional therapy.

## Pharmacokinetic Analysis of Peak Levels

Scheduling does not provide a universal answer for problems in drug selectivity. However, there is one form of acute toxicity that is readily ameliorated by scheduling considerations. Acute cardiovascular or central nervous system side effects can often be caused by high peak levels of drug. The peak levels that are produced by a short bolus infusion can be readily reduced by prolonging the time of infusion. Mathematically, continous infusion therapy provides the lowest peak level of any possible schedule. If the limitation of acute toxicity due to peak levels is overcome, then it is possible to increase the total amount of drug delivered to the target. If target effects depend upon total drug exposure, then the delivery of larger doses will be beneficial. If target effects depend upon length of exposure, infusional therapy offers the surest means for controlling exposure time.

To maintain concentrations within the therapeutic range, repetitive bolus doses are most often used. For each dose, there is a corresponding peak concentration observed in plasma, followed by a decline to a nadir before the next dose. The same type of behavior will be seen in all compartments of the body, although the exact details will differ somewhat from the plasma compartment.[27]

If the same total daily dose is given, the peak concentration can be lowered and the nadir raised if the frequency of dosing is increased. In the mathematical limit, delivery of the drug by continuous infusion smooths out the peaks and valleys in drug levels, which are observed following bolus doses. For linear pharmacokinetics, infusional therapy offers the advantage of lower peak concentrations for the same overall dose and same overall exposure (CxT). In other words, continuous infusion therapy alters the pattern of drug exposure, but does not change the total drug exposure (CxT or AUC) for plasma or any tissue.

These kinetic concepts are illustrated in Figure 1. In panel A the concentration versus time behavior is presented for a drug with a half-life of 2 hours. For repetitive bolus delivery once per day, peak levels exceed 8 units and decline to near zero before the next dose. Continuous infusion of the same daily dose yields a steady-state value of about 1.5 units, which is reached in less than half a day. Linear, single-compartment kinetics are assumed. The total drug exposure is identical for both schedules, but the peak levels are

---

**Figure 1:** Comparison of concentration versus time profiles for a five-day continuous infusion compared with five daily bolus doses. **A.** For a drug with a half-life of 2 hours. **B.** For a drug with a half-life of 24 hours.

A

t_1/2=2 Hours
Concentration
Time (Days)

B

T_1/2=24 Hours
Concentration
Time (Days)

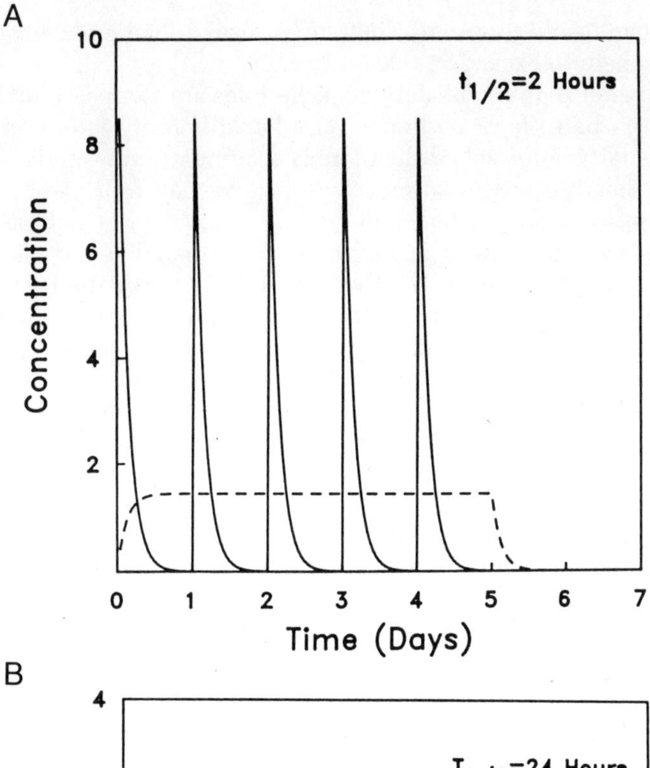

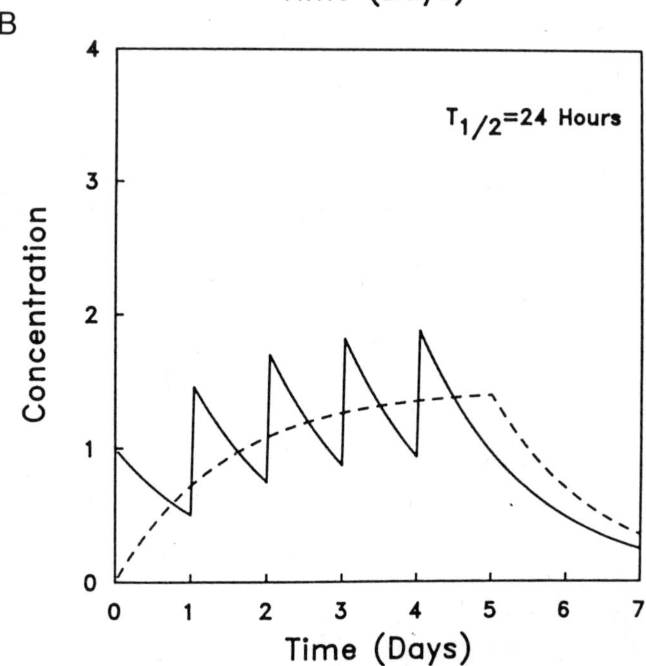

more than 5-fold different. The ratio of peak to valley levels for the bolus schedule exceeds 1,000.

In panel B, the same delivery schedules are compared for a drug that has a half-life of 24 hours. A rather different pattern emerges. For the daily bolus schedule, there is accumulation from day-to-day until a steady-state situation is reached by day four. The peak to valley ratio is only a factor of two. Infusional drug delivery also reaches a steady-state near day four. As in panel A the total drug exposure is identical for the two schedules. Unlike the first panel, the time courses for the two schedules are not radically different.

Thus, the pharmacokinetic optimization of drug therapy is rather straightforward for drugs with a long half-life. There should be no therapeutic advantage for continuous versus intermittent delivery schedules. Additional pharmacodynamic information is not required. Our recent pharmacokinetic study of the antiparasitic agent suramin revealed an extreme example of continuous coverage with intermittent therapy.[28] Since the half-life of this drug is 40 to 50 days, a bolus injection once per month is quite adequate for maintaining continuous exposure.

On the other hand, the pharmacokinetic answer is less definitive for drugs with short half-lives. The pharmacokinetic pattern suggests that it is worthwhile to consider an infusional approach. However, some additional information is needed. If the parent drug is converted to an active form, then the half-life of the active species should be used to determine scheduling. Also, additional data (such as the pharmacodynamic relationship between peak levels and toxicity or efficacy) are usually required.

## Rationale for Regional Drug Delivery

The general goal of selective therapy is to deliver the drug to the desired target while sparing other, possibly sensitive, tissues. Rubbing a cream containing a relatively nonabsorbable antibiotic onto a sore is a common example of a physical approach to drug selectivity. Another common example is the use of oral laxatives, which remain confined to the gastrointestinal tract. The general strategy is known as regional drug delivery, and there are many detailed descriptions of the pharmacologic rationale for this approach.[29-32]

Table 3 lists the various approaches that have been used for regional drug delivery. These can be divided into two categories: di-

**Table 3**
**Routes for Regional Drug Delivery**

| Intravascular | Intracavitary |
|---|---|
| Intraarterial | Intraperitoneal |
| Intra-portal Vein | Intrathecal |
| | Intravesical |

rect injection into an organ's blood supply (intravascular), or direct injection into extracellular fluid spaces in the vicinity of the target tissue (intracavitary). Although intrathecal delivery is used for certain extreme cases of meningeal infections, these types of regional drug delivery are rarely used outside of oncology.

Intraarterial therapy has been extensively analyzed, both in terms of general principles[33-35] and specific locations in the body.[36,37] Similarly, intracavitary therapy has been described in general[38] and for specific sites, such as intraperitoneal[39,40] and intraventricular.[41] Also, there is increasing use of technological advances such as implantable infusion systems for regional delivery.[42]

Regional drug delivery is only appropriate for a narrow set of therapeutic circumstances (Table 4). The most important condition is that the target must be compartmentalized in an accessible region of the body. For example, regional drug delivery cannot be expected to have substantial value in anticancer therapy if the tumor is widely metastatic throughout the body. If intravascular therapy is used, the target must be completely supplied by the infused blood vessel. If intracavitary therapy is used, only target cells in close contact with the injected fluid will experience higher drug levels.[43-45]

Next, the drug of choice must have a very narrow therapeutic index. Otherwise, simply increasing the dose will not be a successful approach to delivering the drug to the target in adequate amounts. Also, the pharmacokinetic properties of the drug of choice and the regional delivery site must offer the opportunity for substantially higher local concentrations than are achieved in the rest of the body.

Finally, the increased risks of these procedures must be balanced by the anticipated improvement in therapeutic index. As a result of this narrow set of specifications, as well as the technical expertise required for successful procedures, regional drug delivery has been limited to a relatively small niche in anticancer drug therapy. Recent advances in both the technical details of the procedures and

---

**Table 4**
**Conditions for Regional Drug Delivery**

---

Target is compartmentalized and accessible.
Drug has narrow therapeutic index.
Substantially higher concentrations must be generated.
Improvements in therapeutic index must outweigh added risks.

---

an understanding of the most appropriate targets have generated a substantial reawakening of interest and activity in this field.

The concepts of "dose-response" and "therapeutic index" are central to an understanding of regional drug delivery. Figure 2 provides a sample set of dose-response curves. It would be preferable to construct and name such diagrams as "concentration−response" curves, but the commonly-used terminology is deeply rooted. The general shape of these curves is sigmoidal and has three areas of interest. At very low concentrations, there is essentially no response produced. Thus, the increased effects caused by higher concentrations are hard to measure versus background. Then, the curve rises more steeply until a maximal response is obtained. We are often uncertain about where we are in a particular clinical application, but the most promising part of the curve is the middle area. For different drugs and different diseases, the slope of this relatively favorable area will range from shallow (not very useful) to very steep (an opportunity to be explored). We always deal with a set of curves rather than a single curve, due to the constraints of normal host tissue toxicity. The therapeutic index of a drug can be expressed as either the horizontal or the vertical difference between these curves, i.e., the differential response of host and target tissues.

Regional drug delivery provides a powerful tool for discovering the in vivo dose response. In the ideal setting, the investigator would know the dose-response curve prior to attempting regional delivery. Indeed, this type of pharmacodynamic information is an important part of the rationale for regional delivery. However, knowledge of dose-response characteristics is often derived from model systems and needs validation in the specific clinical situation for which the therapy is intended.

Once the in vivo dose response from regional therapy has been learned, the approach to therapeutic development can be modified. If the dose-response curve is broad, it is unproductive to pursue either regional drug delivery or aggressive systemic therapy. If the

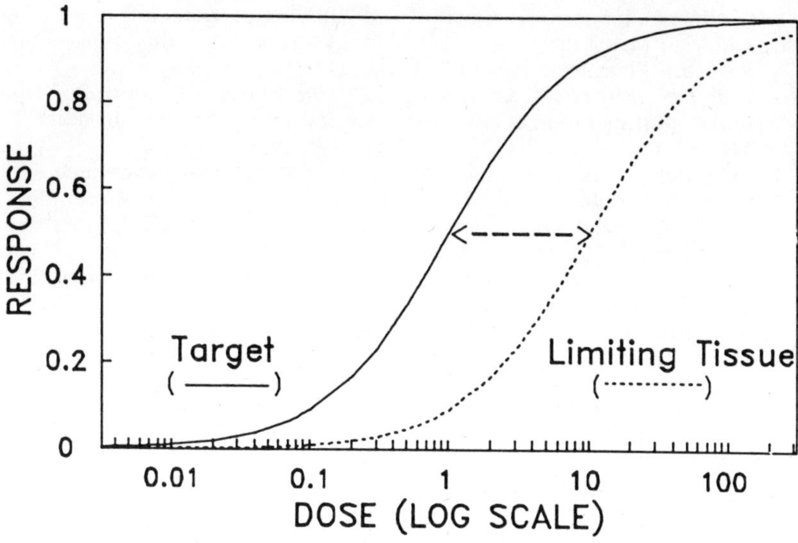


**Figure 2:** Dose response curves for target (solid line) and limiting tissue (dotted line). The horizontal dashed line is one indication of the therapeutic index.

dose-response information is promising, then clearly we are encouraged to pursue regional approaches. But we are also encouraged to more vigorously pursue systemic therapy.

The level of acceptable toxicity depends upon the anticipated benefit. If the therapeutic dose-response curve is steep, then added toxicity might be accepted. If the curve is shallow, pushing the systemic dose is unlikely to be justified. Also, exceptional measures such as autologous marrow repopulation cannot be pursued for every drug and every disease, but only when there is substantial evidence of improved response. Finally, development of antidotes for toxicity or development of new analogs with lessened toxicity are most worthy of pursuit when the dose-response curve is steep.

## References

1. Kleinboesem CH, van Harten J, de Leede LGJ, et al. (1984). Nifedipine kinetics and dynamics during rectal infusion to steady state with an osmotic system. *Clin Pharmacol Ther* 36:396.

2. Graffner C, Johnsson G, Sjogren J. (1975). Pharmacokinetics of procainamide intravenously and orally as conventional and slow-release tablets. *Clin Pharmacol Ther* 17:414.
3. Rutter PC, Murphy F, Dudley HAF. (1980). Morphine: Controlled trial of different methods of administration for postoperative pain relief. *Br Med J* 1:12.
4. Schuttler J, Soecket H, Schwilden H. (1985). Clinical experience with interactive rate control of intravenous anaesthesia. In: Prescott LF, Nimmo WS eds, *Rate Control in Drug Therapy*, Churchill Livingstone, Edinburgh, p 232.
5. Laufer LR, DeFazio JL, Lu JKH et al. (1983). Estrogen replacement therapy by transdermal estradiol administration. *Am J Obstet Gyn* 146:533.
6. Jorgensen A, Overo KF. (1980). Clopenthixol and flupenthixol depot preparations in outpatient schizophrenics. III. Serum levels. *Acta Psychiatr Scand* 61, Suppl 279:41.
7. Weinberger MM, Hendeles L, Wong L. (1981). Relationship of formulation and dosing interval to fluctuation of serum theophylline concentration in children with chronic asthma. *J Pediatr* 99:145.
8. Brown HS, Meltzer G, Merrill RC, et al. (1976). Visual effects of pilocarpine in glaucoma. Comparative study of administration by eyedrops or by ocular therapeutic systems. *Arch Ophth* 94:1716.
9. Carlson RW, Sikic BI. (1983). Continuous infusion or bolus injection in cancer chemotherapy. *Ann Int Med* 99:823.
10. Gerber AU, Craig WA, Brugger HP, et al. (1983). Impact of dosing intervals on activity of gentamicin and ticarcillin against pseudomonas aeruginosa in neutropenic mice. *J Infect Dis* 147:910.
11. Collins JM. (1985). Site-selective and rate-controlled drug delivery by implantable infusion pumps. In Breimer DD, Speiser P eds, *Topics in Pharmaceutical Sciences 1985*, Elsevier, Amsterdam, p 133.
12. Curt GA, Grygiel JJ, Corden BJ, et al. (1983). A phase I and pharmacokinetic study of carboplatinum (CBDCA) NSC 241240. *Cancer Res* 43:4470.
13. Curt GA, Kelley JA, Fine RL, et al. (1985). A phase I and pharmacokinetic study of dihydro-5-azacytidine (NSC-264880). *Cancer Res* 45:3359.
14. Batist G, Klecker RW Jr, Jayaram HN, et al. (1985). Phase I and pharmacokinetic study of tiazofurin (TCAR, NSC 286193) administered by continuous infusion. *Inv New Drugs* 3:349.
15. Balch CM, Urist MM, Soong SJ, McGregor M. (1983). A prospective Phase II clinical trial of continuous FUDR regional chemotherapy for colorectal metastases to the liver using a totally implanted drug infusion pump. *Ann Surg* 198:567.
16. Daly JM, Kemeny N. (1986). Therapy of colorectal hepatic metastases. In DeVita VT, Hellman S, Rosenberg SA ed, *Important Advances in Oncology*, Lippincott, Philadelphia, p 251.
17. Kinsella TJ, Mitchell JB, Russo A, et al. (1984). Continuous intravenous infusion of bromodeoxyuridine as a clinical radiosensitizer. *J Clin Oncol* 2:1144.
18. Kinsella TJ, Russo A, Mitchell JB, et al. (1985). A phase I study of intravenous iododeoxyuridine as a clinical radiosensitizer. *Int J Radiat Oncol Biol Phys* 11:1941.

19. Caballero GA, Ausman RK, Quebbeman EJ. (1985). Long-term, ambulatory, continuous iv infusion of 5-FU for the treatment of advanced adenocarcinomas. *Cancer Treat Rep* 69:13.

20. Lokich JJ. (1986). Epipodophyllotoxin and cisplatin on continuous infusion schedules. In Rosenthal CJ, Rotman M, eds, *Clinical Applications of Continuous Infusion Chemotherapy and Concomitant Radiation Therapy*, Plenum Press, New York, p 43.

21. Egorin MJ, Sigman LM, Van Echo DA, et al. (1987). Phase I clinical and pharmacokinetic study of hexamethylene bisacetamide (NSC95580) administered as a five-day continuous infusion. *Cancer Res* 47:617.

22. Rowinsky EK, Ettinger DS, Grochow LB, et al. (1986). Phase I and pharmacologic study of hexamethylene bisacetamide in patients with advanced cancer. *J Clin Oncol* 4:1835.

23. Legha SS, Benjamin RS, Mackay B, et al. (1982). Reduction of doxorubicin cardiotoxicity by prolonged continuous intravenous infusion. *Ann Intern Med* 96:133.

24. Sikic BI, Collins JM, Mimnaugh EG, Gram TE. (1978). Improved therapeutic index of bleomycin when administered by continuous infusion in mice. *Cancer Treat Rep* 62:2011.

25. McCormack JJ, Heusner JJ, Hacker MP, Mathews LA. (1981). Further pharmacological studies of 2,4-diamino-5-methyl-6-[(3,4,5-trimethoxyanilino) methyl] quinazoline (NSC249008; TMQ). *Proc Am Assoc Cancer Res* 22:245.

26. Lin JT, Cashmore AR, Baker M, et al. (1987). Phase I studies with trimetrexate: Clinical pharmacology, analytical methodology, and pharmacokinetics. *Cancer Res* 47:609.

27. Gibaldi M, Perrier D. (1982). *Pharmacokinetics*, Marcel Dekker. New York.

28. Collins JM, Klecker RW, Yarchoan R, et al. (1986). Clinical pharmacokinetics of suramin in patients with HTLV-III/LAV infection. *J Clin Pharmacol* 26:22.

29. Ensminger WD, Gyves JW. (1984). Regional cancer chemotherapy. *Cancer Treat Rep* 68:101.

30. Collins JM. (1984). Pharmacologic rationale for regional drug delivery. *J Clin Oncol* 2:498.

31. Collins JM, Dedrick RL. (1982). Pharmacokinetics of anticancer drugs. In: Chabner BA, ed, *Pharmacologic Principles of Cancer Treatment*, W.B. Saunders, Philadelphia, p 77.

32. Collins JM. (1987). Regional therapy: An overview. In Poplack DG, Massimo L, Cornaglia-Ferraris P eds, *Pharmacology in Pediatric Oncology*, Martinus Nijhoff, Boston, p. 125.

33. Eckman WW, Patlak CS, Fenstermacher JD. (1974). A critical evaluation of the principles governing the advantages of intraarterial infusions. *J Pharmacokinet Biopharm* 2:257.

34. Chen HSG, Gross JF. (1980). Intra-arterial infusion of anticancer drugs: Theoretic aspects of drug delivery and review of responses. *Cancer Treat Rep* 64:31.

35. Collins JM. (1985). Pharmacokinetic rationale for intraarterial therapy. In Howell SB, ed, *Intra-Arterial and Intracavitary Cancer Chemotherapy*, M Nijhoff, Boston, p 1.

36. Collins JM. (1986). Pharmacologic rationale for hepatic arterial therapy. *Recent Results in Cancer Research* 100:140.
37. Fenstermacher JD, Cowles AL. (1977). Theoretic limitations of intracarotid infusions in brain tumor chemotherapy. *Cancer Treat Rep* 61:519.
38. Collins JM. (1985). Pharmacokinetic rationale for intracavitary therapy. In Howell SB ed, *Intra-Arterial and Intracavitary Cancer Chemotherapy*, M. Nijhoff, Boston, p 41.
39. Dedrick RL, Myers CE, Bungay PM, DeVita VT. (1978). Pharmacokinetic rationale for peritoneal drug administration in the treatment of ovarian cancer. *Cancer Treat Rep* 62:1.
40. Markman M, Cleary S, Lucas WE, Howell SB. (1985). Intraperitoneal chemotherapy with high-dose cisplatin and cytosine arabinoside for refractory ovarian carcinoma and other malignancies principally involving the peritoneal cavity. *J Clin Oncol* 3:925.
41. Collins JM. (1983). Pharmacokinetics of intraventricular administration. *J Neuro-Oncology* 1:283.
42. Gyves JW, Ensminger WD, Stetson P, et al. (1984). Constant intraperitoneal infusion of 5-fluorouracil via a totally implanted system. *Clin Pharmacol Ther* 35:83.
43. Dedrick RL, Flessner MF, Collins JM, Schultz JS. (1986). A distributed model of peritoneal transport. Frontiers in Peritoneal Dialysis. Maher JF, Winchester JF, eds. Field, Rich, and Associates, New York, p 31.
44. Collins JM, Dedrick RL. (1983). Distributed model for drug delivery to the CSF and brain tissue. *Am J Physiol* 245:R303.
45. Blasberg R, Patlak CS, Fenstermacher JD. (1975). Intrathecal chemotherapy: Brain tissue profiles after ventriculocisternal perfusion. *J Pharmacol Exp Ther* 195:73.

# Chapter 2

# The Development of an Implantable Infusion Pump: Historical Aspects, Current Status, and Future Prospects

Perry J. Blackshear

## Introduction

Several types of novel drug delivery systems have been designed in recent years in an attempt to overcome some of the inadequacies of conventional forms of drug delivery. This chapter represents a highly personal, historical view of the development of one such drug delivery system, a totally implantable drug infusion pump for use in animals and humans. My goals are to describe the historical aspects of the device conception and development, then briefly summarize its current clinical status and my views of its future prospects.

A brief chronology of device development includes its conception in August 1969, at the University of Minnesota; the first public description of the device, its design, and initial experimental results at the American College of Surgeons in Chicago in November 1970; an option to license the patent for this device, as applied for by the University of Minnesota, to Metal Bellows Corporation of Sharon, Massachusetts, in April 1971; issue of the patent to the University

*From:* Ensminger WD, Selam JL (eds): *Infusion Systems in Medicine.* Mount Kisco, NY, Futura Publishing Co., Inc.,©1987.

of Minnesota in May 1973; the first clinical implantation of the device in October 1975, for heparin infusion; subsequent human implantation in June 1977, and September 1981, for chemotherapeutic agent infusion and insulin infusion, respectively, also at the University of Minnesota; and a license agreement between the University of Minnesota and Metal Bellows Corporation, executed October 1980. The device, now known as the Infusaid implantable infusion pump, was approved by the Food and Drug Administration (FDA) for the delivery of heparin in patients with refractory thromboembolic diseases, and for the intraarterial infusion of the chemotherapeutic agent 5-fluorodeoxyuridine (FUDR) in March 1982. It was later approved by the FDA for the delivery of several other cancer chemotherapeutic agents, intraspinal morphine for refractory pain of malignant origin, and antibiotics for treatment of refractory osteomyelitis. In October 1980, the pump development division of the Metal Bellows Corporation formed a separate company, the Infusaid Corporation, located in Norwood, Massachusetts. This company has been owned sequentially by Intermedics, Inc. and Pfizer, Inc., and is now a subsidiary of Pfizer operating under the name of Shiley Infusaid, Inc. According to company sources, the current status of overall human implantations worldwide is approximately 20,000 patients as of April 1987. We have recently reviewed the current status of this and related devices.[1]

## Origin

The idea for the development of a drug delivery device of this type was not new; attempts at implanting drug dispensing devices in both human and animal bodies had been carried out since the early 1930s (reviewed in Reference 2). However, these devices were not useful for delivering macroscopic quantities of commercially available drugs into the human body. Rather, they generally consisted of erodible pellets, which would gradually break down over time to release drug into the subcutaneous space or other tissue spaces, or semipermeable polymeric capsules, which would allow slow diffusion of minute quantities of drug into the same tissue spaces. The need for a larger, implantable drug delivery device was initially identified by Dr. Richard L. Varco, then professor of surgery at the University of Minnesota and subsequently one of the pump's inventors. At that time, a prevailing theory held that heparin, a naturally-derived anticoagulant substance with a long history of usage as a drug in humans, if delivered slowly and continuously over long periods of time, might prevent or delay the development of atherosclerosis in susceptible individuals. Dr. Varco reasoned that if one could develop a means of infusing heparin into the ambulatory, i.e., nonhospitalized, patient for long periods of time, one might be able to achieve these beneficial effects on the development of atherosclerosis without the need for continuous hospitalization. His idea was to use one of the methods developed by Dr. Judah Folkman, which involved diffusion of anesthetic agents and other drugs through silicone rubber barriers, by means of, for example, an arteriovenous shunt.

At that time (June 1969), I was hired to work as a summer student in Dr. Varco's laboratory, with my assignment being to investigate the use of these silicone rubber polymers and other diffusion systems then available as a means of delivering heparin continuously at a steady rate into an ambulatory animal or patient. After a series of initial experiments, it became obvious that heparin, because of its large size and powerful negative charge, could not be induced to diffuse through silicone rubber. Other attempts to measure the diffusion of this substance through other polymeric membranes also failed. It became evident that for drugs such as heparin with unusual size and charge properties, a macroscopic drug delivery device such as an infusion pump might be the best way to accomplish the usage requirements. At that point, in discussions with Dr. Henry Buchwald, in whose laboratory I was carrying out these experiments, Dr. Varco, Dr. Perry L. Blackshear, Jr. (my father), a professor of mechanical engineering at the University of Minnesota, and Frank D. Dorman, another mechanial engineer, the idea of a totally implantable drug infusion pump was born.

Out of these preliminary discussions arose essentially all of the ideas for the components of the first prototypes and indeed the eventual commercial device. The major concept making the device possible was the simple physical principle that a vapor in equilibrium with its liquid phase exerts a constant vapor pressure on its surroundings regardless of the enclosing volume. This simple idea, and the fact that the temperature of the human body is maintained at a very constant level under normal circumstances, provided the concept of the pump's vapor–liquid chemical power source. One technical necessity was a chemical substance that produced a sufficient vapor pressure at body temperature to overcome the variability imposed by changes in venous and arterial blood pressure, yet was still nontoxic and noncorrosive to the pump components. Several agents were tried in initial prototype devices, including diethel ether and tetramethyl silane, but by late 1970 the use of a nontoxic, noncorrosive fluorocarbon as the driving vapor pressure had become established.

Another major technical development that made the pump possible was related to this chemical power source. Since the power source was a vapor–liquid mixture, it would clearly have to be separated from the drug reservoir against which it exerted pressure by a totally impermeable barrier. Many forms of collapsible barriers were discussed and then discarded such as polymeric, plastic or rubber membranes, because over time, gas from the power source might diffuse into the drug chamber with resulting change in its properties and loss of driving vapor pressure, or drug might diffuse into the chemical power source chamber. In other words, over the expected life of the pump, which even in the earliest stages of development was envisioned as many years, an absolute permeability barrier between the power source and the drug chamber was mandatory. The concept that made this possible was that of a collapsible metal bellows, which would have the collapsibility characteristic of a rubber membrane but still be totally impermeable to both gas and liquid and not subject to corrosive influences from either. The requirement for such a bellows led us to investigate the current manufacturers of such components in the United States. This led us eventually to the Metal Bellows Corporation of Sharon, Massachusetts, which at that time was one of the few manufacturers of precision welded bellows in this country. Welded bellows were deemed necessary because of the low, constant spring rate that they have, in comparison to formed or molded bellows. The first pump prototypes, therefore, were built with off-the-shelf stock bellows from this company; more on their eventual involvement in the device development below.

Other technical developments that were necessary to complete the device design were the use of a self-sealing silicone rubber/teflon stopper or septum—which was available from commercial sources—use of a special needle to permit puncture of the septum many times without causing damage to the septum, and a long, narrow bore stainless steel or titanium capillary tube, which would serve as the flow regulating resistance element. These components, as well as biocompatible metals and silicone rubber polymers for use in long-term implantation in the body, were already commercially available at the time of the device development, and made possible a biocompatible and functioning prototype in the very earliest stages.

So, armed with these components, the first prototypes were built and tested in vitro at the University of Minnesota in September 1969, and the first animal implantations were performed there in January 1970. It became clear from the earliest bench tests and animal studies that this device was capable of providing reasonably constant drug infusion rates at constant temperatures, such as those prevailing under the skin of an animal or human patient. It was also evident that the uses of such a device for the drug treatment of various disease states in humans were myriad, and we thought that it was appropriate to patent this device and begin a search for possible commercial licensees.

Therefore, in the fall and winter of 1969 and the spring of 1970, when the first prototypes were built in the mechanical engineering shops at the University of Minnesota and later in the hospital machine shop at the University of Minnesota Hospitals, no commercial company had yet been involved in device development except to supply stock component parts for the device. Going from the concept of the device to the first functioning prototypes was not particularly difficult, given the engineering expertise and experience with biocompatible materials of Mr. Dorman and Professor Blackshear, the awareness of the surgical requirements of such a device by Drs. Buchwald and Varco, and ability to test the initial prototypes in the dog laboratories in the Department of Surgery at the University of Minnesota. Thus, once we had identified commercial sources of the various components and decided which off-the-shelf components might be appropriate for use in such a device, the development and testing of the first prototypes proceeded without much difficulty. By that time, I had been hired as a technician at the University of Minnesota while finishing my junior and senior years of college, and the other inventors were already salaried staff members at the University of Minnesota. Other financing for the development of prototypes came from a variety of sources, including Minnesota Medical Foundation Scholarships, private Department of Surgery sources, and some federal grant money for research into the prevention of atherosclerosis awarded to Drs. Buchwald and Varco.

## Development

The patent disclosure for a totally implantable drug delivery device was filed through the University of Minnesota in May 1970.

By this time, it had become clear that the device could deliver heparin at a constant rate into the vascular system of animals, and potentially of man, for long periods of time, and thus might be a useful therapeutic tool. Since this was the first device of its type of which we were aware, it also became evident that a much wider range of drug therapies might be useful using this pump as a drug delivery vehicle. On the basis of these early results, in response to informal contacts within the medical community, and on the basis of the response to the first scientific presentation of our data at the American College of Surgeons meeting in November 1970,[3] it was thought to be advisable to proceed with possible commercialization of the device. We had no interest at that time in forming a company to manufacture and distribute the pump. It had also become clear that a very long research and development period would be necessary before the first clinical implantations of the device would be possible. For this reason, we began looking for companies that would be willing to expend a large research and development effort for many years without expecting a profit in the near term. At this stage the patent disclosure and application had been filed through the University of Minnesota, and it was thought that the time was appropriate to begin making commercial contacts for the possible eventual marketing of a clinically usable device. Thus, the decision to proceed beyond prototype development and into possible eventual commercial usage was made as a more or less consensual agreement among the inventors, the patent officials at the University of Minnesota, and informal advisors.

At that time, we instituted contacts with several medical device organizations. Lengthy discussions were held with Medtronic, Inc., a large Minneapolis pacemaker firm, because of their proximity and their long experience with marketing implantable medical devices. However, on the basis of a marketing survey and other considerations, they decided against becoming involved with pump development at that time (late 1970). One or two other pacemaker firms were approached with equal lack of success. I then wrote to the Metal Bellows Corporation, with whom we had enjoyed an amicable relationship based upon our use of their standard off-the-shelf bellows for prototype construction. This letter was brought to the attention of the president, Mr. Raymond Shamie, who became intrigued with the possibility of manufacturing a medical device based on welded bellows technology and contacted us immediately. A series of discussions ensued among the University of Minnesota, the inventors, and the Metal Bellows Corporation. The University of Minnesota and Metal Bellows Corporation signed an option agreement in April 1971, in which the company agreed to provide certain funds for research and development during the early animal and clinical phases of device development at the University of Minnesota, in return for future exclusive manufacturing rights. At that time, Metal Bellows Corporation did not have any medical device manufacturing or marketing expertise, but the company's feeling was that this could be acquired during the (predicted) long research and development phase.

During the next four years, from 1971–1975, the pump was refined as a joint effort between the University of Minnesota, under the direction of Henry Buchwald, and the Metal Bellows Corporation. The initial prototype construction was improved to accomplish several design requirements, including ease of implantation, decrease of the bellows spring rate, decrease of the flow rate, inclusion of a biologically compatible chemical power source, and other modifications. In addition, during these four years, extensive long-term animal trials, involving the infusion of intravenous heparin or saline into approximately 30 dogs, were carried out at the University of Minnesota Hospitals.[4,5] These studies were performed to test the safety and effectiveness of the device before proceeding with clinical implantation of the device for heparin infusion. In addition, preliminary animal studies were carried out using the pump as a means of delivering the chemotherapeutic agent FUDR into the hepatic artery for the eventual treatment of inoperable liver cancer, and as a means of infusing intravenous insulin in the treatment of patients with diabetes mellitus. During this initial research and development phase, no federal funds were directly involved in the testing of the device, although federal funds were later acquired during some of the clinical trials. As mentioned previously, a patent was issued to the University of Minnesota in 1973.

In 1975, after several years of experience in animals in which both heparin and bacteriostatic water had been infused intravenously with success,[5] the decision was made to proceed to the first clinical implantation of the pump. This was done at the University of Minnesota Hospitals on October 22, 1975, by Dr. Henry Buchwald and his staff. The first patient was a middle-aged woman with severe thromboembolic disease with recurrent pulmonary embolization refractory to therapy with warfarin, an oral anticoagulant. The surgical implantation was uneventful, and the pump functioned perfectly for the duration of this implantation, which was of one year's duration.[6] The pump was removed after one year because of significant weight loss on the part of the patient and evidence that her refractory clotting problem was no longer active after one year of treatment. When it became obvious that the first patient was doing well with the implanted pump, a number of patients with refractory clotting problems underwent pump implantation for the infusion of heparin. These studies were continued for several years and were published in 1980.[7] These studies established in humans, as the animal studies had indicated previously, that the pump could be implanted under the skin safely and without significant morbidity, that it could be left in place for at least several years, that continuous, constant rate drug infusions could be carried out by this means, that the refills could be accomplished at reasonable intervals with minimal patient discomfort, and, in short, that this pump could be used as a totally implantable drug delivery system in man.

Very quickly thereafter, the device research and development effort branched into several new categories. The heparin study was expanded to include patients with severe arterial clotting problems, especially those of the cerebral circulation. After extensive animal testing involving the use of the pump as a means of infusing the chemotherapeutic agent 5-fluorodeoxyuridine (FUDR) into the canine arterial circulation, a grant was applied for and obtained from the National Cancer Institute to support testing of this device as a means of providing intraarterial infusion chemotherapy in patients with inoperable, primary or secondary liver cancer. Accordingly, a series of five patients received implanted infusion pumps for the infusion of FUDR into the hepatic artery at the University of Minnesota Hospitals beginning in 1977.[8] These studies demonstrated that the pump could be used as a means of providing FUDR infusion in these patients with minimal patient morbidity associated with the device itself. This application of the device has become its major clinical use at the present time. Finally, a large series of animal tests were begun and continued to the present time, with the ultimate aim being to demonstrate the usefulness of this device as a means of insulin infusion into animals and eventually human patients with diabetes mellitus. Again, most of the research and development costs during this phase of testing were borne by the Metal Bellows Corporation, although as mentioned previously, the initial clinical trial involving cancer patients was funded by the National Cancer Institute.

During these early studies, the U.S. Food and Drug Administration (FDA) was involved through the mechanism of the Investigational Device Exemption (IDE). The Infusaid Corporation (now Shiley Infusaid) has since acquired premarket approval from the FDA for clinical marketing of the device as an infusion pump for heparin, FUDR, and other cancer chemotherapeutic agents, morphine, and certain antibiotics.

## Current Clinical Status

During its approximately 12 years of clinical use, the Infusaid pump has been implanted in human patients for a wide variety of clinical indications. We have recently reviewed in detail the current clinical status of this pump,[1,9,10] and that of several other newer devices with different pumping mechanisms that seek to provide drug delivery of the same type; no attempt will therefore be made here to review exhaustively the clinical applications now under study. Instead, I will briefly mention some of the types of clinical uses to which this device has been put and discuss briefly the prospects for future drug delivery using devices of this type.

As of April 1987, Shiley Infusaid estimated that about 20,000 devices had been shipped for clinical use. By far the largest use in this country, representing approximately 16,000 patients, has been for the intraarterial, intravenous, or combined intraarterial and intravenous infusion of cancer chemotherapeutic agents such as 5-fluorodeoxyuridine (FUDR) in the treatment of unresectable metastatic hepatic carcinoma, usually from primary tumors of the colon or rectum. The reader is referred to several recent studies concerning the use of this device in this application.[8,11–18] Intraarterial infusion of chemotherapeutic agents is an excellent example of the site-specific drug delivery, which can be achieved using devices of this type. FUDR is quite toxic when administered systemically; delivery directly into the artery supplying the tumor-bearing organ, in this case the liver, maximizes the antitumor effect of the drug while minimizing systemic toxicity. This application also illustrates one of the limitations of devices of this type as far as commercially available approved drugs are concerned; for years, conventional therapy of hepatic metastases from colon and rectal primary carcinomas was the systemic intravenous administration of 5-fluorouracil. However, this drug, which has a reasonable toxicity profile when given in this manner, proved to be too dilute in commercially available formulations to make its use practical in implantable infusion devices of this type.

In addition to this major use of the pump, a wide variety of other unresectable tumors has been treated experimentally by this means. These include cancer of the brain, treated with intraventricular infusions of chemotherapeutic agents, another good example of site specific drug delivery; infusion into the spinal fluid for the treatment of carcinomatous meningitis; localized infusion to other solid tumors; and use of radiosensitizers instead of chemotherapeutic agents as a means of preparing tumors for eventual radiotherapy.

Another major use of this device in this country has been the intraspinal infusion of morphine, generally in a preservative-free preparation, for the treatment of refractory pain from cancer. In this indication, the drug is infused directly into the intrathecal or subdural space, where it serves to provide localized analgesia to the appropriate part of the body, without the profound systemic toxicities of morphine, which include central nervous sytem and respiratory depression. Approximately 2,500 patients have been treated in this manner,[19-24] which represents another excellent example of site-specific drug delivery.

The original clinical application of this pump—treatment of refractory thromboembolic problems with continuous intravenous heparin—has remained a limited use of the device, probably because of the relative rarity of this condition. However, despite the fact that long-term high-dose heparin administration often causes a form of osteopenia, this treatment has been useful in a number of patients with severe clotting problems of the venous or arterial circulation. Two to three hundred patients have received heparin by this means (see References 6, 7, and 25).

A major experimental use of the device has been in the delivery of insulin to patients with diabetes. These studies have, in general, lagged far behind the studies with other drugs because of the serious problem of insulin aggregation in implantable delivery systems of this type, leading to precipitation of the protein and occlusion of delivery tubes and catheters (discussed in Reference 26). Several years ago, we managed to prevent most of this from occurring by using high concentrations of glycerol mixed with insulin,[27] a mixture which has made clinical studies possible. Both continuous basal rate intravenous and intraperitoneal infusions of insulin have been tried; examples of such studies, involving approximately

200 patients to this time, are described in References 28 through 31. Although clinical studies have been possible using the glycerol—insulin mixture, in some cases with pump patency rate up to five years, studies still have been plagued by a high rate of catheter occlusion from insulin precipitates, as well as a predictable rate of loss of insulin bioactivity after incubation in the body at 37° C, both of which have contributed to high dropout rates in the clinical studies. A number of newer insulin formulations are under animal and early clinical investigation at this time, and it is hoped that these new formulations will obviate the problem of insulin precipitation and cathether plugging, and make more widespread clinical studies of this device in the treatment of diabetes practical.

Many other types of clinical uses are being attempted in experimental settings, or with limited numbers of patients. Another example of the application of site-specific drug delivery is in the treatment of refractory osteomyelitis with antibiotics, in which the drugs can be delivered directly to the site of bone infection, resulting in very high local levels of antibiotics while minimizing the profound systemic toxicities of some of these agents. A similar approach might be possible for other localized and refractory infections. Among the experimental treatments still under study are infusion of drugs directly into the cerebrospinal fluid either at the level of the cerebral ventricles or at the spinal level, for treatment of spasticity, amyotrophic lateral sclerosis and Alzheimer's disease, and other degenerative neurological problems. These illustrate the advantages of site-specific drug delivery with an additional wrinkle; that is, some drugs which will not pass the blood—brain barrier can be delivered directly into the central nervous system, which minimizes systemic effects and enhances local drug concentration.

## Future Prospects

Since our device was tested and approved by the FDA for a variety of clinical applications, a number of other macroscopic implantable infusion pumps have been developed to deliver drugs in the same way, although most of them have different internal design principles and are somewhat more sophisticated in terms of variability of drug delivery and other monitoring functions. These devices, which can be viewed as second and third generation devices, with the Infusaid pump representing the first generation, have been reviewed in detail recently.[1] However, in addition to the advantages over conventional drug delivery of the simple Infusaid pump which have been enumerated previously, many of these newer devices offer increased flexibility in dosage adjustment and regulation, telemetered status reports on device function and drug flow rate, and other more sophisticated functions. With this added complexity comes increased expense of the device and ancillary equipment, as well as an increase in the sophistication needed for the operator; it is also possible that this increase in complexity will make the devices more failure-prone in the long-term implanted state. Obviously, once the device is in place under the skin, adjustments, revisions, battery replacements, and device replacements are much more difficult than with most types of conventional drug therapy. My view is that each type of device will be particularly well suited for certain types of indications, and that a spectrum of devices will be usable in the future. For example, a simple but reliable basal rate delivery device such as the Infusaid might be indicated when single infusion rates are required; examples of such applications might include continuous intravenous heparin infusion, intraarterial infusion chemotherapy, other forms of chemotherapy, intraspinal delivery of morphine, and other applications where complex blood profiles are not required. On the other hand, the treatment of Type I diabetes is an excellent example of an application in which a variable flow rate device might be optimal. In addition, the hazards of over- and underinsulinization are such that telemetered feedback is a desirable component of such devices for insulin infusion.

What does the future hold for such devices? Are they merely technical curiosities, or will they become established as new classes of drug delivery devices which will supplant and improve upon conventional forms of drug delivery for the indefinite future? I cannot answer these questions, but my feeling is that for certain types of outpatient drug delivery, where long-term continuous and reliable drug delivery is necessary, these devices will have a secure niche. For example, many new peptide and protein drugs are being devised and can be manufactured in bulk using recombinant DNA technology, which might be suitable for long-term delivery to appropriate patients and for which no good route of administration is currently available. Examples that spring to mind are, besides insulin, recombinant human growth hormone, insulin-like growth factor I, calcitonin, parathyroid hormone or its antagonists, numerous other pituitary and hypothalamic hormones, a wide variety of lymphokine agonists and antagonists, suitably protected enzymes for the treatment of enzyme deficiency diseases, and many others. Once general approaches to the protection of peptide drugs and hormones from the device and from the bloodstream can be perfected, then I think these applications will represent a major use of implantable infusion pumps in the future.

*Acknowledgment*: Portions of this chapter are taken from a report to the U.S. Government Office of Technology Assessment, as part of an investigation into development of innovative devices. I would also like to thank my many colleagues at the University of Minnesota, the Massachusetts General Hospital, and Infusaid Corporation for their help in many aspects of the studies referred to here. I am grateful to Mr. Vincent Bucci of the Shiley Infusaid Corporation for the data on the current clinical uses of the pump, and I thank Lessie Detwiler for typing the manuscript.

---

# References

1. Rohde TD, Buchwald H, Blackshear PJ. (1987). Implantable infusion pumps. In: Tyle P ed, *Drug Delivery Devices: Pharmaceutical and Biological Applications*, New York, Marcel Dekker, Inc.
2. Blackshear PJ. (1979). Implantable drug delivery systems. *Scientific Am* 241:149.
3. Blackshear PJ, Dorman FD, Blackshear PL Jr, et al. (1970). Permanently implantable, self-recycling low flow, constant rate multi-purpose infusion pump of simple design. *Surgical Form* 21:136.
4. Blackshear PJ, Dorman FD, Blackshear PL Jr, et al. (1972). The design and initial testing of an implantable infusion pump. *Surg Gynecol Obstet* 134:51.
5. Blackshear PJ, Rohde TD, Varco RL, et al. (1975). One year of continuous heparinization in the dog using a totally implantable infusion pump. *Surg Gynecol Obstet* 141:176.
6. Rohde TD, Blackshear PJ, Varco RL, et al. (1977). One year of heparin anticoagulation in an ambulatory subject using a totally implantable infusion pump. *Minn Med* Oct: 719.
7. Buchwald H, Rohde TD, Varco RL, et al. (1980). Long-term continuous heparin administration by an implantable infusion pump in ambulatory patients with recurrent venous thrombosis. *Surgery* 88:507.
8. Buchwald H, Grage TB, Vassilopoulos RP, et al. (1980). Intra-arterial infusion chemotherapy for hepatic carcinoma using a totally implantable infusion pump. *Cancer* 45:866.
9. Blackshear PJ. (1985). Implantable infusion pumps: Clinical applications. In Colowick SP, Kaplan NO, eds, *Methods in Enzymology, Drug and Enzyme Targeting*, New York, Academic Press, p 520.

10. Blackshear PJ, Wigness BD, Roussell AM, et al. (1985). Implantable infusion pumps: Practical aspects. In Colowick SP, Kaplan NO, eds, *Methods in Enzymology, Drug and Enzyme Targeting*, New York, Academic Press, p 530.
11. Cohen AM, Wood WC, Greenfield A, et al. (1980). Transbrachial hepatic arterial chemotherapy using an implantable infusion pump. *Dis Colon Rectum* 23:223.
12. Ensminger W, Niederhuber J, Dakhil S, et al. (1981). Totally implanted drug delivery system for hepatic arterial chemotherapy. *Cancer Treat Rep* 65:393.
13. Barone RM, Byfeld JE, Goldfarb PB, et al. (1982). Intra-arterial chemotherapy using an implantable infusion pump and liver radiation for the treatment of hepatic metastases. *Cancer* 50:850.
14. Balch CM, Urist MM, Soong S, et al. (1983). A prospective phase II clinical trial of continuous FUDR regional chemotherapy for colorectal metastases of the liver using a totally implantable drug infusion pump. *Ann Surg* 198:567.
15. Niederhuber JE, Ensminger W, Gyves J, et al. (1984). Regional chemotherapy of colorectal cancer metastatic to the liver. *Cancer* 53:1336.
16. Schwartz SI, Jones LS, McCune CS. (1985). Assessment of treatment of intrahepatic malignancies using chemotherapy via an implantable pump. *Ann Surg* 201:560.
17. Kemeny MM, Goldberg D, Beatty JD, et al. (1986). Results of a prospective randomized trial for continuous regional chemotherapy and hepatic resection as treatment of hepatic metastases from colorectal primaries. *Cancer* 57:492.
18. Kaplan WD, Come SE, Takvorian RW, et al. (1984). Pulmonary uptake of technetium 99m macroaggregated albumen: A predictor of gastrointestinal toxicity during hepatic artery perfusion. *J Clin Oncol* 11:1266.
19. Onofrio NM, Yaksh TL, Arnold PG. (1981). Continuous low-dose intrathecal morphine administration in the treatment of chronic pain of malignant origin. *Mayo Clin Proc* 56:516.
20. Greenberg HS, Taren J, Ensminger WD, et al. (1982). Benefit from and tolerance to continued intrathecal infusion of morphine for intractable cancer pain. *J Neurosurg* 57:360.
21. Harbaugh RE, Coombs DW, Saunders RL, et al. (1982) Implanted continuous epidural morphine infusion system, *J Neurosurg* 56:803.
22. Coombs DW, Saunders RL, Gaylor M, et al. (1981). Continuous epidural analgesia via implanted morphine reservoirs. *Lancet* 2:425.
23. Coombs DW, Saunders RL, Pageau MG. (1982). Continuous intraspinal narcotic analgesia—technical aspects of an implantable infusion system. *Reg Anesthesiol* 7:110.
24. Coombs DW, Saunders RL, Gaylor MS, et al. (1983). Relief of continuous chronic pain by intraspinal narcotic infusion via an implantable reservoir. *JAMA* 250:2336.
25. Chapleau LE, Robertson JT. (1981). Spontaneous cervical carotid artery dissection: Outpatient treatment with continuous heparin infusion using a totally implantable infusion device. *Neurosurgery* 8:83.
26. Blackshear PJ, Rohde TD. (1983). Modern methods of insulin delivery

in the treatment of patients with diabetes. In Bruck SD, ed, *Controlled Drug Delivery*, Boca Raton, CRC Press Inc. Vol II.

27. Blackshear PJ, Rohde TD, Palmer JL, et al. (1983). Glycerol prevents insulin precipitation and interruption of flow in an implantable insulin infusion pump. *Diabetes Care* 6:387.
28. Irsigler K, Kritz H, Lovett RG. (1985). Controlled drug delivery in the treatment of diabetes mellitus. *CRC Crit Rev Ther Drug Carrier Syst* 1:189.
29. Buchwald H, Barbosa J, Varco RL, et al. (1981). Treatment of a type II diabetic by a totally implantable insulin infusion device. *Lancet* 1:1233.
30. Rupp WM, Barbosa JJ, Blackshear PJ, et al. (1982). The use of an implantable insulin pump in the treatment of Type II diabetes. *N Engl J Med* 307:265.
31. Blackshear PJ, Shulman GI, Roussell AM, et al. (1985). Metabolic response to three years of continuous, basal rate intravenous insulin infusion in type II diabetic patients. *J Clin Endocrinol Metabol* 61:753.

# Devices and Biocompatibility

# Chapter 3

# Fundamental Aspects of Biocompatibility

D. F. Williams

## Introduction

Many materials of both natural and synthetic origin are utilized in the construction of medical devices. Traditionally, the word *biomaterial* is used to describe such materials. The exact definition of biomaterial has been a matter of controversy for many years, but the following definition has recently achieved some consensus[1]: "A biomaterial is a non-viable material used in a medical device, intended to interact with biological systems." Included within this definition, therefore, are all those devices that are implanted in tissues. The performance of any such device and of the materials used in its construction is dependent on many properties and features. Some of these naturally relate to the functional requirements of the device, including intrinsic mechanical or physical properties. In most circumstances, however, the single most important feature controlling performance is the biocompatibility of the material under the circumstances in which the device is operating. Even if a material has the desired biofunctionality in respect to the initial performance criteria, without adequate biocompatibility, the material may

*From:* Ensminger WD, Selam JL (eds): *Infusion Systems in Medicine.* Mount Kisco, NY, Futura Publishing Co., Inc.,©1987.

not be able to offer those properties for an appropriate length of time.

## Definition of Biocompatibility

Biocompatibility may be defined as[1]: "The ability of a material to perform with an appropriate host response in a specific application." This definition takes into account a number of features of its interaction between implanted materials and tissues, which have not hitherto been appreciated. First, the emphasis is on an active ability of a material to perform. We are no longer merely concerned with a passive existence of a material that has been designed to be as inert as possible in its tissue location. There is no such thing as a material that is completely inert within physiological environments; there will always be some interaction. Therefore, biocompatibility refers to the ability to perform with the most appropriate interaction with the tissues.

Second, biocompatibility has often been construed to mean the reaction of the tissues to the material. This is not the case; biocompatibility refers to the totality of the interfacial reaction, including both the effects of the material on the tissue and of the tissue on the material. This interfacial reaction is a two-way process that is mutually interdependent. The manifestation of a lack of biocompatibility is usually seen in terms of an adverse tissue reaction, but this is frequently dependent upon a release from the implant of chemical species, this release being induced or caused by the specific features of that environment. Thus, we refer to the ability to perform with an appropriate host reponse in order to reflect the importance of the host response in determining the success of the biomaterial or device and the importance of the entire interfacial reaction in allowing the material to perform with the desired host response.

Third, biocompatibility is qualified by reference to the specific application. What might be an appropriate host response in one situation may not be the appropriate response in another; moreover, the ability to perform with a specified response in one location and under one set of conditions may not apply in a different location and under different circumstances. There is no such thing as a biocompatible material; the property of biocompatibility has to be qualified by the circumstances to which this property pertains.

When considering this interfacial reaction and its consequences, four broad phenomena must be taken into account.

## Immediate Physicochemical Interactions

A biomaterial may be regarded as a solid substance that is placed within an essentially fluid environment that contains, in solution, suspension, or colloidal state, a complex variety of species. Classical laws of physical chemistry dictate that some interfacial reaction will take place such that components from the fluid environment may be adsorbed onto the solid surface. This is the first stage in the interfacial reaction. Under some circumstances, for example, when materials are placed in flowing blood, the adsorption of proteins or other species onto the surface has been demonstrated as a very influential phase in determining the overall biocompatibility. In other situations, for example, implantation into soft connective tissue, similar events certainly occur, but their significance has not yet been clearly demonstrated.

## Material Degradation

Biomaterials have traditionally been selected on the basis of inertness. We now know that all materials will interact to some extent with the tissues, and most will exhibit some form of structural change: metals may corrode, polymers degrade or release leachables, ceramics may dissolve. The kinetics and mechanisms of these processes are extremely important parameters of biocompatibility. It is also very important to appreciate that the physiological environment is as complex as it is hostile, and that many of its constituent species may be involved in the corrosion processes. Thus, proteins may influence metallic corrosion, enzymes cause polymer degradation, cells bring about ceramic degradation by phagocytosis, and so on. In vitro testing in saline solutions is no longer sufficient to determine the stability of biomaterials.

## Local Host Response

The most obvious sequel to an interfacial reaction between biomaterial and host is the response of that host tissue. The nature of this response will depend on many features, relating to material variables, device variables, and host variables, but in concept it may be viewed as a modification of a wound-healing process. Whenever a material is implanted in tissues, those tissues are injured by the process of implantation. The normal wound-healing process is a sequence of events leading through acute inflammation and chronic inflammation to repair, the end result being an area of reparative collagenous tissue. If an implant is present, we may regard it as a persistent stimulus to inflammation so that the usual subsidence of the cellular inflammation in favor of fibroblastic repair will not as readily take place. There is, therefore, a competition between inflammation and repair, with minimal interaction; then repair dominates, leading to the generation of a thin capsule of fibrous tissue around the implants. With a greater interaction, which may be mediated by many mechanisms, the inflammation may persist such that eventually the repair process succeeds but only after it has been forced into excessible fibrosis or alternatively a granuloma, or chronic focus, or inflammation persists.

## Systemic Host Response

The products of the interfacial reaction may not be confined to the local tissue. Released metal ions, corrosion products, leachables, and other debris may gain access to the systemic circulation (vascular or lymphatic). Some may readily be excreted; others may be stored within distant tissues or organs. This systemic distribution can, at least in theory, lead to a number of problems, which may not be readily identifiable with the source of the material. Little is known about the incidence of systemic effects resulting from the use of implanted biomaterials, but such possibilities do find cause for concern.

In summary, our knowledge of biocompatibility is increasing rapidly, and there is now widespread agreement on the nature of the problems concerning biocompatibility. The nature of the interfacial reactions between biomaterials and tissues in their entirety constitute the most important aspect of implantable devices, including the infusion systems that are the subject of this symposium. The specific features relating to the types of material used and their location within the tissue need to be seriously addressed.

---

## Reference


1. Williams DF (forthcoming). European Society for Biomaterials, Consensus Conference on "Definitions in Biomaterials," March 1986, Chester, U.K. To be published by Elsevier Science Publishers, Amsterdam, The Netherlands.

# Chapter 4

# Improvements to Constant Flow Infusion Pumps

Anthony Bailey
Paul Burke
Jim Sluetz

## Introduction

Since its commercial introduction in 1982, the implantable constant flow pump has found wide acceptance in a variety of drug delivery applications. More than 15,000 have been implanted in the five years since its introduction.

During this time, the design of the constant flow pump has remained relatively unchanged. This is primarily due to the high degree of safety and effectiveness experienced with the initial design. For example, implantable constant flow pumps have been reported to have a significantly lower device complication rate than external ambulatory pumps.[1,2]

Notwithstanding the proven reliability of the existing design, there are impetuses for a second generation of the device. The new components and configuration changes discussed here are the results of investigations into improving the implantable constant flow pump.

From: Ensminger WD, Selam JL (eds): *Infusion Systems in Medicine*. Mount Kisco, NY, Futura Publishing Co., Inc., ©1987.

## Current Design

The current pump looks essentially like a disc-shaped titanium can with an elastomer band wrapped around the circumference. A silicone rubber catheter exits the elastomer band tangentially from the side of the pump. The existing pump, with a 50 ml reservoir, is approximately 87 millimeters in diameter, 28 millimeters thick, and weighs 165 grams when empty.

Inside the titanium can is a collapsible titanium bellows, which comprises the drug reservoir. The space between this reservoir and the outer can is filled with a mixture of liquid and vapor phase freon. At constant temperature, the freon vapor exerts a constant pressure on the bellows reservoir, forcing the drug through the filtered outlet in the lid.

The lid also contains a central inlet port, used to refill periodically the drug reservoir via percutaneous injections. This port is capped by a self-sealing silicone rubber septum. There is an additional access port at the outer edge of the pump, providing direct percutaneous access to the catheter.

Roughly 18 meters of 0.08 millimeter internal diameter capillary tubing is connected to the filtered outlet and coiled around the circumference of the pump beneath the elastomer band. The capillary tubing provides flow restriction, thus determining the pump's flow rate.

## Proposed Second Generation Design

The proposed second generation constant flow pump is also disc-shaped; however, it has much smoother, more biocompatible contours. While incorporating more features than the first generation device, it will still be roughly the same size and weight.

The basic configuration of the device has been modified from the earlier can/lid configuration to a "clam shell" configuration, which allows more efficient use of the existing volume.

The new configuration internalizes all flow control components and the sideport. This would eliminate the need for the bulky elastomer band and the sideport protrusion of the previous design.

It also adds an additional degree of reliability to the pump by hermetically enclosing, in an intermediate chamber, all points in the fluid path that are upstream from the flow restriction. In this way, in the unlikely event of an "upstream" connection failure, any unrestricted flow would be "trapped" or contained in the upper chamber.

Several new components have also been added to the pump in this new configuration; namely, a catheter connector, a silicon restrictor, and a flow regulator.

## Catheter Connector

Different drug delivery applications can require different catheter materials and/or configurations. A catheter connector has been investigated for the new constant flow pump configuration in order to provide catheter options at the time of implant.

The configuration of the connector is quite similar to that of a pacemaker lead connection. The proximal end of the catheter terminates in a silicone rubber strain relief, which surrounds a titanium fitting. This fitting plugs into the pump outlet and is retained via a miniature captive setscrew. The setscrew is tightened using a custom torque release wrench, supplied with the catheter.

When implanted, the connector will be exposed to nominal differential pressures of approximately 41 to 55 kPa. The connection may also experience some minimal tension or side loading. The proposed catheter connector has been tested in stepped stress tests up to 207 kPa with both straight and side loads up to 1.1 kg with no discernible leaks. The connection has also been pressure tested with no load up to 690 kPa with the same results.

## Silicon Restrictor (Figs. 1−3)

Photochemically-etched silicon restrictors have been investigated as alternatives in future constant flow pump designs. In the final configuration, the silicon restrictor would be significantly smaller, less expensive, with a potentially broader range of drug compatibility than the current stainless steel capillary tube restrictor.

Three configurations of silicon restrictors are currently being tested for flow accuracy, particulate susceptibility, and drug compatibility. The configurations consist of small, medium, and large fluid diameters with proportional lengths such that all three configurations should provide the same flow restriction.

## PROPOSED CONSTANT FLOW PUMP- FLOW SCHEMATIC

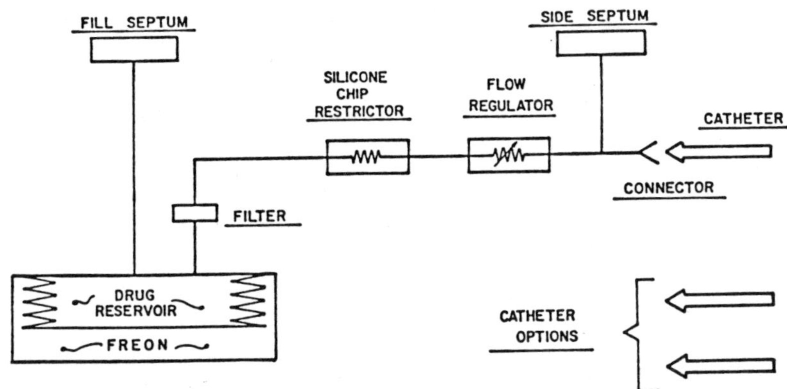



Figure 1.

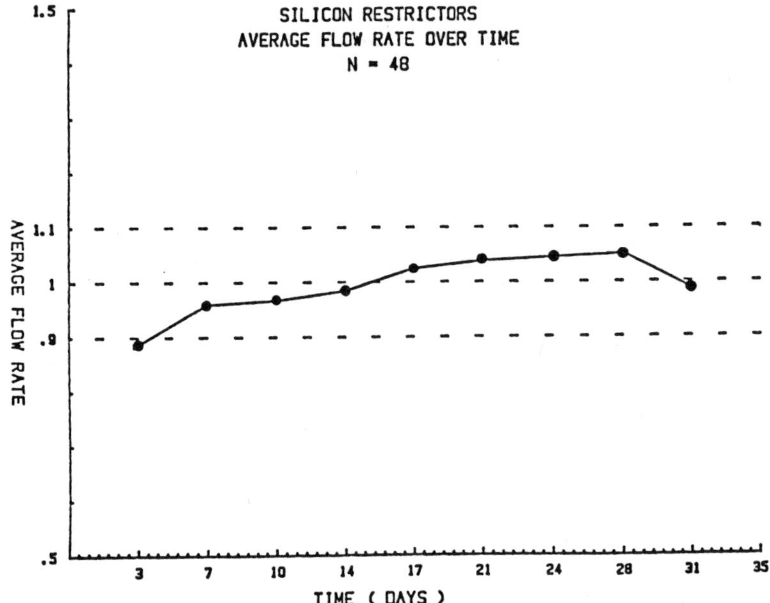



Figure 2.

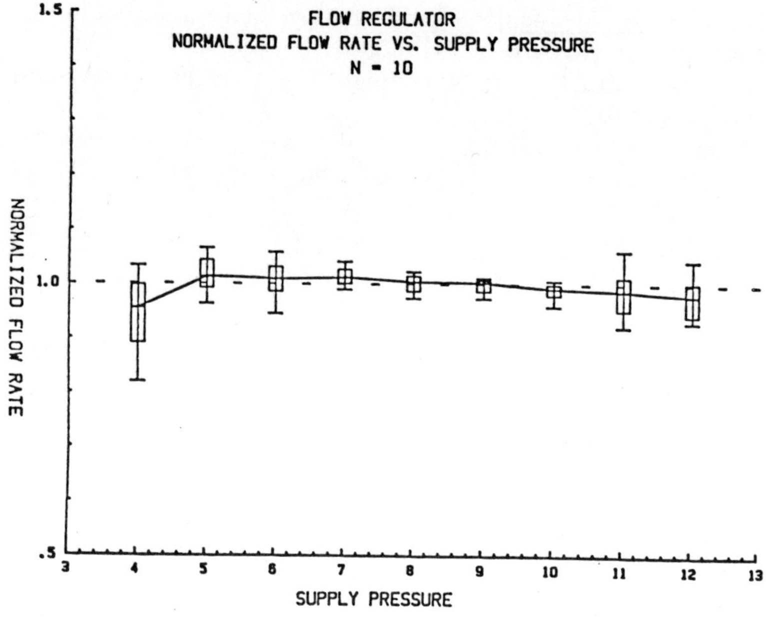


**Figure 3.**

No significant difference in flow accuracy or repeatability was found among the three configurations. Furthermore, accuracy and repeatability of all three configurations were found to be as good as that experienced with capillary tube restrictors.

## Flow Regulator

The existing pump's flow accuracy, as measured in patients by standard pump refill techniques, has been generally reported in the literature as better than ± 10%.[3,4] This has proven quite acceptable for most existing applications.

However, in the current design, flow rates can vary significantly due to extreme changes in temperature and ambient pressure. Therefore, increased flow accuracy has been investigated as a means of easing patient constraints and enabling the pump's use in drug delivery applications where extremely precise doses are critical (such as drugs with a narrow therapeutic to toxic range).

A patented flow regulator has been designed and tested for this purpose. In its most recent configuration, the device has been miniaturized so that it can be adapted to any of the existing constant flow pumps.

Tests demonstrate better than ± 6% flow regulation with this device over the entire range of environmental extremes. Under more typical patient conditions, this would translate to less than ± 2% flow variations.

## Summary

In considering the second-generation implantable constant flow pump, design changes have been investigated that would improve size, shape, flow accuracy, versatility, patient constraints, and manufacturability.

In considering these improvements, maintenance of the integrity and reliability exhibited by the existing design has been of primary importance.

## References


1. Bucci Vincent A, Reiss John B. (1985). The Food and Drug Administration's Regulation of Implantable Infusion Pumps. *Food Drug Cosmetic Law Journal* 40(No.2):245.
2. von Roemeling R, MacDonald M, Langevin T, et al. (1986). Chemotherapy via implanted infusion pump: New perspective for delivery of long-term continuous treatment. *Oncology Nursing Forum* 13(No. 2):19.
3. Penn RD, Paice JA, Gottschalk W, et al. (1984). Cancer pain relief using chronic morphine infusion. *J Neurosurg* 61:305.
4. Ensminger W, Niederhuber J, Dakhil S, et al. (1981). Totally implanted drug delivery system for hepatic arterial chemotherapy. *Cancer Treat Rep* 65(No.5–6):393.

# Chapter 5

# Intraperitoneal (IP) Biocompatible Implants


R.L. Stephen
D. Gregonis
B.K. Hanover


## Introduction

Access to the peritoneal cavity for therapeutic purposes has a surprisingly long history, probably beginning with Warrick, who introduced pure Bristol water and Cohore claret into the abdomen of a patient suffering ascites.[1] In the late 19th century, first Wegner[2] and then Starling established bidirectional solute and water flux when solutions were introduced into the peritoneal cavities of animals.[3] In 1918, Blackfan and Maxcy[4] introduced fluids into the peritoneal cavity as treatment for dehydrated children, and then Ganter undertook the first tentative peritoneal dialyses in 1923.[5] In the 1950s, peritoneal dialysis was accepted as therapy for acute renal failure[6]; and in the 1960s, long-term peritoneal dialysis as renal replacement therapy was established.[7,8] Experience gained in the field of chronic peritoneal dialysis led to the peritoneal delivery of insulin for persons with diabetes[9–11] and chemotherapeutic agents for disseminated abdominal cancers.[12,13]


From: Ensminger WD, Selam JL (eds): *Infusion Systems in Medicine*. Mount Kisco, NY, Futura Publishing Co., Inc., ©1987.

Obviously, there is a need for long-term trouble-free access to the peritoneal cavity, but this has not yet been achieved. Intraperitoneally, difficulties have arisen with fibrin plugging, omental wrapping, and displacement of catheters. However, the most intractable problem is mesothelial overgrowth and sheathing of the IP catheter.[14-16] Cognizant of these difficulties, investigators at the University of Utah investigated new designs and materials for peritoneal access devices.

## Methods

Following a thorough analysis of the survival and reasons for failure of 97 subcutaneous and 56 percutaneous peritoneal catheters,[17] our group designed and fabricated a subcutaneous peritoneal access device for infusion of medications and/or fluids. Design criteria were: subcutaneous in order to avoid exit site problems, and for cosmetic reasons; as large a subcutaneous surface area as is consistent with reconciling ease of needle insertion, relative inconspicuousness and absence of discomfort for patients; a penetrable dome underlying the skin and an impenetrable bowl underlying the dome; the dome and bowl of the access device to be separated by a depth allowing consistent ease of needle insertions (including bevels) up to size 16 gauge and yet to minimize the internal volume; the extraperitoneal section covered with Dacron® velour to insure tissue ingrowth, consequent fixation of the device and sealing of punctures following needle insertion; a short tubular section leading just into the peritoneal cavity; a retaining flange for intraperitoneal fixation; and no intraperitoneal tubular sector (catheter) in order to avoid problems of fibrin plugs, omental wrapping, displacement and intraperitoneal trauma.

Fifty-one of these peritoneal access devices were implanted in 30 patients with insulin-dependent diabetes mellitus (IDDM) and IP insulin was administered by the multiple injection technique. Because of the appearance of mesothelial overgrowth causing device obstruction, different materials were used in the following sequence: polyurethane (14 devices); silicone (18 devices); polyethylene glycol polyurethane, (PuPEG) (19 devices).

Concurrently, discs of the following materials were implanted into the peritoneal cavities of mice: Pellethane 2363-80A; polyvinyl pyrrolidone-coated Pellethane; PuPEG; Pyrolytic-carbon-coated Pellethane. The discs were removed and examined for omental and cellular adhesion at intervals of one week, one month, and three months. Full details have been described.[18]

## Results

### Animal Experiments

Of the materials tested within the peritoneal cavities of mice, PuPEG and polyvinyl pyrrolidone (PVP)-polyurethane demonstrated the most desirable characteristics in terms of absence of omental adhesion and minimal cellular adhesion. However, PVP-polyurethane demonstrated toxic properties when tested by inhibition of cell growth (probably leaching of monomeric vinyl pyrrolidone), whereas the PuPEG was shown to be nontoxic.

### Clinical Studies

Actuarial survival results of access devices using three different intraperitoneal surfaces (Pellethane®, silicone, and PuPEG) are shown in Figure 1. Differences in survival among the three types of devices at 3, 6, 9, and 12 months are statistically significant with PuPEG easily demonstrating the most superior results.

The prime reason for failures occurring with some PuPEG-coated devices has been the appearance of a new form of obstruction. A sac-like composite of omentum lined with mesothelium has become associated with several of these peritoneal access devices (Figure 2). Attachment of this sac is to the section of parietal peritoneum adjacent to the rim of the intraperitoneal flange of the device. Animal experiments with dogs conducted by investigators at the Zentralinstitut fur Diabetes, Karlsburg, have shed some light on this problem. Soon after implantation of the peritoneal access device, there was attachment of omentum to this region, which frequently coalesced to form a sac-like structure. On all occasions, the flange itself remained virtually free of cellular overgrowth, and the parietal peritoneum overlying all of the flange, except that section at the rim, remained free of inflammation. The tentative consensus is that the IP flange is of insufficient mechanical compliance, and irritation of parietal peritoneum at the rim of the flange sets in motion a chain of events that results in an obstructed reservoir: mechanical incompatibility rather than bioincompatibility.

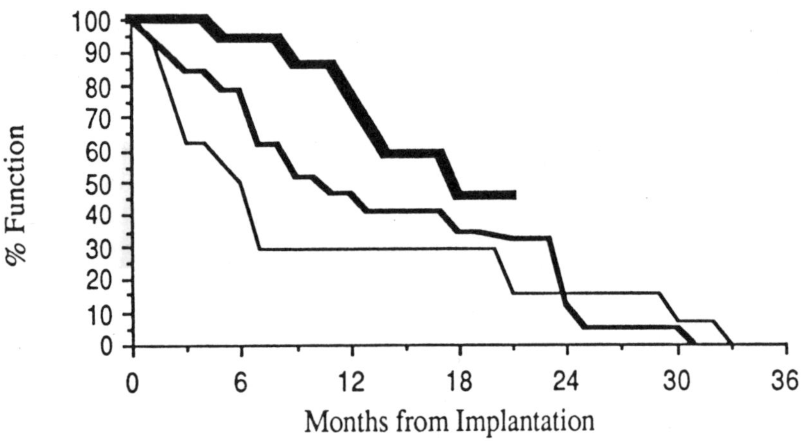


**Figure 1.**

## Conclusion

Satisfactory (>90% for one year) survival of peritoneal access devices is a goal yet to be achieved by investigators working in this field. The best material for intraperitoneal devices used so far at the University of Utah is PuPEG, which combines the desirable structural characteristics of polyurethanes with the biocompatible surface properties of a hydrogel (PEG). It is also important that materials implanted intraperitonally assume a mechanical compliance as close to that of surrounding tissues as possible; otherwise, an "irritative" incompatibility becomes manifest with the same obstructive end result as bioincompatibility.

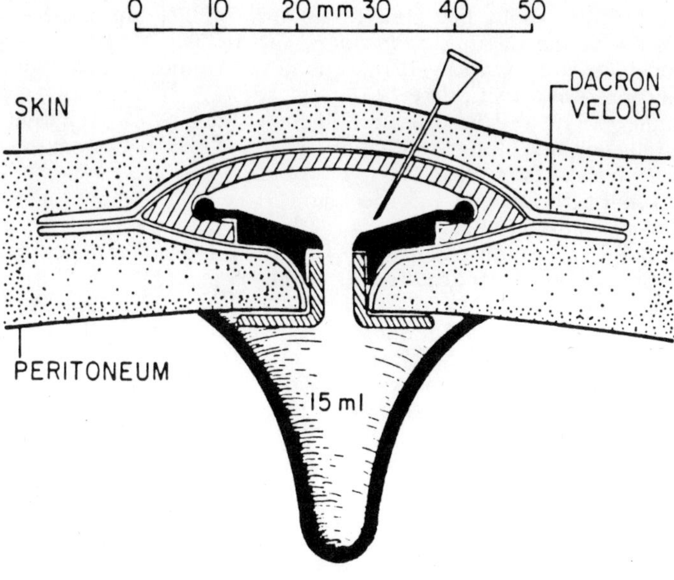


**Figure 2.**

Acknowledgment: The authors wish to thank the staff of the Research Institute at the Zentralinstitut fur Diabetes, Karlsburg, German Democratic Republic, for their cooperation in these investigations.

# References

1. Warrick C. (1744−1745). An Improvement on the Practice of Tapping; by Which That Operation Instead of a Relief for Symptoms, Becomes an Absolute Cure for an Ascites. *Philos Trans R Soc Lond (Biol)* 43:5.
2. Wegner G. (1877). Chirurgische Bermerkungen Uber Die Peritoneal-hohle Mot Besonderer Seruchsichtigung Der Ovariotomie (Surgical Considerations Regarding the Peritoneal Cavity with Special Attention to Ovariotomy). *Langenbects Arch Chir* 20:51.

3. Starling EH, Tubby EH. (1895). On Absorption From and Secretions into the Serous Cavities. *J Physiol (Lond)* 18:106.
4. Blackfan KD, Maxcy KF. (1918). The Intraperitoneal Injection of Saline Solution. *Am J Dis Child* 2:1257.
5. Ganter G. (1923). Uber Die Beseitigung Giftiger Stoffe Aus Dem Blute Durch Dialyse (On the Elimination of Toxic Substances from the Blood by Dialysis). *MMW* 70:1478.
6. Maxwell MH, Rockney RE, Kleeman CR, Twiss MR. (1959). Peritoneal Dialysis.*JAMA* 170:917.
7. Palmer RA, Quinton WE, Gray JE. (1964). Prolonged Peritoneal Dialysis for Chronic Renal Failure. *Lancet* 1:700.
8. Tenckhoff H, Schechter H. (1968). A Bacteriologically Safe Peritoneal Access Device. *Trans Am Soc Art Int Organs* 14:181–186.
9. Schade DS, Eaton RP, Spencer W, et al. (1979). The Peritoneal Absorption of Insulin in Diabetic Man: A Potential Site for a Mechanical Insulin Delivery System. *Metab* 28(3):195.
10. Irsigler K, Kritz H, Hagmuller G, Franetzki M, Prestele K, Thurow H, Geisen K. (1981). Long-Term Continuous Intraperitoneal Insulin Infusion with an Implanted Remote-Controlled Insulin Infusion Device. *Diabetes* 30:1072–1075.
11. Stephen RL, Jacobsen SC, Maxwell JG, Kablitz C, Maddock Jr RK, Tyler FH. (1982). Long-Term Intraperitoneal Insulin Treatment: Preliminary Studies in 12 Diabetic Patients. *Diabetic Renal–Retinal Syndrome* 2(4):447–461, Section: *Prevention and Management* (eds) E.A. Friedman, F.A., L'Esperance, Jr.,: Grune and Stratton, Inc.
12. Dedrick RL, Myers CE, Bungay RM, DeVita Jr VT. (1978). Pharmacolokinetic Rationale for Peritoneal Drug Administration in the Treatment of Ovarian Cancer. *Canc Treat Rep* 62:11–19.
13. Sugarbaker PH, Gianola FJ, Speyer JC, Wesley R, Barofsky I, Meyers CE. Prospective, Randomized Trial of Intravenous Intraperitoneal 5-Fluorouracil in Patients with Advanced Primary Colon or Rectal Cancer. *Surgery* 98(3):414–422.
14. Ponce SP, Pierratos A, Izatt S, Mathews R, Khanna R, Zellerman G, Oreopoulos OG. (1982). Comparison of the Survival and Complications of Three Permanent Peritoneal Dialysis Catheters. *Peritoneal Dial Bul* 2(2):82–86.
15. Selam JL, Giraud P, Mirouze J, Saeidi S, Hedon B, Slingeneyer A, Lapinski H, Humeau C. (1985). Continuous Peritoneal Insulin Infusion with Portable Pumps: Factors Affecting the Operating Life of the Chronic Catheter. *Diab Care* 8:34–38.
16. Pfeifle CE, Howell SB, Markham M, Lucas WE. (1984). Totally Implantable System for Peritoneal Access. *J Clin Oncol* 2(11):1277–1280.
17. Kablitz C, Hanover BK, Maxwell JG, Nelson EW, Harrow JJ, Stephen RL, Jacobsen SC. (1984). Intraperitoneal Access Survival. *Trans Am Soc Artif Int Organs* XXX:652–656.
18. Hunter SK, Gregonis DE, Coleman DL, Hanover BK, Stephen RL, Jacobsen SC. (1983). Surface Modification of Polyurethane to Promote Long-Term Patency of Peritoneal Access Devices. *ASAIO Trans* XXIX:250–254.

# Clinical Applications in Diabetes Mellitus and Endocrinology

# Chapter 6

# Towards the Implantable Artificial Pancreas

Jean-Louis Selam

## Introduction

The pathogenesis of long-term complications associated with insulin dependent diabetes mellitus (IDDM) remains a contentious issue between two schools of thought: either accelerated macro-angiopathy, microangiopathy, and neuropathy are genetically determined and independent of biochemical derangements; or they result from metabolic abnormalities. Although this issue is not yet decided, proponents of the "metabolic" theory have gathered impressive clinical evidence,[1-4] confirmatory data from animal models,[5,6] and demonstrable histologic changes,[7-12] which correlate with metabolic abnormalities.[13-18] Conversely, there are other reports[19-24] either directly opposing or questioning this published evidence. Nevertheless, at present it is a reasonable assumption that long-term diabetic abnormalities with genetic factors play a modifying role.

Hyperglycemia is the most important, but not the only[25] metabolic abnormality potentially responsible for long-term complication. Even hypoglycemia might aggravate the complications of diabetes.[26] Conventional insulin therapy has been unable to normalize both blood glucose[27-29] and other metabolic and hormonal abnor-

From: Ensminger WD, Selam JL (eds): *Infusion Systems in Medicine.* Mount Kisco, NY, Futura Publishing Co., Inc., ©1987.

malities.[30] In an ongoing National Survey in France, insulin-treated diabetics have been found to have a mean blood glucose of about 200 mg/dL and a normal hemoglobin Alc in less than 10% of the cases.[31]

Thus, newer methods of intensified intermittent subcutaneous insulin injection (ISII) treatment have been used to achieve normal blood glucose levels in insulin-dependent or type 1 diabetes.[32-35] This treatment modality requires intensive patient and provider activity, including multiple injections of insulin daily, multiple self-blood glucose measurements daily, and frequent clinic visits. Intensive subcutaneous insulin treatment includes multiple insulin delivery strategies, one of which is continuous subcutaneous insulin infusion (CSII), without continuous feedback control ("open loop" system).

The effectiveness of intensive ISII and CSII in studies using relatively smaller experimental groups of diabetic patients studied for a year or less indicate that both intensive methods, i.e., ISII or CSII, can normalize glycosylated hemoglobin levels.[35-39] In larger nonresearch patient populations, however, the long-term safety and effectiveness of intensive ISII and CSII treatment appear unclear since glycosylated hemoglobin levels are not reduced into the normal range, and significant treatment-related complications are reported.[40-50] The frequency of severe hypoglycemic events using CSII has been reported to be higher,[45,48] equal,[46-47] or lower[41,51] when compared with ISII. Treatment with CSII, however, has been associated with an increased frequency (2-17.5 fold) of ketoacidosis when compared with nonCSII treated patients.[43-46,52]

Two novel approaches to regulate blood glucose are under intensive evaluation: pancreatic transplantation and mechanical devices that control blood glucose concentration by means of feedback controlled ("closed loop") insulin delivery. The latter has been unproperly called "artificial pancreas."[53]

Basically, a so-called artificial pancreas or artificial beta-cell consists of three basic components: a glucose sensor, insulin pump, and a computer controller that regulates the administration of insulin based on a measured amount of glucose. Ideally, such a device should be small enough to offer the potential for implantatory. No such device is currently available. The present state of the art was reviewed in terms of the individual components of the system and the recent progress and applications of these devices.

We exclude from the above definition the "biological artificial pancreas" in which pancreatic cells are used in place of the sensor and delivery pump, inserted either within a chamber (extravascular bioartificial pancreas)[55,56] or are just separated from the blood-stream by a membrane (vascular bioartificial pancreas).[57–61] We also exclude from the above definition the "chemical artificial pancreas" in which insulin is fixed on a carrier and delivered according to the ambient blood glucose.[62] Both systems are at an early experimental phase and have to face specific problems different from those of a mechanical system.

From an historical point of view, the term and the concept artificial pancreas have been first employed in the early 1970s by Albisser[54] and others.[55] However, predecessors like Mirouze in 1962 for his pioneering work on blood glucose monitoring,[63] Kadish in 1964[64] for having described the first servo-controlled insulin infusion system, Metcalf in 1934[65] for having been the first to propose to administer insulin via a pump also deserved to be cited.

## Glucose Sensor

Blood glucose has been chosen as the parameter to regulate in the implantable artificial pancreas. However, it must be remembered that (1) tissue glucose concentration—especially in the subcutaneous space—might be different from blood, and even might vary from one point to another of the body.[66] (2) Blood glucose is not physiologically only regulated by insulin along a single loop but by several hormones, and some insulin reactions are even totally independent from blood glucose, as the anticipatory insulin secretion triggered by meal ingestion before any glucose rise (cephalic phase).[67]

Although the development of glucose sensors has been tackled for more than 10 years, a sensor stable even for a few days only has not yet become available for wide clinical use.

### The Enzyme Electrode Sensor

Pioneers in the development of the enzyme electrode glucose sensor were Clark and Lyons.[69] Their sensor used a glucose oxidase solution sandwiched between semipermeable polymeric membranes to catalyze the reaction between glucose and oxygen to form gluconic acid and hydrogen peroxide. Initially, a pH electrode measured glucose concentration as a function of hydrogen ion concentration change, which resulted from the formation of gluconic acid. Later versions used an oxygen electrode, also designed by Clark[70] to potentiometrically measure glucose concentration as a function of oxygen depletion.

In an attempt to refine the enzyme electrode design to make it suitable for use in an implantable artificial beta cell, Bessman and Schultz[71] modified the original design of Clark by immobilizing and stabilizing the glucose oxidase by intra- and intermolecular cross-linkages in a cloth matrix. Disks of the cloth matrix were cemented over the plastic membrane of a polarographic oxygen electrode.

The most advanced version of enzyme electrode glucose sensor is that developed by Miles Laboratories for their Biostator Glucose Controlled Insulin Infusion System, and external version, version of the artificial pancreas. As described by Clarke and Santiago,[72] this sensor consists of a membrane 1 cm in diameter, made up of solid-phase glucose oxidase sandwiched between polyacrylamide and polycarbonate membranes. In contrast, previous versions measured hydrogen peroxide polarographically. Double-layered protective membranes with differential pore sizes protect the hydrogen peroxide electrode from substances that might interface with the measurement.

Although designed for extracorporeal use, the Biostator glucose sensor is relatively small (4 × 2.5 cm). It is accurate and stable with a useful operating range of 0 to 600 g/dL and has a response time of less than 1 min.

While this type of sensor obviously works well in an extracorporeal device, it has several drawbacks when considered for implantable uses. First, the length of time during which an enzyme electrode sensor retains its sensitivity and stability is short. Second, it shares the problem with other types of implantable sensors developed to date, namely, of becoming encapsulated by fibrotic tissue and its communication with surrounding blood and body fluid disrupted shortly after implantation. With the sensors designed as needles and applied SC.[73] service times of up to one week are reported.[74] The development is still in the laboratory stage with individually produced prototypes of electrodes. The problems of reproducible and cheap manufacture which, as experience with other sensors teaches, should represent the central problem, still oppose wide application. Furthermore, the problems of storing the electrodes and their possible pretreatment before application must be solved. They must be in steady state when applied.

## The Electrochemical Sensor

One way to avoid the problem of rapid degradation of enzyme electrodes is to design a sensor that can operate without enzymes. Noble metals such as platinum can be substituted for glucose oxidase to catalyze the oxidation of glucose. Several modes of operation are possible using this approach, including fuel cell, polarographic, potentiometric, and potentiodynamic systems. Although the polarographic approach was taken by many other investigators in the field, Chang et al.[75] of Soeldner's group chose to use a fuel cell sensor in their initial experiments. The fuel cell consists of nonconsumable catalytic anode and cathode, an electrolyte, and a system of membranes to maintain the disparate anodic and cathodic environments. Since the fuel cell measures the electrical energy generated by the electrochemical oxidation of glucose, the system needs no applied current nor reference electrode, thereby reducing the problem of oxide formation and eliminating the problem of reference electrode degradation.

One difficulty with the electrochemical sensor is that it is relatively nonspecific, responding to a variety of endogenous substances such as ethanol, urea, monosaccharides other than glucose, and amino acids. In addition to affecting the accuracy of the response, these substances can cause deactivation of the platinum electrode. Selective membranes have been used to protect the electrode from these substances, but these have not been entirely successful because of the small size of the interfering molecules. Additionally, these membranes increase the response time of the sensor.

Both the enzyme electrode and electrochemical sensors have yet to solve the problem of how to prevent the sensor from encapsulation once it is implanted.

## The Optical Sensor

Laser absorption spectrometry is based on the fact that the glucose concentration in the aqueous humor of a human eye can be determined by the degree to which it causes rotation of the plane of a laser beam of light, and that there is a good correlation between blood glucose and glucose concentration in the anterior chamber. This method is a noninvasive technique for measuring glucose concentration.[76] Encouraging results in animals have been achieved recently by Rabinovitch et al.[77-79] It remains to be seen whether this device can be miniaturized enough to make it practical.

### Affinity Sensors

These sensors are based on the affinity of glucose and a fluorescein-labeled analog for receptor sites specific to carbohydrate. They have only been tested in vitro so far. Concanavalin A is immobilized on the inner surface of a hollow fiber, which holds fluorescent dextran but allows diffusion of glucose into the fiber. Then an optical probe is inserted into the fiber to determine the quantity of dextran that remains unbound to the fiber walls. As glucose diffuses into the fiber, it displaces dextran, and the resulting change in fluid composition is detected and reported by the probe. Advantages of this system are that there is no membrane to create problems and that it can be tested with extremely small quantities of the mixture.[80]

## The Computer Controller

The function of the computer controller is to regulate the administration of insulin based on measured amounts of glucose and using a special *algorithm*. An algorithm can be defined as a rule of procedure needed to solve a repetitious mathematical problem. Algorithms form the pattern by which a closed-loop insulin infusion system mimics the complex process of insulin secretion by a normal beta cell. It is based on glucose measurements alone rather than on the host of physiologic mediators of insulin release.

### Glucose Predictions with Rising Glucose Concentrations

It was clear from early studies that a 5- or 10-min. delay between blood withdrawal and glucose measurement introduced an inherent error or delay in closed-loop controls.[53,81] Because of the delay in glucose measurement and insulin delivery, algorithms were developed so that insulin administration was based on an extrapolated or predicted glucose concentration. This prediction was a function of the actual glucose concentration and its rate of change over the previous few minutes.

## Glucose Predictions with Declining Glucose Concentrations

The selection of projected glucose concentrations to control insulin delivery when blood glucose concentrations are declining rapidly have been designed so that insulin delivery can be blunted well before the onset of hypoglycemia. An alternate approach would be to activate a counterregulatory system, such as a dextrose or glucagon infusion, as blood glucose concentrations fall below a given value. Both approaches were studied by the Toronto group[54,82–84] although our experience was that activation of a glucose or glucagon infusion is seldom needed to avert hypoglycemia after meals when appropriate algorithms are selected.[81,85]

## Selection of the Glucose Concentration–Insulin Infusion Rate Relationship

It became clear soon after development of the radioimmunoassay for insulin that the relationship between glucose concentrations and insulin secretory rates was not linear.[86] Foster developed a mathematical model that simulates an intravenous glucose tolerance test with a computer[87] to produce acceptable glucose disappearance rates while it averts postprandial hypoglycemia during a simulated IVGTT. The algorithms selected contained elements of proportionate control that varied in sensitivity at different glucose levels and had a preselected limit to the insulin infusion rate. The term saturation control was used to describe these algorithms.

In 1973, the Toronto Group[88] proposed an algorithm for computer-controlled insulin delivery based on a hyperbolic tangent function. A dynamic control element was achieved through the calculation and use of a predicted glucose concentration, based on the average rate of change over the prior four minutes, applied to an exponential equation. The glucose-control algorithms were similar to those for insulin control except that they were proportionate to the measured rather than to the predicted glucose concentration.

A.H. Clemens and associates developed a series of control algorithms and control programs throughout the evolution of the Biostator GCIIS.[89]

The Miles algorithms differed from those of the Toronto group in one aspect—they no longer used the hyperbolic tangent equation for the control of the static insulin release but introduced a biquadratic and, subsequently, a quadratic function, with the advantage that the new control constants could be selected in physiologically meaningful terms, such as the desired (basal) blood glucose level and the desired basal insulin infusion rate. The hyperbolic tangent function used in the Toronto approach has the theoretic advantage of resembling more closely the sigmoidal pattern of insulin secretion at high glucose levels in the isolated rat pancreas perfused with glucose. While the Miles algorithm closely resembled the hyperbolic tangent control curve in the lower (physiologic) range, its maximal insulin release was limited by an operator-selected value. During the same period, we developed our own artificial pancreas using several personal algorithms without,[81] then with, projected functions.[85] Algorithms for subcutaneous[90] and intraperitoneal[91] insulin infusion have also been described. In both cases, the onset of hypoglycemic effect is delayed and the action is prolonged,[92-95] which makes the feedback control difficult. For the IP route "hybrid" control, including a preprogrammed early infusion and a pure feedback control, infusion has been proposed, and shown to be infusion in a pure feedback control algorithm. The preprogrammed infusion stimulates the important cephalic phase,[67] and the time variant control characteristics provide the nonlinear biphasic response to a blood glucose in a normal pancreas.[96] We have shown that even with the IV route, this preprogrammed early injection may be beneficial.[81]

## Insulin Pump

This is the most technically advanced part of the artificial pancreas. External pumps have been widely used in diabetes since the pioneering works of Slama (IV)[97] and Pickup (SC).[98] The rate of the pump is usually adapted manually according to intermittent blood glucose testings ("open-loop," or better "semiclosed-loop" system).

## Externally Portable Devices

Approximately 30 different devices are commercially offered for insulin delivery alone. The majority are motor-driven syringes. The syringes are in part commercially available disposable plastic products with a volume of 1 to 3 ml (for one to three days supply), in part plungers or cylinders that are specially designed to achieve high accuracy or for reasons of pump drive design. With one model, the syringes are supplied prefilled as cartridges (Nordisk-Infuser). The second pump principle to be encountered is the peristaltic or roller pump.

Pumps with electromagnetically driven pistons and two passive valves and a prefilled plastic insulin reservoir have not yet reached the commercial stage. The technical data of the various types cannot be discussed here individually. Reference is made to what currently must be considered the most comprehensive survey on this topic.[99]

With the general trend toward miniaturization of the devices, the reservoirs (syringes) are reduced more and more in size. Nearly all devices are suitable only for the SC route.

## Implantable Devices

### Devices

With implantable devices, the number of active companies is clearly lower than with the external devices because of the greater technical complexity.

*Devices with Fixed Rates.* Only one company offers implants commercially for human use at present (Infusaid-Intermedics USA). This product is a purely mechanical pump. A titanium bellows is filled with the infusion liquid through a pierceable septum and is pressurized by means of an evaporating fluid (freon)[30] (Fig. 1). The fluid is driven out through a capillary flow resistor into a suitably placed catheter. According to the Hagen-Poisseuille law, the supply rate depends upon the differential pressure between the bellows interior and the catheter tip and viscosity of the fluid, in addition to the fixed dimensions of the capillary. The pressure in the bel-

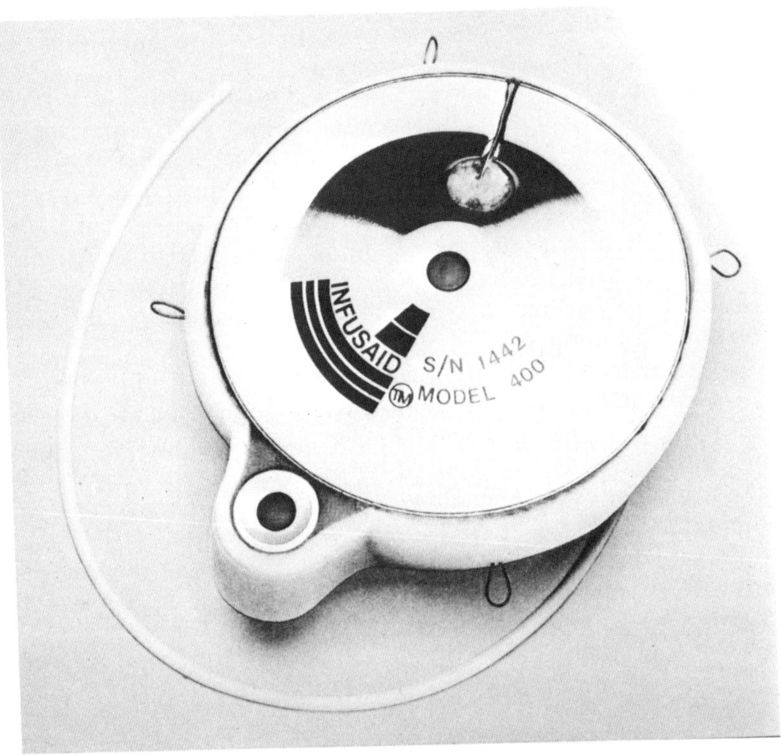


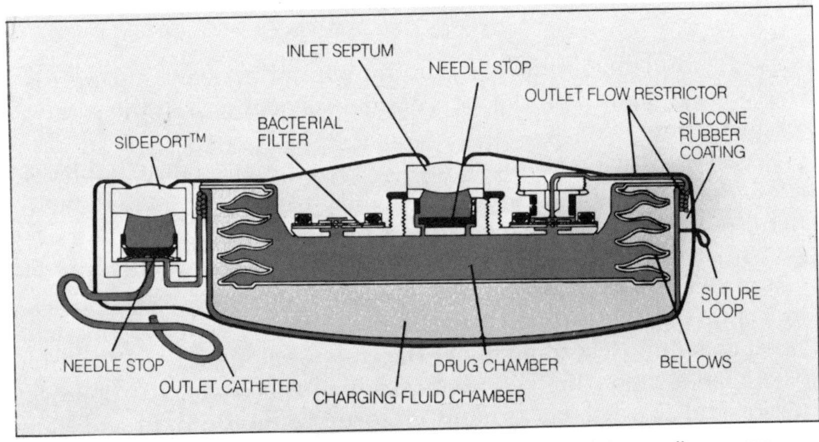


**Figure 1:** View (A) and diagram (B) of the Infusaid−Intermedics pump.

lows interior varies considerably with temperature and filling condition (because of the recoil force of the bellows). A change of 1° C induces a change of the internal pressure (and thus the rate) of approximately 4%, and temperature fluctuations of 5° C can be easily imagined to occur 1 cm below the skin. The variability of the rate as a function of the filling level, fully compared with empty, amounts to approximately 7%. The pressure at the catheter tip fluctuates with the barometric pressure (height above sea-level), which is superimposed upon the physiological pressure at the site of application (e.g., in the vein or in the peritoneum). The viscosity is a function of the temperature. The viscosity is selected as high as possible with insulin infusions in order to achieve the desired low flow rate with the largest possible capillary lumen (minimization of the risk of clogging because of possibly precipitated insulin). Apparently users of the devices can cope with these fluctuations by special precautionary measures when flying, moutaineering, in the sauna, with fever, etc.

The rates of these devices can only be changed on a long-term basis by replenishment and therefore are only conditionally suitable for diabetes therapy. This statement concerns the commercially available devises. Naturally, a rate control by valves is conceivable, but because of the risk of large quantities of the drug flowing into the body in the case of a leaking valve (the drug is pressurized), this has not yet been used in humans.

*Devices with Controllable Variable Rates.* They are necessarily electromechanical. The information transfer from the external programming or control device takes place electromagnetically or magnetically; storage in the implant occurs electronically. The drug delivery itself is necessarily a mechanical process.

Sandia Laboratory pump. A prototype of the Sandia pump was first implanted by Schade et al.[101] in January 1981; it functioned for five months. The main difference between it and the Siemens pump is that the Sandia pump has its reservoir outside the pump capsule. To date, only Schade has implanted this pump, and no prototypes have been available for testing at other centers.

Siemens pump (Fig. 2). It was first implanted in 1981 in a human being by Irsigler et al.[102] at Vienna-Lainz by the Mehnert's group[103−105] in Munich and by Selam et al.[107] at Montpellier. Due to electronic defects the pump at Lainz was replaced eight months later. After an additional four months, the second pump was explanted due to a catheter break. The other pumps functioned

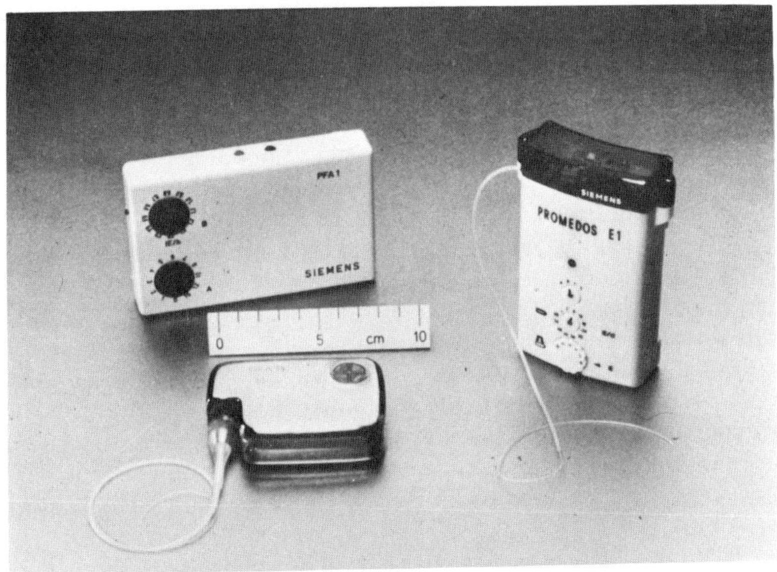


A

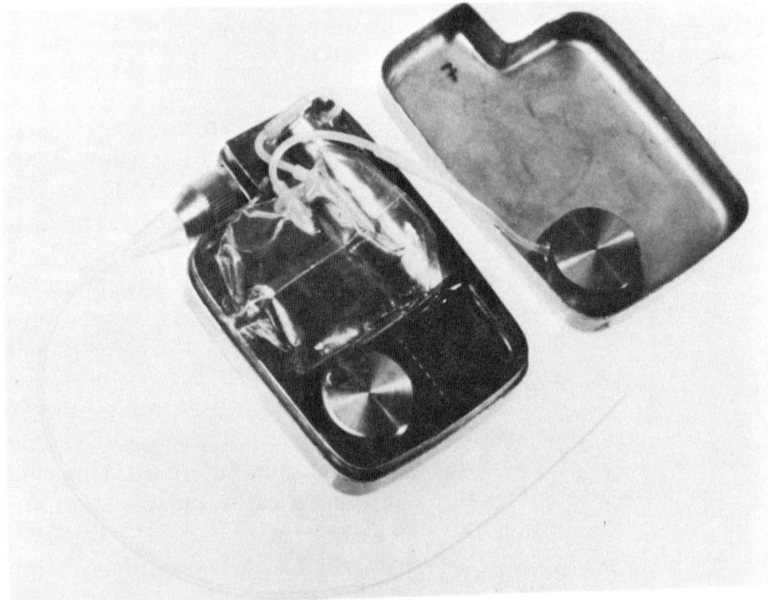

B

**Figure 2:** Siemens implantable pump (A, B) with its remote controller (left A). Right A: portable peristaltic pump (Siemens, Promedos E1).

for about 12 months each. The continued problem of insulin instability seen in animal experimentation has prevented any further human implantation. The influence of mechanical shear forces on insulin used in roller pumps or the so-called diffusion forces present with synthetic reservoirs and tubing may have had additional effects upon insulin stability. There have been too few systematic studies to date to determine the real causes of the problem. In the meantime, the electronic switching system has been reworked.

Medtronic pump (Fig. 3). It was first used in humans to deliver morphine, and has been implanted in dogs for insulin delivery[108].

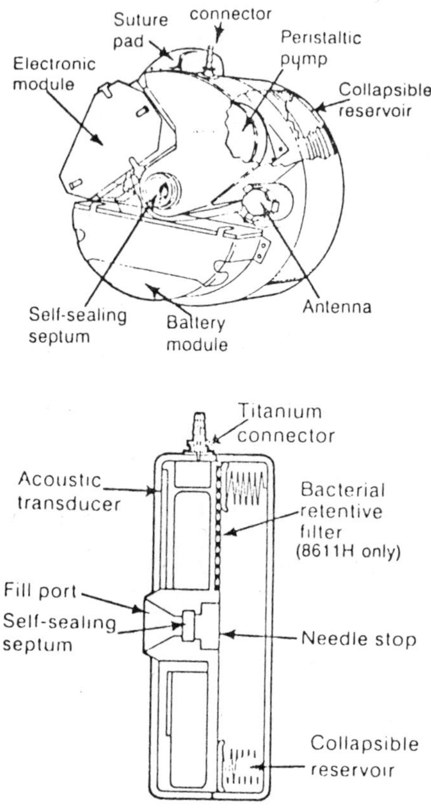


**Figure 3** (*continued*)

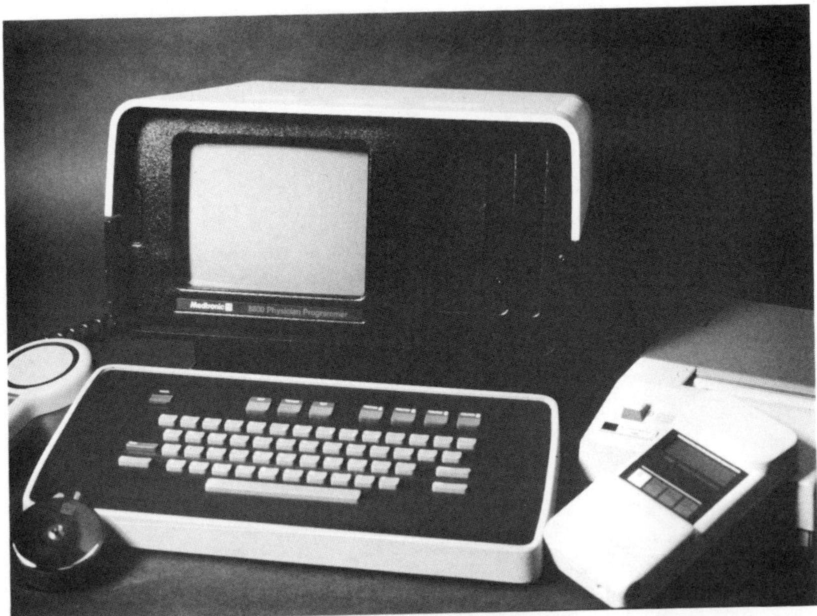

**Figure 3:** Medtronic Drug Administration System. The Medtronic Drug Administration System consists of an implantable infusion pump (DAD) (A) a variety of implantable catheters, an implantable access port, and a clinician's programmer. (B) The programmer can noninvasively program the implanted infusion pump to a specific prescription.

Human implantation is planned as soon as problems with insulin aggregation are solved. The Medtronic pump works on a peristaltic principle. A special feature is its programmability by patient and physician using a computer terminal. Figure 13 shows the physician's programming unit (left and center), the pump (left foreground), the printer (right rear), and the patient's portable programming unit (right front).

Pacesetter-Minimed pump (Fig. 4). The pump was developed at the Johns Hopkins University,[109] and the prototype was built by Pacesetter Systems. Noteworthy is the use of the diaphragm. Freon gases used in the pump to create a negative pressure so that there is no risk that insulin can leak out into the body. The pump is powered by a lithium battery. Reprogramming of the pump over a telephone and computer modem has already been carried out with dogs.

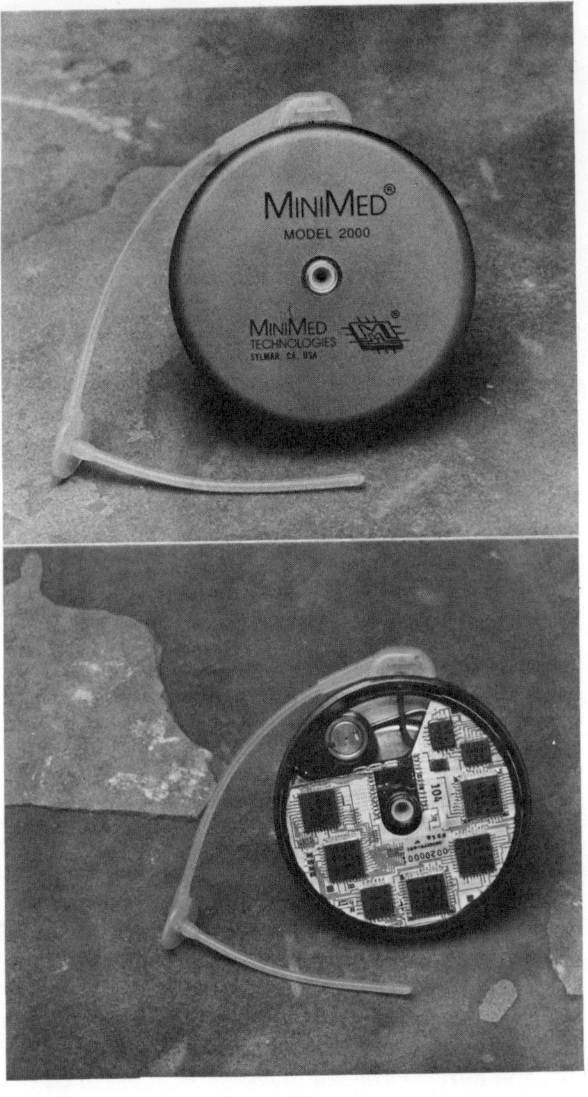

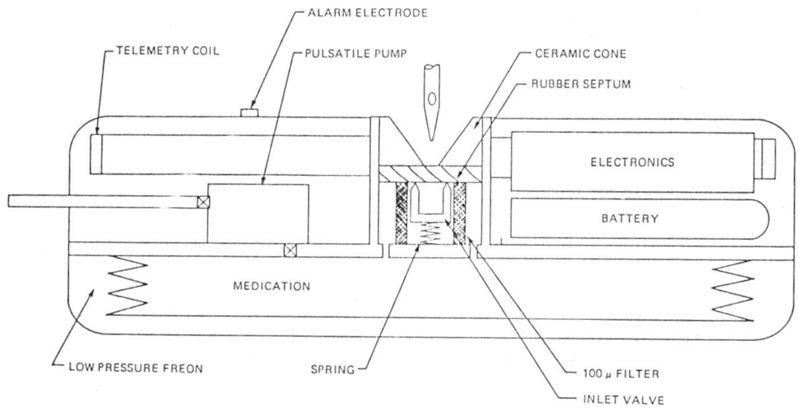


**Figure 4:** View (A) and diagram (B) of the Pacesetter (Minimed Technologies) implantable pump.

Individual pumps have functioned successfully in diabetic dogs for more than three years.[110] The insulin used in this system only comes in contact with metal, just as the Infusaid pump. This pump has recently received FDA approval for human testings in the United States, by Johns Hopkins and our group.

*Other Approaches.* The valve-piston principle ranks among the earliest designs for drug delivery, with Bessman reporting on animal experiments as early as 1975.[111] This approach was discontinued. The same happened to another design[142] where the valve and piston were integrated in a plate of piezoelectric material. Already in the early 1970s and more recently, other groups were experimenting with the pumps that operate according to the electro-osmotic principle[113–115]—nevertheless still in a very early development phase—and yet others with magnetic pellets.[116] The latter consist of implantable plastic matrices in which the drug is distributed as in depot preparations. Iron particles are embedded additionally. The administration rate can be influenced by applying an external magnetic alternating field.

## Advantages and Disadvantages of the Different Mechanisms

*Magnetic Pellets.* The rate control is not yet satisfactorily solved. This technique is in the early development stage.

*Electro-Osmotic Pump.* The problem of the consumption of the electrodes as well as the replenishment of the reservoir are not satisfactorily solved.

*Vapor-Pressure Pumps.* Because of the simplicity of these bellow-capillary pumps, they are well proven for noncritical drugs that can be administered at predetermined rates with some variability as a result of varying external conditions.

For controlled drug delivery at variable rates, pumps of this type are not yet available, since the required totally leakproof valves are still lacking.

*Syringe Pumps.* While in widespread use for external devices and SC infusion, they are technically difficult to realize for implantable devices (plunger return, replenishment valve); this approach has apparently not yet been attempted.

*Valve-Piston and Diaphragm Pumps.* The central problem is the susceptibility of the pumps to air bubbles located in or arising from the drug solution: gas in the pump chamber hampers the aspiration of further liquid because of its compressibility. The pulsated (nonphysiological) delivery can also be a disadvantage with this principle when applied to the IV catheter route.

*Peristaltic Pumps (e.g., Roller Pumps).* The quasicontinuous delivery that is also insensitive to bubbles and external influences permits a broad rate and application range. These pumps have been already used clinically as external devices; with implants, only higher stability requirements for the insulin preparation prevent their widespread use.

## Insulin

The physiochemical tendency of insulin to form macromolecular aggregates or fibrils seemed to cause no problem during the early years of insulin treatment but constitute a major problem for the development for insulin pumps.

Schade et al.[117] differentiate between the formation of macromolecular aggregation due to the association of insulin hexamers and the association of multiple insulin fibrils with macromolecules arranged along a central axis. In contrast to crystals, insulin fibrils in an aqueous medium are extremely stable and biologically inactive.

Both the tendency toward aggregation and that toward fibril formation are aggravated by movement and body temperature, a fact that was not considered during bench tests for early pumps. The situation first became critical when pumps were worn by humans, and test groups were faced with catheter stoppage and aggregation in insulin reservoirs.

When the residual insulin is withdrawn from a pump reservoir prior to refill, high-pressure liquid chromatography (HPLC) shows that, in addition to aggregation, there are changes in the insulin monomer and the formation of dimers and plymers (Fig.5).[118,119] The monomer is the active form of insulin, so that biological effectiveness is reduced at polymerization.

Today, six years after the appearance of these problems, more insight has been gained, but there are still no definitive answers. Compromise solutions have been the changing of the milieu to an acidic pH or the addition of highly concentrated glycerol or other additives, which have made the further development of pump therapy possible. All the other trials were unsuccessful or unapplicable in vivo.


## Acidic Insulin

When hydrochloric acid is used to change the pH level from 7.2 to the isoelectric point of 5.5 (where the number of positive and negative charges is equal), soluble zinc insulin rapidly crystallizes.[117] Commercially available insulin solutions, therefore, have a pH value clearly above or below 5.5. In 1978 the only insulin that could pass a simple shake test without aggregation was the acid insulin from Hoechst AG. It has been used by our research team[94,120−122] and by others[124−126] in portable externally worn devices ever since, for it has shown itself to be dependably more stable than any of its competitors to date.[123] Our group and Vienna-Lainz group has used acid insulin for more than 250 diabetics with portable external devices equipped with insulin reservoirs with a three-week capacity. During a total of more than 200 patient years, both groups have not observed a single instance of catheter stoppage or aggregation in tubing or reservoir. However, this solution was rejected "a priori" by the major companies, arguing that acidic insulin in pumps is transformed in an unacceptably high percentage of multiple derivatives.[127] We were unable to demonstrate any transformation using an experimental acidic insulin (Organon), except desamidation,[128] which has been shown to be innocuous[129] and almost as effective

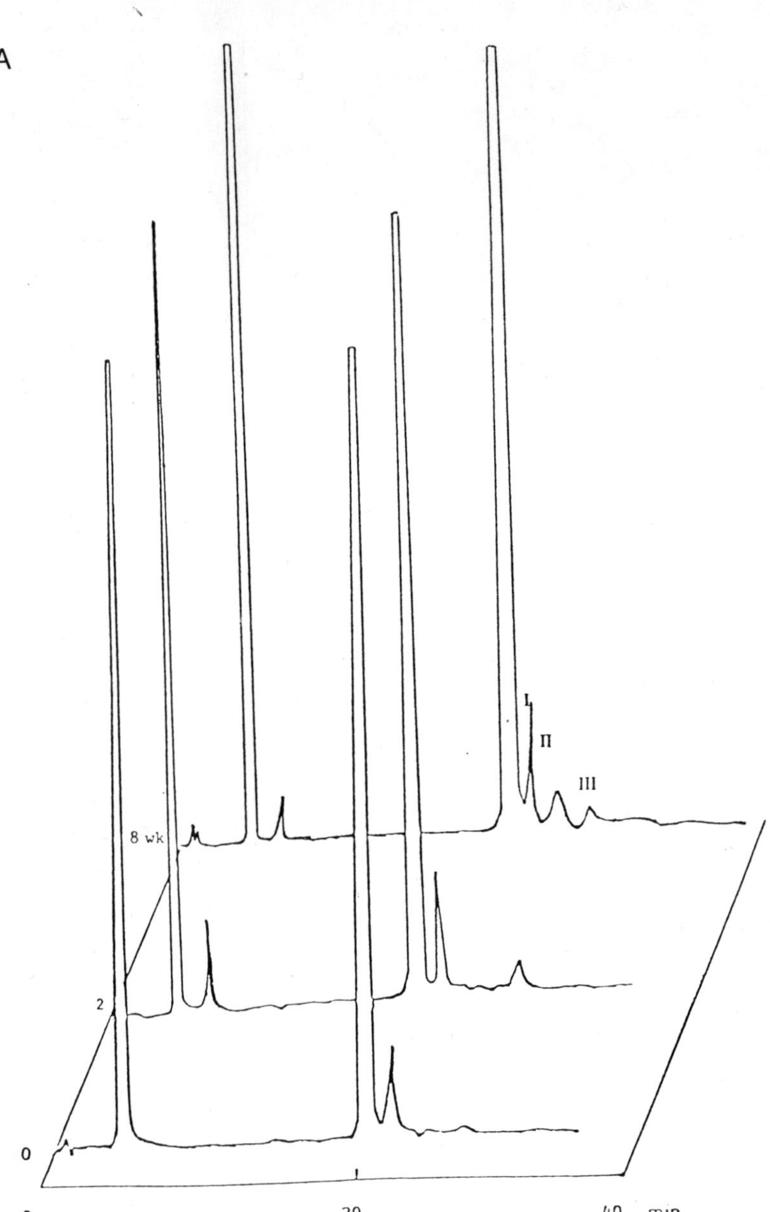


**Figure 5:** HPLC of neutral (A) and acidic (B) Organon insulin after eight weeks of 37C agitation in pump. Peaks (from left to right) represent preservative, insulin (at 20 min), desamido insulin and secondary peaks (dimers and polymers).

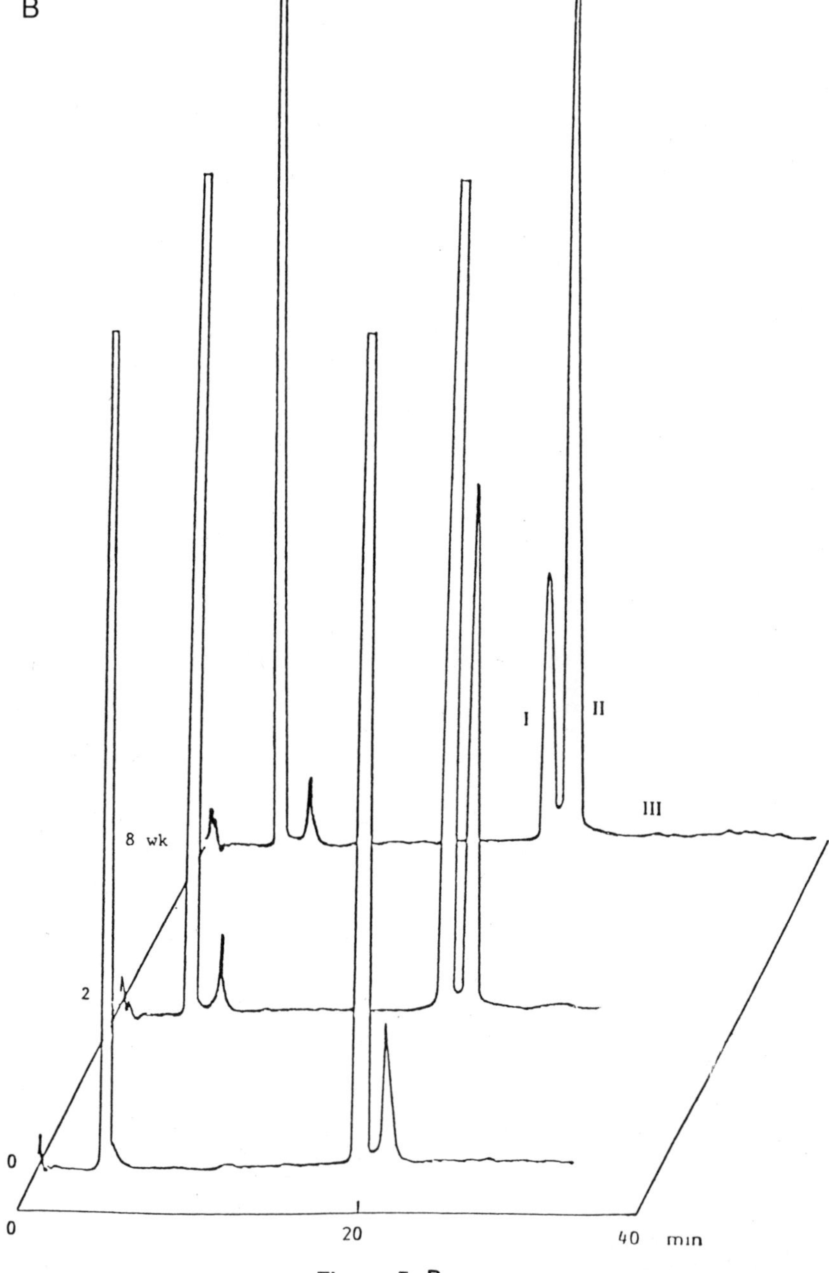


**Figure 5 B**

as the native insulin.[130] The risk of corrosion of metal parts of pumps due to acidity also remains to be demonstrated, as there was no corrosion reported with morphine, although it was acidic, too.

## Addition of Surface-Active Substances

Hoechst sought an additive for neutral insulin which would hinder aggregation, and chose the surface active product, Genapol, a pluronic polyol. (Pluronic polyols are polymers that can be chemically described as copolymers of polyoxypropylene and polyoxyethylene, with molecular weights between 1,000 and 15,000.)

The first programmable implants used in humans, the Siemens Promedos II, had a reservoir with a refill interval of 3 to 4 weeks, and used an insulin–Genapol solution. During a two-year period in which four of these devices were used, not a single case of aggregation was observed.

Although this insulin–Genapol combination showed itself stable during intensive shake testing and in implanted pumps, when used in portable external devices massive aggregation was occasionally seen and led Hoechst to postpone further implantations and to undergo additional intensive testing in dogs using implanted programmable pumps.[131–133] In addition to the Promedos II, developed especially for implantation by Siemens, the pumps from Medtronic and Pacesetter were also tested with Genapol–insulin.[127] The results led Hoeschst to produce two different types of insulin, the original one for the nonperistaltic pumps, and a new, although still Genapol-added, insulin for the peristaltic pumps.

## Addition of Glycerol

Buchwald et al.[134] and Rupp et al.[135] sought to solve the problem of insulin aggregation by adding highly concentrated glycerol (80% to 85%) to the insulin. The combination is continuously infused into the organism with a gas pressure Model 100 Infusion pump, which has a metal container and a silicone catheter.

Brange and Havelund[119] showed in 1981 that the addition of carbohydrates, such as fructose or glycerol, could prevent aggregation, but that when higher concentrations were used, there was a lessening of chemical stability and the growth of higher dimer and polymerization products.

Using the two-dimensional HPLC method developed by Havelund and used by Brange, it was possible to determine polymerization products in the same analysis as degradation products. The glycerol–insulin mixture was examined at the time the pump was filled and again three weeks later when the reservoir was emptied prior to refill. It was discovered that, in addition to 8% to 12% insulin dimers and polymers, there were a considerable number of modified molecules in the monomer fraction. These monomers showed a diminution of biological activity in the mouse convulsion test, but surprisingly, no evidence of diminished biological activity had been observed in the metabolic control of the patients from whose pumps the insulin had been withdrawn. In addition, reduction of flow rate has been recently reported, leading to Buchwald's group to reduce their refill period to one week [135,136] and to propose methods for restoring correct flow.[137]

## Catheter

The catheter is probably the weakest part of the system. In addition to the risk of insulin deposition and catheter occlusion, it carries the risk of bioincompatibility, with, as a consequence, fibrin deposition (Fig. 6), tissue growth (Fig. 7) and, again occlusion[121,122] (Fig. 8). Therefore, factors such as chemical comparison and geometry are of a major importance.

### Geometry

In an uncontrolled in vivo follow-up, we have noted that long (10–15 cm) catheters were better accepted than short ones (5–10 cm).[115,138] Diameter, sharpness of the extremity,[139] and shape[140] of the catheters may also play a role.

### Chemistry

#### Titanium

Titanium is often used for the capsule of implantable pumps (e.g., Siemens, Infusaid, Medtronic, and Pacesetter) and for the insulin reservoir (e.g., Infusaid and Pacesetter pumps). Titanium bio-

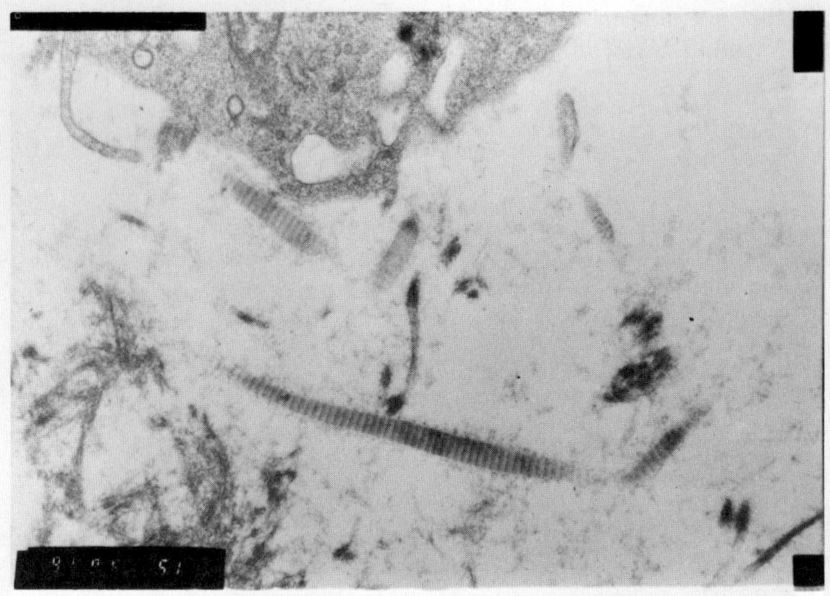

**Figure 6:** Transmission electron microscopy of a chronic peritoneal insulin catheter obstructed by Fibrin products. Note a giant cell (top) and col lagen fibers.

compatibility has already been demonstrated in the pacemaker field, where it has had long-term usage for human implantation. The optimum surface characteristics and the elimination of the diffusion problem help to explain its problem-free usage in the manufacture of insulin reservoirs.

## Silicone Rubber

Silicone rubber distinguishes itself by its high degree of elasticity and its limited thrombogenicity. The elasticity makes it an ideal material for the connective tubing between reservoir and catheter, particularly in peristaltic pumps, where this elasticity is exactly the characteristic desired.

Unfortunately, silicone has a tendency toward diffusion of both liquids and gases, so that special methods of pump encapsulation have had to be developed for use in implantable pumps.[141]

The tissue biocompatibility of silicone rubber is almost as good as that of titanium, although Eaton et al.[142] and the research group at Vienna-Lainz[143] have seen peritoneal adhesions in individual cases.

## Polyurethane

Developers of glucose sensors favor polyurethane for its first-class diffusion characteristics, together with the minimal tissue reaction that it causes. However, it is this tendency toward diffusion that makes polyurethane unsuitable for the production of insulin catheters and reservoirs.

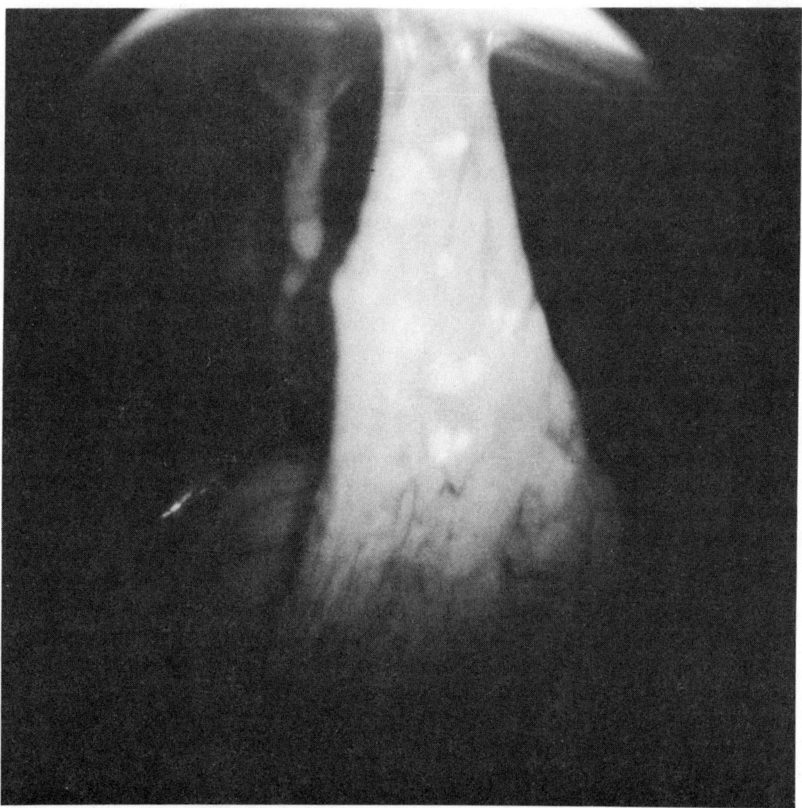

**Figure 7:** Laparoscopic view of chronic peritoneal catheters obstructed by omental adhesion (A) and fibrin mode (B). (*continued*)

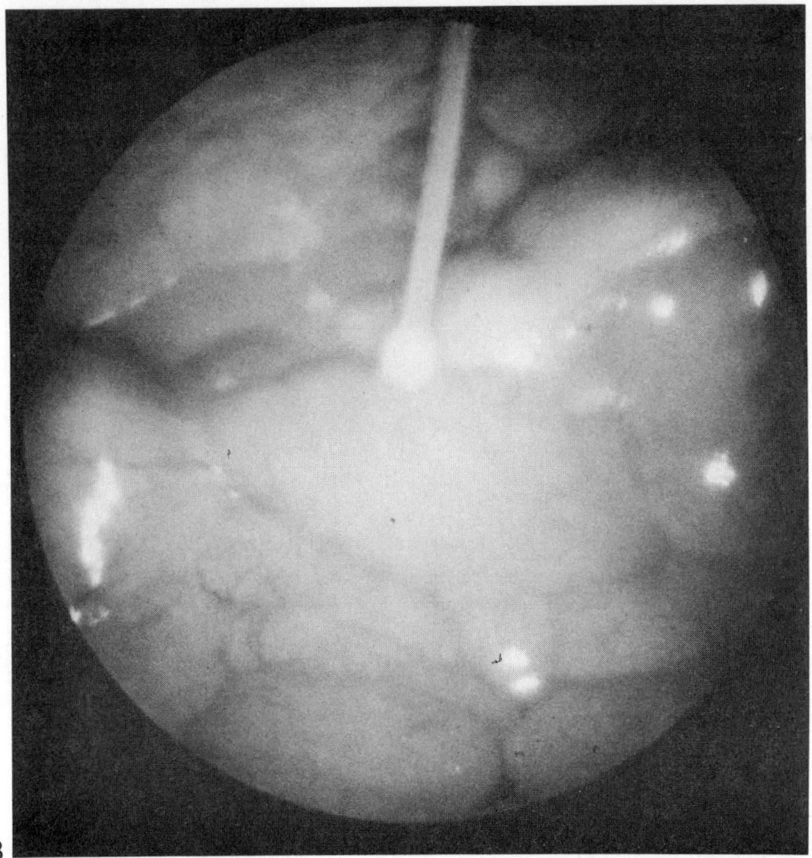

**Figure 7B.**

The thrombogenicity of polyurethane makes it a poor choice for IV use. To date, we have no reports of any IP applications.

## Polyethylene

Polyethylene catheters have been generally regarded to be thrombogenic unless irrigated.[144] However, several researchers have reported success when they were used for insulin delivery.

We have used such catheters externally covered with Silastic

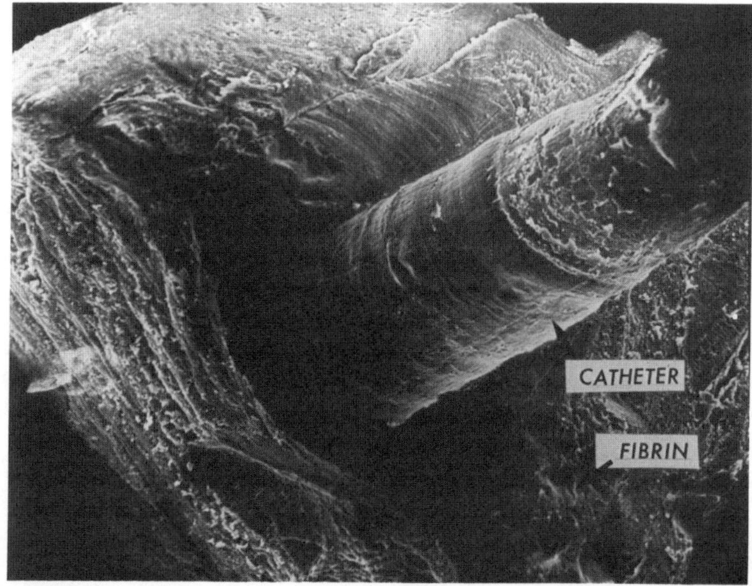


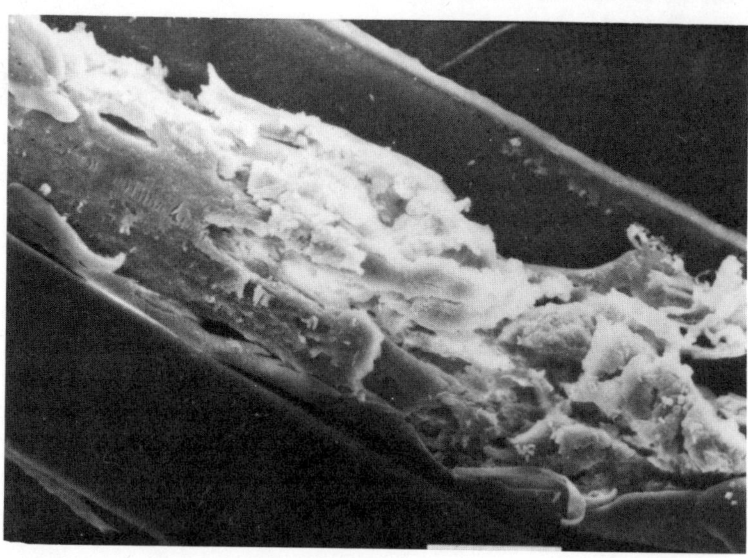


**Figure 8:** (A) Scanning electron microscopy of the tip of the catheter shown on Figure 7. (B) Scanning electron microscopy of an obstructed IP catheter.

(Siemens) for IP infusion without reaction at the point of entrance or in the skin tunnel, and without any thrombotic complications. Catheters examined endoscopically in the IP cavity appeared to be free-floating, although in individual cases some tissue growth had led to adhesions.[121,122,138] During laparoscopic examinations, the Vienna Group found no difference in the number of omental or parietal adhesions in connection with either silicone or polyethylene catheters.

The greatest drawback of polyethylene is its limited ability to withstand stress and torque. Under mechanical stress, such a catheter can be irreversibly twisted out of shape or actually broken.

Where polyethylene catheters were used with implantable insulin delivery devices, several pumps had to be explanted due to catheter breakage some months after implantation. By contast, there has not been a single report to the Registry sponsored by the International Study Group on Implantable Insulin Infusion Devices (ISGIID) of a silicone catheter being explanted due to breakage.[145]

## Routes of Infusion

### The Subcutaneous Route

#### Physiology

Although reduced when compared with conventional injections, local degradation of insulin persists after subcutaneous infusion, still variable and resulting in a 20–50% unpredictable loss of activity in certain individuals.[146] Moreover, the kinetics of resorption are not greatly different from those from subcutaneous injections. A mean delay of 136 min. for the plasma insulin peak following a 1-h square wave of 6 U and a persistent hyperinsulinemia still 4 h after the bolus, under a 1-U/h basal infusion, were observed.[122,147] The peak delay is shortened by 15–30 min.[148,149] if the bolus is given in a few minutes. However, the return to baseline is in any case sluggish, approximating 6–8 h.

#### Efficiency

The real superiority of continuous subcutaneous insulin infusion (CSII) over injections has been questioned.[150] In the authors' opinion, the response is not ubiquitous. CSII is probably ineffective in brittle and insulin-resistant diabetes because it does not bypass the subcutaneous tissue, the poor resorption of which is probably involved in the mechanism of such forms of diabetes.[151] CSII is probably superior to injections in highly insulin-sensitive, low dose-requiring patients (pancreatectomized, hypophysectomized diabetics). In the average diabetic patient, it seems that CSII may be superior to twice-daily conventional insulin injections but not to multiple dose programs.[154]

## Feasibility

The technique of CSII is easy to handle and does not require sophisticated pumps nor highly stable insulin because the reservoirs and catheters are changed frequently.

The risks and problems are limited to accidental under- or overdosage and local subcutaneous reactions. However, long-term acceptability is poorer than expected with a nonnegligible dropout rate.[146,152] Unverifiable intermittent disconnections from pump must also be accounted for.

Finally, the authors recommend the subcutaneous route only for CSII in nonbrittle, insulin-dependent, but poorly controlled diabetes and only if the patients wish to avoid multiple injections or fixed mealtimes. This route is definitely not adapted to a feedback controlled system.

## The Intravenous Route

### Physiology

The physiology of intravenously infused insulin was extensively investigated in the 1970s, as it was the route for insulin from the artificial pancreas. The intravenous infusion gives the fastest insulin response: Plasma insulin reaches its maximum and returns to baseline values in <30 min. following a bolus.[92] However, this route invariably produces hyperinsulinemia.[153,154]

### Efficiency

The efficiency of the intravenous route has been proven,[153] even in the most severe forms of diabetes.[147] However, this advantage is balanced by the risk of rapid glucose rise in case of pump discontinuation[155] and rapid glucose fall during physical exercise.[156]

### Feasibility

The procedure for catheter insertion in a central vein is difficult and not innocuous. Technical requirements and patient constraints under portable intravenous pumps are as important as with the intraperitoneal route (see below). The risks of infection may be minimized by severe asepsy precautions, but not the risk of catheter obstruction by blood clotting, which was the mode of termination of the authors' only two chronic intravenous catheters after eight and six months of constant infusion.[94,157] However, results with totally implanted devices appear more encouraging.[134,135]

## The Intramuscular Route

The intramuscular route has been proposed as an intermediate between the subcutaneous and intravenous routes, as it bypasses the subcutaneous barrier and has intermediate kinetics of absorption.[158]

Encouraging results with the intramuscular route have been noted by some authors in insulin-resistant and brittle diabetes. However, the intramuscular route was rapidly abandoned because of very poor long-term feasibility: Pain, muscle fibrosis, and abscesses were not infrequent.

## The Portal Route

The portal route is theoretically the ideal route, as insulin is delivered primarily to the liver, thus reproducing the physiological portoperipheral insulin gradient.[159]

So far, the portal route has been tested only in animals, with conflicting results.[154,160–162]

Owing to the potential risks of thrombosis and infection, it seems unlikely, at least with portable systems, that human testing will be ethically valid, unless the clear superiority and advantages of portal over peripheral infusion are definitely proven in long-term animal studies.

## The Intraperitoneal Route

### *Physiology*

Like the intravenous route, the intraperitoneal route bypasses the subcutaneous tissue and thus may be beneficial in patients with subcutaneously related problems (instability, insulin resistance), with the further advantage of a larger surface of resorption and no risk of catheter obstruction by clots.

The two major physiological advantages are a rapid insulin resorption[92,95] and a partial portal uptake.[163,164] The plasma-free insulin in 28 chronically pumped insulin-dependent diabetics (IDD) and six normal subjects were measured during 4 h after a standardized breakfast.[95] In the IDDs, insulin was infused as a 1-U/h basal rate and a 1-h superimposed meal dose intraperitoneally ($n = 20$) or subcutaneously ($n = 8$). The fasting plasma-free insulin level was lower, and bolus peaks occurred earlier in intraperitoneally than in subcutaneously treated patients (70 ± 6 versus 136 ± 28 min., respectively). Intraperitoneal values tended to return to baseline within the normal time (<3 h), whereas subcutaneous values were still elevated after 4 h (Fig. 9). Many factors may affect the intraperitoneal insulin kinetics: High insulin concentrations[164] and instant boluses[164,165] instead of square waves seem to increase the rapidity of absorption. In the same way, higher bolus-induced peaks were observed when the intraperitoneal catheter was situated in the mid rather than the low abdomen,[138] confirming for the first time that, as for the solutes, the peritoneum absorbs insulin better in the higher abdominal regions, probably owing to a lower pressure and more important venous and lymphatic circulations, especially in the diaphragmatic areas.[166]

According to Schade et al.,[164] up to 50% of intraperitoneally administered insulin is absorbed through the portal circulation, reproducing the normal portoperipheral insulin gradient. However, further experiments are needed to confirm those results and to demonstrate that the relative peripheral hypoinsulinemia also observed by the authors[95] is not due simply to partial in situ insulin degradation.

### *Efficiency*

The efficiency of the intraperitoneal route appears for most[94,167−169] but not all[170] of the authors superior to the sub-

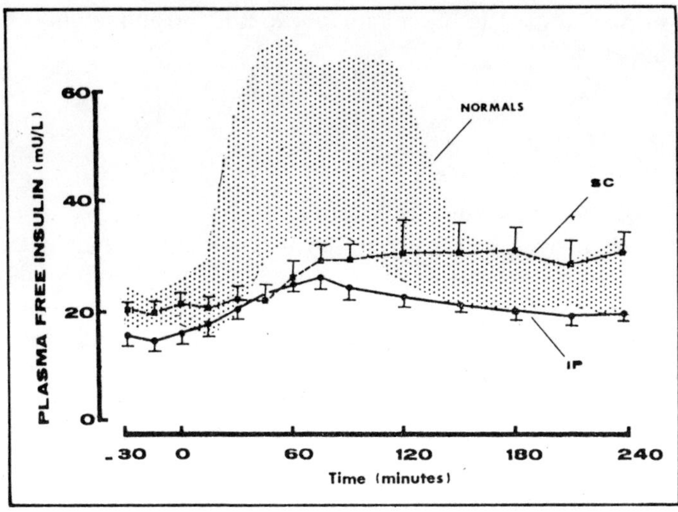


**Figure 9:** Plasma insulin kinetics following a bolus of insulin of 7U at time 0 and a basal infusion of 1U/h from −30 to +240 min. Solid line: IP infusion, dotted line SC infusion, shaded area: normal insulin response after a meal.

cutaneous and similar to the intravenous infusion of insulin. The authors' group conducted a short-term[94] and a long-term[121,122] protocol for evaluation of the efficacy of intraperitoneal insulin. The short-term protocol consisted of three randomized one-month periods of infusion in six brittle IDDs via a chronic catheter delivering insulin subcutaneously, intravenously, and intraperitoneally. The two last routes gave similar results, with significantly fewer hyperglycemic episodes and lower insulin requirements than observed with subcutaneous infusion. The long-term study was the follow-up of 40 chronically intraperitoneally pumped patients (present experience up to 1986, 80 patients). All patients had been poorly controlled by two to four daily subcutaneous injections. Mean CBG reached 127 ± 24 versus 192 ± 48 mg/mL before CPII and hemoglobin $A_1$ 8.1 ± 1.1 versus 10.6 ± 2.4% before CPII. The results did not drift with time (1−27 months of continuous intraperitoneal infusion; mean 13 months). Daily insulin doses decreased from 63 ± 4 U/24 h before to 45 ± 3 U/24 h after three months of CPII. However, it still remains to be demonstrated that the IP route is able to normalize the other metabolite and hormone abnormalities of diabetes.[171]

## Feasibility

The authors' experience[122] confirms that of Irsigler et al.,[171] the only other group with a long-term wide experience with the intraperitoneal route through either portable or implantable pumps. In the present population treated with portable intraperitoneal pumps, the method was judged satisfactory by 90% of the patients, a result usually not attained by CSII.[146]

The technical requirements for CPII via portable pumps include a reliable pump with long-duration insulin reservoir, to avoid too frequent manipulations and thus limit the risk of infection. The pump must be compact, robust, and of a sufficient impermeability (at least for showers), as it cannot be removed on any occasion for safety reasons. The insulin must remain stable in the reservoir and must not precipitate in the permanently placed tubings. Preferentially, the authors are using the Promedos peristaltic pump (Siemens AG, Erlangem, F.R.G.) equipped with a disposable polyethylene reservoir of 30 mL, filled with acidic U40 insulin (CS21; Hoechst AG, Frankfurt F.R.G.). Stabilized U100 neutral insulins (Hoechst, F.R.G. and Organon, France) have also been tested, with more variable results in Nordisk pumps. Technical requirements also include a robust, compatible, thin, chronic peritoneal catheter. A polyethylene catheter covered by silicon rubber (Siemens), was chosen by the authors. The technique of catheter insertion must be safe and simple. Thus, a nonsurgical procedure using a blind needle technique was developed,[94] which was used successfully for >80 catheter insertions.

The medical requirements include severe criteria for selection of the patients. Patients should be both poorly controlled (to provide a good biological advantages-to-constraints ratio) and reasonably motivated and reliable. Intensive education, severe asepsy instructions, free delivery of pumps and accessories, monthly consultation, 24 hour/day technical and medical backup given by a specialized staff through an individualized unit are also of the utmost importance. In the authors' opinion, all of the above precautions are a sine qua non condition for the technique to be ethically acceptable.

Indeed, the most threatening clinical risk with intraperitoneal infusion is peritonitis. Only one case of local peritonitis, which was cured by antibiotics and surgical drainage, was observed by the authors. On the other hand, local infections at the skin exit were not rare: A mean of one infection every 35 patient-months, i.e., in 18 of the 71 catheters implanted, was obtained. Seven of the infected catheters had to be explanted because of persisting infection. Severe metabolic disorders were rare and never life threatening (one hypoglycemic coma and one severe ketoacidosis every 39 and 67 patient-months, respectively). Catheter-related problems were not rare, although breakages were usually repaired. Obstructions were usually irreversible, and led to six catheter explantations and a 50% survival rate of the catheters of 16 months. Intraluminal fibrin growth was noted in three cases, whereas enclosure of the catheter in a peritoneal adhesion was seen in the other three cases. In no case did precipitation of acidic insulin appear to be the primary cause of obstruction.

Finally, most of the problems and those constraints can be bypassed by implantable devices. The intraperitoneal route was used successfully by several groups[147] for insulin administration through totally implanted pumps. Peritoneal infections were never encountered, and the reasons for occasional premature termination of the experience were in most cases technical, i.e., pump or catheter related.

## Conclusion

Contrary to the optimistic predictions of scientists in the 1970s, the implantable artificial pancreas is still not available. However, bedside and even wearable feedback-controlled devices are in use, and the pumping part of the system has been implanted in humans with success.

Before a complete and safe device can be developed, the remaining problems of long-term reliability of insulin, reliability of the glucose sensor, and biocompatibility of the catheter for longer life must be solved.

It is wise to avoid predictions after the slow progress during the 1970s and 1980s, but we believe that it will probably take decades rather than years before this technique will routinely replace conventional injections unless transplantation progresses faster and wins the competition. In the meantime, implantable insulin pumps represent the alternative of choice and thus are promised wide application.

---

## References


1. Johnsson S. (1960). Retinopathy and nephropathy in diabetes mellitus. Comparison of the effects of two forms of treatment. *Diabetes* 9:1−8.
2. Pirart J. (1978). Diabetes mellitus and its degenerative complications: A prospective study of 4,400 patients observed between 1947 and 1973. *Diabetes Care* 1:168−188.
3. Job D, Eschwege E, Guyot-Argenton C, et al. (1976). Effect of multiple daily insulin injections on the course of diabetic retinopathy. *Diabetes* 25:463−469.
4. Eschwege E, Job D, Guyot-Argenton C, et al. (1979). Delayed progression diabetic retinopathy by divided insulin administration: A further follow up. *Diabetologia* 16:13−15.
5. Engerman R, Bloodworth JMB Jr, Nelson S. (1977). Relationship of microvascular disease in diabetes to metabolic control. *Diabetes* 26:760−769.
6. Mauer SM, Stettes MW, Michael AF, et al. (1976). Studies of diabetic nephropathy in animals and man. *Diabetes* 25(2):850−857.
7. Kilo C, Vogler N, Williamson JR. (1972). Muscle capillary basement membrane changes related to aging and diabetes mellitus. *Diabetes* 21:881−890.
8. Karam J, Rosenthal M, O'Donnell J, et al. (1976). Discordance of diabetic microangiopathy in identical twins. *Diabetes* 25:24−28.
9. Gander OP, Soeldner JS, Gleason RE, et al. (1977). Monozygotic triplets with discordance for diabetes mellitus and diabetic microangiopathy. *Diabetes* 26:469−479.
10. Osterby R. (1975). Early phases in the development of diabetic glomerulopathy. *Acta Med Scand* (Suppl) 574:1−82.
11. Mauer SM, Barbosa J, Vernier RL, et al. (1976). Development of diabetic vascular lesions in normal kidney transplants into patients with diabetes mellitus. *N Engl J Med* 295:916−920.
12. Mauer SM, Miller K, Goetz FC, et al. (1976). Immunopathology of renal extracellular membranes in kidneys transplanted into patients with diabetes mellitus. *Diabetes* 25:709−712.
13. Beisswenger PJ, Spiro RG. (1970). Human glomerular basement membrane: Chemical alteration in diabetes mellitus. *Science* 168:596−598.
14. Gabbay KH. (1975). Hyperglycemia, polypol metabolism and complications of diabetes mellitus. *Ann Rev Med* 26:521−536.
15. Spritz N. (1978). Nerve disease in diabetes mellitus. *Med Clin North Am* 62:787−798.

16. Brownlee M, Cerami A. (1981). The biochemistry of the complications of diabetes mellitus. *Ann Rev Biochem* 50:385−423.
17. Merimee TJ. (1978). A follow-up study of vascular disease in growth hormone deficient dwarfs with diabetes. *N Engl J Med* 298:1217−1222.
18. Wolinky H, Goldfischer S, Capron L, et al. (1978). Hydrolase activities in the rat aorta. I. Effects of diabetes mellitus and insulin treatment. *Circ Res* 42:831.
19. Ashikaga T, Borodic G, Sims EA. (1978). Multiple daily insulin injections in the treatment of diabetic retinopathy. The job study revisited. *Diabetes* 27:592−596.
20. Knowles H. (1971). Long-term juvenile diabetes treated with unmeasured diet. *Trans Assoc Am Physicians* 84:95−101.
21. Siperstein M, Foster DW, Knowles HC Jr, et al. (1977). Control of blood glucose and diabetic vascular disease. (editorial). *N Eng J Med* 296:1060−1063.
22. Siperstein M, Unger RH, Madison LL. (1968). Studies of muscle capillary basement membranes in normal subjects, diabetic and prediabetic patients. *J Clin Invest* 47:1973−1999.
23. Kalant N. (1978). Diabetic glomerulosclerosis. Current status. *Can Med Assoc J* 119:146−153.
24. Clements RS Jr. (1979). Diabetic neuropathy—New concepts of its etiology. *Diabetes* 28:604−611.
25. Pickup JC, Keen H, Parsons JA, Alberti KGMM. (1979). Continuous subcutaneous insulin infusion: Improved blood glucose and intermediary metabolite control in diabetics. *Lancet* 2:1255−1257.
26. Frier BM, Hilsted J. (1985). Does hypoglycemia aggravate the complications of diabetes. *The Lancet* i:1175−1177.
27. Service JS, Molnar GD, Rosevear JE, et al. (1970). Mean amplitude of glycemic excursions, a measure of diabetic instability. *Diabetes* 29:644−655.
28. Malone JI, Hellrung JM, Malphus EWk, et al. (1976). Good diabetic control—A study in mass delusion. *J Pediatr* 88:943−947.
29. Raskin P, Unger RH. (1978). Effect of insulin therapy on the profile of plasma immunoreactive glucagon in juvenile-type and adult-type diabetes. *Diabetes* 27:411−419.
30. Anonymous. (n.d.). Effect of intensive treatment on substrate and hormonal abnormalities. *Intensive insulin therapy*. In: Schade, Santiago Skyler, Rizza, ed, pp 71−87.
31. G.E.F.C.O.D. Unpublished results.
32. Editorial. (1981). Evidence, implications, and corollaries. *Diabetes Care* 4:573−575.
33. Felig P, Bergman M. (1982). Intensive ambulatory treatment of insulin-dependent diabetes. *Ann Intern Med* 97:225−230.
34. Rizza RA, Gerich JE, Haymond MW, et al. (1983). Control of blood sugar in insulin-dependent diabetes: Comparison of an artificial endocrine pancreas, continuous subcutaneous insulin infusion, and intensified conventional insulin therapy. *N Engl J Med* 303:1313−1318.
35. Tamborlane WV, Sherwin RS, Genel M, Felig P. (1980). Outpatient

treatment of juvenile onset diabetes with a preprogrammed portable subcutaneous insulin infusion system. *Am J Med* 68:190–196.

36. Champion MC, Shepherd GAA, Rodger NW, DuPrie J. (1980). Continuous subcutaneous infusion of insulin in the management of diabetes mellitus. *Diabetes* 29:206–212.

37. Schiffrin A, Colle E, Belmonte M. (1980). Improved control in diabetes with continuous subcutaneous insulin infusion. *Diabetes Care* 3:643–649.

38. Schiffrin A, Belmonte M. (1981). Combined continuous subcutaneous insulin infusion and multiple subcutaneous injections in type 1 diabetic patients. *Diabetes Care* 4:595–600.

39. Home PD, Capaldo B, Burrin JM, Worth R, Alberti KGMM. (1982). A crossover comparison of continuous subcutaneous insulin infusion (CSII) against multiple insulin injections in insulin-dependent diabetic subjects: Improved control with CSII. *Diabetes Care* 5:466–471.

40. Chiasson JL, Ducros F, Poliquin–Hamet M, ′Lopez D, Lecavalier L, Hameet P. (1984). Continuous subcutaneous insulin infusion versus multiple injections in the treatment of insulin dependent diabetes mellitus and the effect of metabolic control on microangiopathy. *Diabetes Care* 7:331–337.

41. Muhlhauser I, Berger M, Sonnenberg G, Koch J, et al. (1985). Incidence and management of severe hypoglycemia in 434 adults with insulin-dependent diabetes mellitus. *Diabetes Care* 8:268–273.

42. Mecklenburg RS, Benson JW Jr, Becker NM, et al. (1982). Clinical use of the insulin infusion pump in 100 patients with Type 1 diabetes. *N Engl J Med* 307:513–518.

43. Peden NR, Bratten JT, McKendry JBR. (1984). Diabetic ketoacidosis during long-term treatment with continuous subcutaneous insulin infusion. *Diabetes Care* 7:1–5.

44. Bending JJ, Pickup JC, Keen H. (1985). Frequency of diabetic ketoacidosis and hypoglycemic coma during treatment with continuous subcutaneous insulin infusion: An audit of medical care. *Am J Med*, cited in leters, *JAMA* 253:No. 18.

45. Teutsch SM, Herman WH, Dwyer DM, Lane JM. (1984). Mortality among diabetic patients using continuous subcutaneous insulin infusion pumps. *N Engl J Med* 310:361–368.

46. Mecklenburg RS, Benson EA, Benson JW Jr, et al. (1984). Acute complications associated with insulin infusion pump therapy. Report of experience with 161 patients. *JAMA* 252:3265–3269.

47. The Kroc Collaborative Study Group. (1984). Blood glucose control and the evolution of diabetic retinopathy and albuminuria. *N Engl J Med* 311:365–372.

48. Unger RH. (1982). Special Comment. Meticulous control of diabetes: Benefits, risks, and precautions. *Diabetes* 31:479–483.

49. White NH, Skor DA, Cryter PE, Levandoski LA, Brier DM, Santiago JV. (1983). Identification of type 1 diabetic patients at increased risk for hypoglycemia during intensive therapy. *N Engl J Med* 308:485–491.

50. Hoeldtke RD, Boden G, Shuman CR, Owen OE. (1982). Reduced epinephrine secretion and hypoglycemia unawareness in diabetic autonomic neuropathy. *Ann Intern Med* 96:459–462.

51. Thorsteinsson B, Pramming S, Lauritzen T, Binder C. (1984). Frequency of biochemical hypoglycemia at different blood glucose levels in conventionally and pump-treated type 1 (insulin-dependent) diabetic patients. *Diabetologia* 27:338 A.

52. Eichner HL, Holleman C, Worcester B, Turner D, Woertz L. Selam JL, Charles MA. Reduction of severe hypoglycemic events in type I diabetic patients using CSII. *Diabetes Care* (submitted).

53. Knight G, Boulton AJM, Ward JD. (1984). Success in reducing the rate of ketoacidosis in patients treated with continuous subcutaneous insulin infusion. European Association for the Study of Diabetes, London Abs. p 297A.

54. Albisser AM, Leibel BS, Ewart TG, Davidovac Z, Botz CK, Wingg W, Schipper H, Gander R. (1974). Clinical control of diabetes by the artificial pancreas. *Diabetes* 23:397−404.

55. Lim F, Sun A. (1980). Microencapsulated islets: bioartificial endocrine pancreas. *Science* 210:908−910.

56. Altmann JJ, Houlbert D, Chollier A, Leduc A, McMillan P, Galletti PM. (1984). Encapsulated human islet transplants in diabetic rats. *Trans Am Soc Artif Intern Organs* 30:3812.

57. Scharp DW, Mason NS, Sparks RE. (1984). Islet immuno-isolation: The use of hybrid artificial organs to prevent islet tissue rejection. *World J Surg* 8:221−229.

58. Reach G, Poussier P, Sausse A, Assan R, Itoh M, Gerich JE. (1981). Functional evaluation of a bio-artificial pancreas using isolated islet perifused with blood ultrafiltrate. *Diabetes* 30:296−301.

59. Reach G, Jaffrin MY, Vanhoutte C, Desjeux JF. (1984). Importance of convective transport in a model of bioartificial pancreas. *Am Soc Artif Intern Organs* 7:85−90.

60. Reach G, Jaffrin MY, Desjeux JF. (1984). A U-shaped bioartifical pancreas with rapid glucose-insulin kinetics: In vitro evaluation and kinetic modelling. *Diabetes* 752:761.

61. Orsetti A, Bouhaddioui N, Crespy S, Perez R. (1981). Analyse critique de la valeur fonctionnelle d'un pancreas bio-artificiel (modele a fibre creuses). *C R Soc Biol* (Paris) 175:228−234.

62. Browlee M, Cerami A. (1983). Glycosylated insulin complexed to concanavalin A: A biochemical basis for a closed-loop insulin delivery system. *Diabetes* 32:499−504.

63. Mirouze J, Jaffiol C, Sany C. (1962). Enregistremene glycemique hycthemeral continu deno le diabete instable. *Rev Fr Endovrinol Clin Miti Metab* 3:337−353.

64. Kadish AH. (1964). Automation control of blood sugar I. A servo-mechanism for glucose monitoring and control. *Am J Med Electron* 3:82.

65. Metcalf J. (1934). The administration of insulin by continuous injection. MB Thesis, University of Cambridge.

66. Kessler M, Hoper J, Volkhor HJ, Sailer D, Demling L. (1985). Tissue measurement of glucose with a new potential electrode in continuous insulin infusion therapy. KD Hepp and R Renner Ed, Schattauer, Stuttgort, New York pp 19−26.

67. Woods SC, Porte D. (1974). Neural control of the endocrine pancreas. *Phys Rev* 54:596−619.
68. Anonymous. (1983). Substrate and hormonal alteration in diabetes mellitus in intensive insulin therapy. Shade DS, Santiago JV, Styler JS and Rizza RA, eds, Excerpta Medica, pp 36−70.
69. Clark LC Jr, Lyons C. (1962). Electrode systems for continuous monitoring in cardiovascular surgery. *Ann N Y Acad Sci* 102:29.
70. Clark LC Jr. (1956). Monitor and control of blood and tissue oxygen tensions. *Trans Am Soc Artif Intern Organs* 2:41.
71. Bessman SP, Schultz RD. (1973). Prototype glucose-oxydase sensor for the artificial pancreas. *Trans Am Soc Artif Intern Organs* 19:361.
72. Clarke WL, Santiago JV. (1977). The characteristics of a new glucose sensor for use in artificial pancreatic beta cell. *Artif Organs* 1:78.
73. Schichiri M, Kawamori R, Yamashki Y, Hakui N, Abe H. (1986). Wearable artificial pancreas with needle-type glucose sensor. *Lancet* 2:1129.
74. Schichiri M, Kawamori R, Goriya Y, Yamasaki Y, Nomura Y. (1983). *Diabetologia* 24:179−184.
75. Chang LW, Aisenberg S, Soeldner JS, Hiebert JM. (1973). Validation of bioengineering aspects of an implantable glucose sensor. *Trans Am Soc Artif Intern Organs* 352:19.
76. March W, Engerman R, Rabinovitch B. (1979). Optical monitor of glucose. *Trans Am Soc Artif Intern Organs* 25:28.
77. Kaiser N. (1977). Laser absorption spectroscopy with an ATR prism: Noninvasive in vivo determination of glucose. *Horm Metabl Res Suppl* 7:72.
78. Rabinovitch B, March W, Adams RL. (1982). Noninvasive glucose monitoring of the aqueous humor of the eye. I. Measurement of very small optical rotations. *Diabetes Care* 5:254.
79. Rabinovitch B, March WF, Adams RL. Noninvasive glucose monitoring of the aqueous humor of the eye. II. Animal studies and the scleroal lens. *Diabetes Care* 5:259.
80. Schultz J, Mansouri S, Goldstein I. (1982). Affinity sensors: A new technique for developing implantable sensors or glucose and other metabolites. *Diabetes Care* 5:245.
81. Mirouze J, Selam JL, Pham TC, Cavadore D. (1977). Evaluation of exogenous insulin homeostasis by the artificial pancreas in insulin-dependent diabetes. *Diabetologia* 13:273−278.
82. Botz CK. (1976). An improved control algorithm for an artificial $\beta$-cell. *IEEE Trans Biomed Eng* 23:252−255.
83. Marliss EB, Murray FT, Stokes EF, Zinman B, Nakhooda AF, Denoga A, Leibel BS, Albisser AM. (1977). Normalization of glycemia in diabetics during meals with insulin and glucagon delivery by the artificial pancreas. *Diabetes* 26:663−672.
84. Albisser AM, Leibel BS, Zinman B, Murray FT, Zingg W, Botz CK, Denoga A, Marliss EB. (1977). Studies with an artificial pancreas. *Arch Intern Med* 137:639−649.
85. Soegijoko S, Selam JL, Ferrand D, Mirouze J. (1980). External artificial pancreas—4th generation and first time. 7th Meeting of the Europ Soc Artif Org Genera.

86. Curry DL, Bennett LL, Grodsky GM. (1968). Dynamics of insulin secretion by the perfused rat pancreas. *Endocrinology* 83:572−584.
87. Foster RO. (1970). The dynamics of blood sugar regulation. M Sc Thesis, Massachusetts Institute of Technology.
88. Ewart TG, Albisser AM, Leibel BS, Davidovac Z, Zingg W. (1973). Computer analog of the endocrine pancreas. Int. Symp. on Dynamics Fluid Controls in Pysiological Systems. Iberall AS, Guyton AC, eds *Am Physiol Soc* pp 509−511.
89. Clemens AH, Chang PH, Myers RW. (1977). The development of bio-stator, a glucose controlled insulin infusion system (GCIIS). *Horm Metabl Res Suppl* 7:22−23.
90. Schichiri M, Kawamori R. (1985). Optimized algorithim for closed-loop glycemic control. In: Computer Systems for Insulin Adjustment in Diabetes Mellitus, J Beyer, et al. Pascienta-Verlag, Hedingen, Switzerland, pp. 171−183.
91. Piwernetz K, Renner R, Hepp KID. Attempt at glucose-controlled feed-back regulatory of intraperitoneal insulin infusion.
92. Schade, DA, Eaton RP, Friedman N, Spencer W. (1979). The intravenous, intraperitoneal, and subcutaneous routes of insulin delivery in diabetic man. *Diabetes* 28:1068−1072.
93. Gyaram H, Bottermann P, Ehrhardt W, Blumel G. (1983). Pharmacokinetics of intraperitoneally injected insulin and the development of a cannula system to facilitate intraperitoneal injection. In: Brunetti P et al eds, *Artificial Systems for Insulin Delivery*, Raven Press, New York.
94. Selam JL, Slingeneyer A, Hedon B, Mares P, Beraud JJ, Mirouze J. (1983). Long-term ambulatory peritoneal insulin infusion of brittle diabetes with portable pumps: Comparison with intravenous and subcutaneous route. *Diabetes Care* 6:105−111.
95. Selam JL, Raymond M, Jacquemin JL, Orsetti A, Richard JL, Mirouze J. (1985). Pharmacokinetics of insulin infected intraperitoneally via portable pumps. *Diab Metab* 11:170−173.
96. Bergmann RN, Bucolo RJ. (1973). Nonlinear metabolic dynamics of the pancreas and liver. *J Dynam Syst Trans ASME* 95:296−900.
97. Slama G, Hautecouverture M, Assan R, Tchobroutsky G. (1974). One to five days of continuous intravenous insulin infusion on seven diabetic patients. *Diabetes* 23:732−738.
98. Pickup JC, Keen H, Parsons JA, Alberti KGMM. (1978). Continuous subcutaneous insulin infusion: An approach to achieving normoglycaemia. *Br Med J* 1:204−207.
99. Novo Industry. (1983). Data on insulin infusion pumps.
100. Carlson GA, Bair REk, Goana JI Jr, Schidknecht HE, Love JT, Urenda R. (1982). An implantable, remotely programmable insulin infusion system. *Med Prog Technol* 9:17.
101. Schade DS, Eaton RP, Edwards WS. (1982). A remotely programmable insulin delivery system: Successful short-term implantation in man. *JAMA* 247:1848.
102. Irsigler K, Kirtz H, Hagmuller G. (1981). Long-term continuous intraperitoneal insulin infusion with an implantable remote controlled insulin infusion device. *Diabetes* 30:1072.

103. Hepp KD, Renner R, Funcke HJ, Mehnert H, Haerten R, Kresse H. (1975). Intravenous insulin therapy under conditions imitating physiological profiles. *Diabetologia* 11(Abstr):349.
104. Hepp KD, Renner R, Funcke HJ, Mehnert H, Haerten R, Kresse H. (1977). Glucose homeostasis under continuous intravenous insulin therapy in diabetics. *Horm Metab Res* (Suppl) 7:72.
105. Hepp KD, Renner R, Piewernetz K, Mehnert H. (1980). Control of insulin-dependent diabetes with portable minaturized infusion systems. *Diabetes Care* 3:309.
106. Walter H, Kemmler W, Kronski D, Franetzki M, Prestele K, Hepp KD, Renner R, Mehnert H. (1983). Implantation of a program-controlled device with intravenous insulin infusion in a patient with Type I diabetes mellitus. In: Brunetti P, Alberti KGMM, Albisser AM, Hepp KD, Massi Benedetti M eds, *Artificial Systems for Insulin Delivery* Serona Symp Publ Vol 6, Raven Press, New York, p 313.
107. Selam JL, Slingeneyer A, Chaptal PA. (1982). Total implantation of a remotely controlled insulin minipump in a human insulin dependent diabetic. *Artif Org* 6:315.
108. Elsberry D, Vadnais K, Bartelt K, VanKampen K. (1984). Abstract in artificial insulin-delivery systems. Workshop of the study group of EASO−Iglo (Austria).
109. Fischell RE, Saudek C. (1983). A programmable implantable medication system: Application to diabetes. 6th Hawaii International Conference on System Sciences.
110. Saudek CD, Fischelle RE, Swindle M, et al. (1986). Preclinical trial of the programmable implantable medication system. *Diabetes* (suppl) 35:82A.
111. Thomas LJ, Bessman SP. (1975). *Trans Am Soc Artif Organs* 21:516−522.
112. Schubert W, Baurschmidt P, Nagel J, Thull R, Schaldacl M. (1980). *Med Biol Eng Comput* 18:527.
113. Kuhl D, Luft G. (1976). Deutsches Patent Nr 2626348.
114. Luft G, Kuhl D, Richter GJ. (1978). *Med & Biol Eng Comput* 16:45−50.
115. Uhlig ELP, Graydon WF. (1983). *Biomed Mater Res* 1:931−943.
116. Hsieh DST, Langer R, Folkman J. (1981). *Proc Nat Acad Sci USA* 78:1863.
117. Schade D, Eaton R, DeLongo J, Saland L, Ladman A, Carlson G. (1982). Electron microscopy of insulin precipitates. *Diabetes Care* 5:25.
118. Blackshear PJ, Rohde TD, Palmer JL, Wigness BD, Rupp WM, Buchwald H. (1983). Glycerol prevents insulin precipitation and interruption of flow in an implantable insulin infusion pump. *Diabetes Care* 6:387.
119. Brange J, Havelund S. (1983). Properties of insulin solutions. In: Brunetti P, Alberti KGM Albisser AM, Hepp KD, Massi Benedetti M, eds, *Artificial Systems for Insulin Delivery*. Serono Symp Publications, Vol 6, Raven Press, New York, p 89.
120. Selam JL, Slingeneyer A, Cahptal PA, Franetzki M, Prestele K, Mirouze J. One year continuous run with the totally-implantable Siemen pump in a human diabetic. In: Irsigler K, Kritz H, Lovett R, eds,

*Diabetes Treatment with Implantable Insulin Infusion Systems*, Urban & Schwarzenberg, Munich, p 119.

121. Selam JL, Giraud P, Mirouze J, Saeidi S. (1985). Continuous peritoneal insulin infusion with portable pumps: Factors affecting the operating life of the chronic catheter. *Diabetes Care* 8:34−38.

122. Selam JL, Slingeneyer A, Saeidi S, Mirouze J, Richard JL, Rodier M, Daynes B, Lapinski H. (1985). Experience with long-term peritoneal insulin infusion from external pumps. *Diab Med* 2:41−44.

123. Selam JL, Mirouze J, Cavalie-Barthez G, Mellet M, Zirinis P, Gagnol JP, Humeau P. (1985). Insulin for portable pumps: Influence of pH on in vitro stability in reservoirs. *Diabetes* 34:200 (a) *Artif Organs* (in press).

124. Hepp KD, Renner R, vonFuncke HF. (1977). Glucose homeostasis under continuous intravenous insulin therapy in diabetics. *Horm Metabol Res Suppl* 7:72.

125. Irsigler K, Kirtz H. (1979). Long-term continuous intravenous insulin therapy with a portable insulin dosage-regulating apparatus. *Diabetes* 28:196.

126. Froesch ER, Blatter G, Morell B. (1979). Optimal blood sugar control in labile diabetics using a portable open-loop insulin infusion system with a flexible program. *Feedback-Controlled and Preprogrammed Insulin Infusion in Diabetes Mellitus*, In: Hepp KRD, Kerner W, Pfeiffer EW, eds, Horm Metabl Res (Suppl 8), Georg Thieme Verlag, Stuttgart, p 198.

127. Grau U. (1985). Chemical stability of insulin in a delivery system environment. *Diabetologia* 28:458−463.

128. Selam JL, Zirinis P, Mellet M, Mirouze J. (1987). A stable insulin for implantable insulin delivery systems—in vitro studies with different containers and solvents. *Diabetes Care* 10:343−347.

129. Kritz H, Najemnik C, Hagmuller G, Leddolter S, Olbert F, Mostbeck A, Denck H, Irsigler K. (1983). Long term results using different routes of infusion; in diabetes treatment with implantable insulin infusion systems. K. Irsigler et al, ed., Urban and Schwartzenberg, Munich, pp 81−102.

130. Brange J, Langljaer L, Havelund S, Sorensen E. (1985). Chemical stability of insulin: Neutral insulin solutions. *Diabetologia* 25:143(A).

131. Geisen K, Gerlach MH, Keil M. (1982). Morphological findings in pancreatectomized dogs with an implanted insulin dosing device: tissue reaction to the pump housing and to the vascular catheter. *Horm Metab Res* 15:180.

132. Geisen K, Jung S, Fiedler B. (1983). Result with a catheterless insulin delivery device implanted in a pancreatectomized dog. *Horm Metabol Res* 15:111.

133. Geisen K, Thurow H, Jung S. (1982). A remote programmable implantable insulin dosing device. II. Results of animal experiments. In: Federlin K, Pfeiffer EF, Raptis S, eds, *Islet-Pancreas Transplantation and Artificial Pancreas*, Georg Thieme, Stuttgart, p 310.

134. Buchwald H, Varco RL, Rupp WM. Treatment of a type II diabetic by a totally implantable insulin device. *Lancet* 6:1233.

135. Rupp WM, Barbosa J, Blackshear PH, McCarthy HB, Rohde TD,

Goldenberg F. (1982). Implantable insulin pump therapy in Type II diabetics. *N Engl J Med* 307:265.

136. Rupp WH, Rohde TD, Wigness BD, Blackshear PH, Buchwald H. Clinical experiences with insulin-glycerol solution in an implantable pump. *Trans Artif Org* (in press).

137. Kernstinek K, Wianess B, Krygeski S, et al. (1986). Restoration of implantable insulin infusion device flow. *Diabetes* (suppl) 35:143A.

138. Selam JL, Giraud P, Hedon B, Saeidi S, Mirouze J, Orsetti A, Slingeneyer A. (1985). Factors affecting the operating life and efficiency of catheters for continuous intraperitoneal insulin infusion. *Continuous Insulin Infusion Therapy Experience From One Decade.* In: Hepp, Renner, eds, Shattauer, Stuttgart, pp 65−73.

139. Selam JL. Personal unpublished results.

140. Lord P. Pacesetter unpublished results.

141. Franetzki M, Prestele K, Kresse H. (1979). Technological problems of minaturized insulin dosing devices and some approaches to clinical trials. In: Hepp KO, Kerner W, Pfeiffer EF, eds, *Feedback-Controlled and Preprogrammed Insulin Infusion in Diabetes Mellitus, Horm Metab Res* (Suppl 8), 58.

142. Eaton RP, Schade DS, Pitcher L. (1983). Catheter encapsulation during prolonged intraperitoneal insulin infusion in a patient with a remote-controlled insulin delivery system. In: Irsigler K, Kritz H, Lovett R eds, *Diabetes Treatment with Implantable Insulin Infusion Systems*, Urban & Schwarzenberg, Munich, p 126.

143. Kritz H, Najemnik C, Hagmuller G, Leodolter S, Olbert F, Mostbeck A, Dench H, Irsigler K. (1983). Long-term results using different routes of insulin infusion. In: Irsigler K, Kritz H, Lovett R, eds, *Diabetes Treatment with Implantable Insulin Infusion Systems*, Urban & Schwarzenberg, Munich, p 81.

144. Williams HF, Jarvis CW, Neal WA, Reynolds JW. (1972). Vascular thromboembolism complicating umbilical artery catheterization. *Am J Roentgenol Radium Ther Nucl Med* 116:475.

145. Knatterud G, Fisher M. (1985). Report from the International Study Group on Implantable Insulin Delivery Devices. *Diabetes Care* 8:308−309.

146. Dupre J, Champion M, Rodger NW. (1982). Advances in insulin delivery in the management of diabetes mellitus. *Clin Endocrinol Metabol* 11:525−549.

147. Selam JL, Mirouze J, Slingeneyer A, Hedon B, Millet P, Chaptal PA, Orsetti A. (1983). Two years experience of ambulatory peritoneal insulin infusion. In: Irsigler K, Kritz H, Lovett R, eds, *Implantable Delivery Systems*, Frankfurt, Urban & Schwartzenberg, pp 132−136.

148. Chisholm DJ, Kraegen EW. (1982). Pharmacokinetics of subcutaneous insulin with reference to pumps. Presented at the Toronto International Workshop on Insulin and Portable Delivery Systems, June 9−11, Toronto, Canada.

149. Home PD, Pickup JC, Keen H, Alberti KGMM, Parson JA, Binder C. (1980). Continuous subcutaneous insulin infusion: Comparison of plasma insulin profiles after infusion or bolus injection of the meal-time dose. *Metabolism* 30:439−442.

150. Schiffrin A, Belmonte MM. (1982). Comparison between continuous subcutaneous insulin infusion and multiple injections of insulin, a one year prospective study. *Diabetes* 31:255−264.
151. Pickup JC, Keen H, Viberti GC, White MC, Kohner EM, Parsons JA, Alberti KGMM. (1980). Continuous subcutaneous insulin infusion in the treatment of diabetes mellitus. *Diabetes Care* 3:290−300.
152. Who-Study on CSII acceptability and efficiency. Unpublished report.
153. Goriya Y, Bahoric A, Marliss EB, Zinman B, Albisser AM. (1979). Glycemic regulation using a programmed insulin delivery device. III: Long-term studies on diabetic dogs. *Diabetes* 28:558−564.
154. Albisser AM, Nomura M, Greenberg GR, McPhedran NT. (1986). Metabolic control in diabetic dogs treated with autotransplants and insulin pumps. *Diabetes* 35:97−100.
155. Miles JM, Rizza RA, Raymond MW, Gerich JD. (1980). Effects of acute insulin deficiency on glucose and ketone body turnover in man. *Diabetes* 29:926−930.
156. Gooch BR, Abumrad NM, Robinson RP, Petrik M, Campbell D, Crofford OB. (1983). Exercise in insulin dependent diabetes mellitus: The effect of continuous infusion using the subcutaneous, intravenous and intraperitoneal sites. *Diabetes Care* 6:122−127.
157. Mirouze J, Selam JL. (1983). Clinical experience in human diabetics with portable and implantable insulin minipumps. *Life Support Syst* 1:39−50.
158. Pickup JC, Home PD, Bilous RW, Alberti KGMM, Keen H. (1981). Management of severely brittle diabetes by continuous and intramuscular insulin infusion: Evidence for a defect in subcutaneous insulin absorption. *Br Med J* 282:347−350.
159. Field JB, Rojdmark S, Harding P, Ishida T, Chou MCY. (1980). Role of liver in insulin physiology. *Diabetes Care* 3:255.
160. Albisser AM, Botz CL, Leibel BS. (1979). Blood glucose regulation using an open-loop insulin delivery system in pancreatectomized dogs given glucose infusion. I: Portal square waves. *Diabetologia* 16:129−133.
161. Riza QA, Westland RE, Hall LD, Patton GS, Haymond MW, Clemens AH, Gerich JE, Service FJ. (1981). Effect of peripheral versus portal venous administration of insulin on postprandial hyperglycemia and glucose turn-over in alloxan, diabetic dogs. *Mayo Clin Proc* 56:434−438.
162. Stevenson RW, Parsons JA, Alberti KGMM. Comparison of the metabolic responses to portal and peripheral infusions of insulin in diabetic dogs. *Metabolism* 30:745−752.
163. Nelson JA, Stephen R, Landau ST, Wilson DE, Tyler FH. (1982). Intraperitoneal insulin administration produces a positive portal-systemic blood insulin gradient in unanaesthetized unrestrained swine. *Metabolism* 31:969−972.
164. Schade DS, Eaton RP, Davis T, Akiya F, Phinnem E, Kubica R, Vaughn EA, Day PW. (1981). The kinetics of peritoneal insulin absorption. *Metabolism* 30:149−153.
165. Renner R, Piwernetz K, Hepp KD. (1983). Continuous intraperitoneal

insulin treatment in type I diabetes: Comparison between square wave infusion and bolus application. *Diabetologia* 25:189A.
166. Kraft AR. (1968), Peritoneal electrolyte absorption, analysis of portal system, venous and lymphatic transport. *Surgery* 64:148.
167. Irsigler K, Kritz H. (1980). Alternate routes of insulin delivery. *Diabetes Care* 3:219–228.
168. Pozza G, Spotti D, Mizossi P, Cristallo M, Melandri M, Piatti PM, Monti LD, Pontirolli AE. (1983). Long-term continuous intraperitoneal insulin treatment in brittle diabetes. *Br Med J* 286:255–256.
169. Marshall SM, Husband DJ, Walford S, Wrigth PD, Alberti KGMM. (1983). Use of intraperitoneal insulin in brittle diabetes. *Diabetologia* 25:179A.
170. Rizza RA, Service JF, Westland RE, Hall RD, Patton GS, Haymond MW, Gerich JE. (1979). Comparison of peripheral venous, portal, subcutaneous and intraperitoneal routes for insulin delivery in diabetic dogs. Presented at the Workshop on Artificial Beta Cells, September 19–29, Heviz, Hungary.
171. Irsigler K, Kritz H, Hagmuller G, Najemmik C, Leddolter S. (1983). Long-term safety of insulin infusion: The intravenous and intraperitoneal route for pump treatment. *Diabetologia* 25:167A.

The reader will find excellent reviews on the subject in the following few references.
Blackshear PJ. (1987). Implantable pumps for insulin delivery. In: *Drug Delivery Systems: Controlled Drug Delivery* Ellis Horwood Pub, England.

Santiago J, Clemens A, Clarke W, Kipnis D. (1979). Closed-loop end open-loop devices for blood glucose control in normal and diabetic subjects. *Diabetes* 28:71–85.

Irsigler K, Kritz H, Lovett RG. (1985). Controlled drug delivery in the treatment of diabetes mellitus. In: *Critical Review in Therapeutic Drug Carrier Systems* 1:189–278.

Franetzki M. (1984). Drug delivery by program or sensor-controlled infusion devices *Pharmaceutical Res*:237–244.

# Chapter 7

# Bioartificial Pancreas as an Approach to Closed-Loop Insulin Delivery

G. Reach
M.Y. Jaffrin

## Definition of a Closed-Loop Insulin Delivery System

Currently, the treatment of insulin-dependent-diabetes mellitus is limited by the fact that insulin is delivered on a programmed basis, taking into account the results of urine and blood glucose monitoring of the previous days. By contrast, insulin secretion by the islets of Langerhans is regulated minute by minute by the concomitant blood glucose concentration. The aim of a closed-loop insulin delivery system is to simulate this basic property of normal insulin secretion. It is expected that such a system would be more efficient in normalizing blood glucose concentration, and therefore in preventing the long-term complications of the disease.

From: Ensminger WD. Selam JL (eds): *Infusion Systems in Medicine*. Mount Kisco, NY, Futura Publishing Co., Inc., © 1987.

## Bioartificial Pancreas as a Potential Closed-Loop Insulin Delivery System

Three kinds of approach are possible. In the electromechanical one (the so-called "artificial pancreas"), a glucose sensor generates a current that is used as a signal to be processed by a computer to control, with appropriate algorithms, the rate of a pump delivering insulin. This approach is limited by the short lifespan of the currently available sensors. In the chemical approach, glycosylated insulin is released by competition with glucose from a support (such as a lectin), which can bind both glucose and the osidic moiety of glycosylated insulin. Thus, insulin would be released as a function of blood glucose concentration. The ability of such systems to correct experimental diabetes in animals remains to be demonstrated. The third approach uses the regulatory properties of living pancreatic tissue. However, pancreas or islet transplantation is limited by immune rejection of the graft. A possible solution is the immunoprotection of the graft by a membrane permeable to glucose and insulin, but not so to immunoglobulins and lymphocytes, in a "bioartificial pancreas." This approach would have the further advantage of overcoming the obstacle of the poor availability of transplantable pancreatic tissue, as xenogenic islets could be used.

Several kinds of bioartificial pancreas have been proposed so far. In extravascular systems, islets are encapsulated either in microcapsules or in a hollow fiber. These systems have been shown to normalize blood glucose concentration in diabetic rats for several months. In vascular systems, the blood of the recipient is allowed to circulate in contact of the membrane, islets being placed on its other side within a closed compartment.

## Development of a Vascular Bioartificial Pancreas Using Convective Transfer of Glucose and Insulin Across the Membrane

A major theoretical obstacle to the development of all these systems is related to the slowness of glucose and insulin diffusion across membranes, which introduces a lag in the response time of the system to glucose and which might not be compatible with the achievement of a closed-loop insulin delivery system. This obstacle can be overcome in vascular systems, in which the hydrodynamic pressure of blood in the blood channel generates a flux of ultrafiltrate from blood to the islet compartment, followed by reabsorption of fluid from the islets to blood. It is possible to set up a kinetic model of this phenomenon and to demonstrate that it can accelerate glucose and insulin transfer in a bioartificial pancreas.[1] We also demonstrated in short-term experiments that islets perfused with blood ultrafiltrate do respond to glucose.[2] A device with a U-shaped blood channel (which accelerates further the response time of the system) was evaluated in vitro[3] and in vivo in rats.[4] The response time to glucose was found to be shorter than 10 min., which should be compatible with the use of this device as a closed-loop insulin delivery system.

## The Problems to be Solved

Presently, this research is still in an experimental stage. To reach the stage of clinical use,[1] it is necessary to develop methods for the large-scale isolation of pure islets of Langerhans. Recent progress in this field indicates that a large number (more than 100,000) islets can be isolated from one pancreas (from beef, dogs, or human beings).[2] It must be demonstrated that the islets can survive in an immunological state for several months. A recent report by Araki[5] demonstrated the survival of 50,000 dog islets placed in a vascular device perfused with a culture medium. The device released up to 10 units of insulin per day for at least 80 days. These results also demonstrate that the properties of the membrane were not altered by a contact with a medium containing 10% of fetal calf serum.[3] The last (but not least) problem to solve will be the prevention of blood clotting inside the device. Thus, the development of hemocompatible materials is required for the full development of this reasearch toward a therapeutic tool.

## References


1. Reach G, Jaffrin MY, Vanhoutte C, Desjeux JF. (1984). Importance of convective transport in a model of bioartificial pancreas. *Am Soc Artif Intern Organs J* 7:85–90.
2. Reach G, Poussier P, Sausse A, Assan R, Itoh M, Gerich JE. (1981). Func-

tional evaluation of a bioartificial pancreas using isolated islets perifused with blood ultrafiltrate. *Diabetes* 30:296−301.
3. Reach G, Jaffrin MY, Desjeux JF. (1984). A U-shaped bioartificial pancreas with rapid glucose-insulin kinetics: In vitro evaluation and kinetic modelling. *Diabetes* 33:752−761.
4. Reach G, Chenard PS, Darquy S, Lepeintre J, Desjeux JF, Cannon R, Jaffrin MY. (in press). Kinetics of insulin delivery by a bioartificial pancreas: In vivo evaluation in conscious normal rats. *Prog Artif Organs*.
5. Araki Y, Solomon BA, Basile RM, Chick WL. (1985). Biohybrid artificial pancreas. Long term insulin secretion by devices seeded with canine islets. *Diabetes* 34:850−854.

# Chapter 8

# Realization of a Bioartificial Pancreas Using New Performant Asymmetric Membrane


A. Orsetti
F. Schue
G. Paleirac
J. Sledz
A. El Harfi
S. Crespy


## Introduction

The degenerative complications of diabetes mellitus can be prevented by precise control of blood glucose.

Among the methods proposed for maintenance of euglycemia—which has received much attention during the ten last years—is the implantation of a "bioartificial pancreas."

To prevent immune rejection of islets of Langerhans, the pan-

*From:* Ensminger WD, Selam JL (eds): *Infusion Systems in Medicine.* Mount Kisco, NY, Futura Publishing Co., Inc., ©1987.

creatic cells are housed in an appropriate chamber, separated from blood by a membrane permeable to glucose and insulin, but impermeable to antibodies and lymphocytes.

Several bioartificial devices were studied and published, working according to the diffusion principle for transferring glucose and insulin across a semipermeable membrane.[1-6]

Experimental studies and mathematical modeling of these types of bioartificial pancreas showed two major defects[7-9]: (1) clotting problems in islet transplantation chambers; and (2) slow glucose insulin kinetics.

## Blood Clotting Problems

Several processes to produce hemocompatible membranes were originated. We have chosen the most performant asymmetric membrane, synthesized with Kariflex transformed in cyclic polymer.

The asymmetric membrane is prepared from a collodion, which is cast as a thick film on a glass plate; then the solvent is allowed to evaporate during a given time, and finally the film is immersed into a gelation bath.

The following conditions are used to prepare the asymmetric membrane:

Polymer/solvent/nonsolvent/porogenic agent: 14,5/65/19,8/0,7 (in weight percentage)

Time of evaporation of the solvent: 5 sec (at 25° C)

Gelation bath: ethanol/water (at 25° C): 4 vol./1 vol.

The structure of the membrane obtained by casting the collodion is evidenced by scanning electron microscopy (Fig. 1). Chemical modification of the membrane with addition of N-Chlorosulfonyl isocyanate introduces heparin active groups ($NHSO_3-$, $COO^-$) into the polymer. This modification affects only slightly the morphology of the membrane.

### Determination of Anticoagulant Activity

The anticoagulant activity is determined by measuring the thrombin clotting time of platelet poor plasma (PPP) incubated with various amounts of membrane.

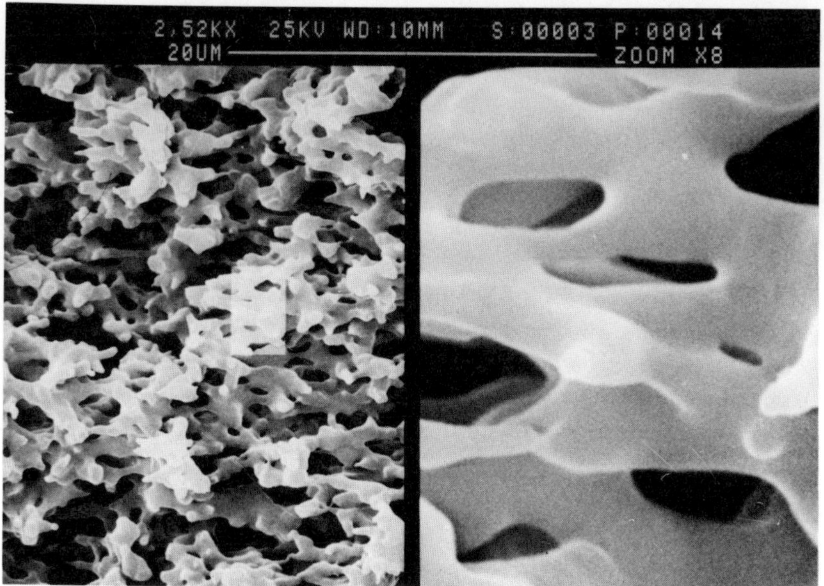


**Figure 1:** Electron micrograph:  structure of the membrane.

Chemical transformation of the membrane with N-Chlorosulfonyl isocyanate during 15 minutes gives the best number of "heparin-like" sites.

The amounts of inactivated thrombin are a function of the suspended membrane:  10 mg of the membrane are able to inactive 60% of thrombin with a solution at 20 U ml$^{-1}$ of thrombin (78% with a solution at 10, 90% with a solution at 5, 94% with a solution at 2). Ten mg of this material corresponds to 1.4 mmole/g of sulfonate group and carboxylate group.

The synthetic material resolves the platelet aggregation problem, studied with a photometric method (measure of the variations of optic transmission of platelet suspension). There is no platelet agregation with the membrane.

## Kinetic Problems

To obtain satisfactory glucose insulin kinetics the mechanic properties of the membrane need to be improved.

### Mechanic Properties

The new membrane can be used at higher pressures than the conventional acrylic copolymer membrane. It has an important pressure strength associated with an exceptionally good deformability.

### Ultrafiltration Characteristics

Permeability and permselectivity of the membrane are followed by ultrafiltration rates of pure solvents (water, methanol, ethanol...) as well as aqueous solutions of dextran of different molecular weights but with low polydispersity (I = 1.02).

The evolution of ultrafiltration rate of distilled water is a function of time.

A high hydraulic permeability is observed: 30,000 l/day − m$^2$ atm = (27 × 10$^{-4}$ ml/min × cm$^2$ × mmHg).

Permselectivity followed by ultrafiltration rate of dextran solution is: mean 50% dextran molecular weight cutoff: 80,000 Daltons. Permeability was followed by ultrafiltration rate of an insulin solution (concentraton = 40 μU/ml) is 16,600 l/day m$^2$ atm.

## Histocompatibility Study

It is important to evaluate the viability of islets cultured on the membrane.

### Isolation of Rat Islets

For the different experiments, islets of Langerhans were isolated from fed male Wistar rats weighing approximately 250 g, by the collagenase digestion method of Lacy and Kostianovsky.[10]

The pancreatic tissue is distended by infusion of Hank's solution through the common duct. After the tissue is chopped and digested with collagenase, the islets are separated by centrifugation on a discontinuous ficoll gradient. Then, islets are hand-picked and washed in a 199 solution.

Twenty rat islets are cultured on the membrane, in ten incubation dishes, in 2 ml 1640 RPMI medium supplemented with 10%

heat inactived fetal calf serum and antibiotics (penicillin 100 μ/mL and streptomycine 100 μg/mL).

The culture dishes are placed in a wet chamber at 37° C and in an atmosphere of 5% $CO_2$ and 95% air.

Control islets are cultured in identical conditions, but without membrane. The islet viability is evaluated by measuring the insulin release three times a week. The results show that the islets cultured on membrane have a dynamic vitality: The quantity of insulin secreted by the islets placed in a membrane is similar to the response observed with the control islets. During one month, rat islets produce 50−90 μU of insulin/islet/day (Fig. 2).

A structural study (SEM) shows that the islets' morphology was kept very well.

## Kinetic Study in a Device Built with the New Membrane

The excellent deformability of the membrane allowed us to develop and to optimize a device, following the indications given by

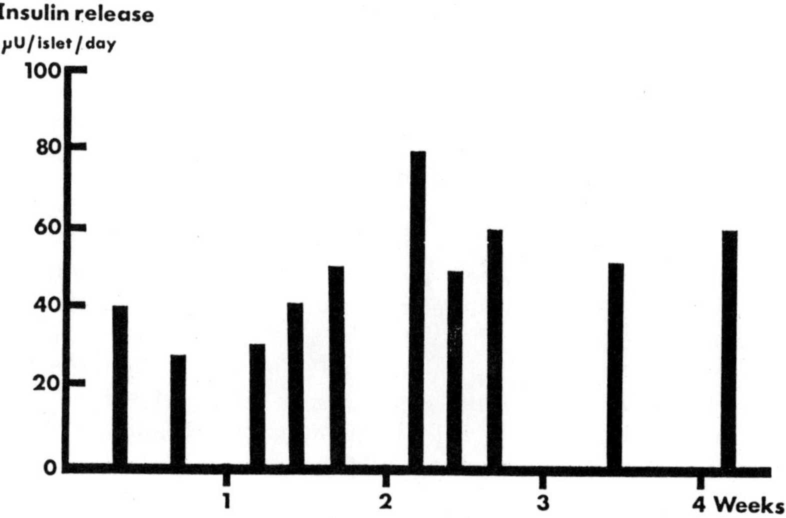


**Figure 2:** Mean insulin release from cultured rat islets in RPMI medium (glucose concentration:  17 mM/L) on the asymmetric membrane, during one month.

our mathematical modeling.[8,9] Simulated endocrine pancreas function showed that certain geometric parameters can be altered to yield a satisfactory insulin response to the glucose stimulus. By reducing the volume of the islets compartment, maintaining a good surface of exchange, we obtained a reduction of the functional inertia.

The islets compartment is built with two rectangular pieces of membrane (1.5 × 0.5 cm) tightened together and glued side to side with the collodion used to prepare the membrane. We introduce the islets in the unit with a very thin catheter, inserted in the chamber by one extremity. Fifty islets of Langerhans are placed in this functional unit, within approximately 50 μl RPMI 1640 medium. This end is closed with collodion. In such a two-membrane unit, the islets are working in a genuine virtual space. Consequently, by reducing the volume of the islet compartment, it must be possible to increase the glucose insulin transfers through the membrane. The islets unit prepared according to a helical geometry is placed in a tubular reservoir (vol.: 1 mL). The two extremities of the reservoir are ended by a short little tube (Fig. 3).

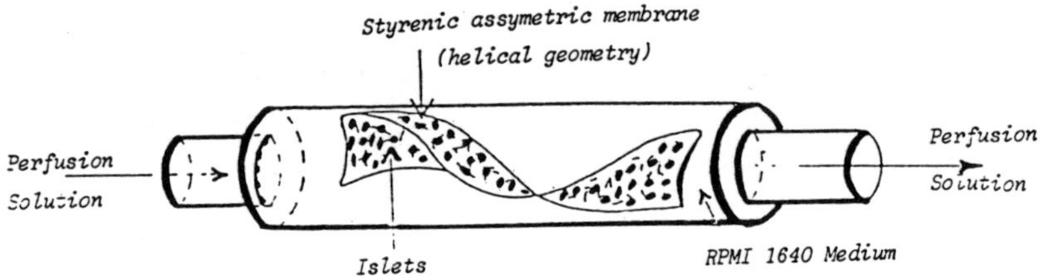


**Figure 3:** Bioartificial pancreas.

At the end of a 10 min. preperfusion period with a 199 solution, the prepared device is perfused with RPMI 1640 medium for a rate of 0.2 mL/min. at different glucose concentrations: 11 mM/L, 22 mM/L and again 11 mM/L. The RPMI medium is maintained near pH 7.4 by bubbling within a mixture of 5% $CO_2$ and 95% air. Effluent from the bioartificial pancreas is sampled for insulin determinations double antibody (radio immunoassays): aliquots of 5 min. periods (1 mL) are stored at −20° C.

## Results (Fig. 4):

During the three 5 min.-periods perfusion with RPMI 1640 medium at a 11 mM/L glucose concentration, the insulin release re-

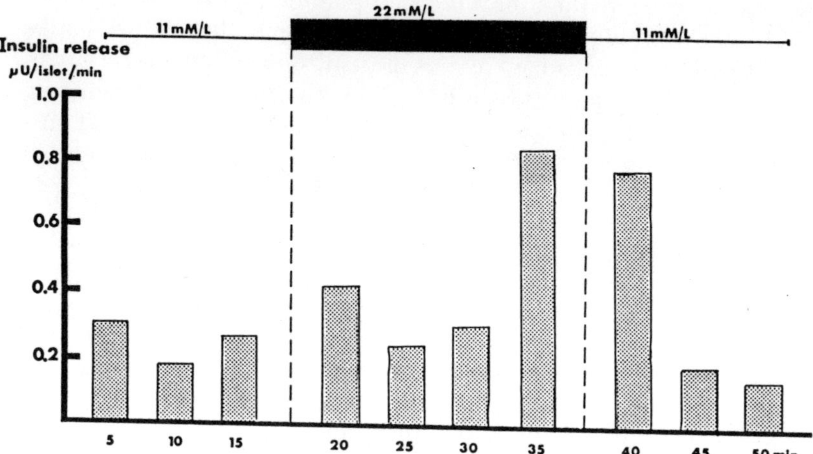


**Figure 4:** Insulin release from the bioartificial pancreas during a 3-period perfusion test with RPMI solution (0.2 ml/min.) at different glucose concentrations (the insulin values are the means of three tests).

mains at a relatively stable level (mean value: 0.25 μU/islet/min.). When the concentration of glucose in the perfusing solution is increased to 22 mM/L, the insulin release rises according to a biphasic insulin secretion curve: during the first 5 min. period of this 22 mM/L phase, insulin production reaches 0.5 μU/islet/min.; then it decreases at a mean value of 0.2 μ/islet/min. during the ten following minutes, and increases again to 0.8 μU/islet/min. during the last 10 minutes.

When the glucose concentration is lowered to 11 mM, insulin release decreases and returns to basal level (0.2 μU/islet/min.) 15 minutes after the end of stimulation.

All insulin values are the means of three tests.

## Conclusion

The results of this work show a new asymmetric membrane very performant, characterized by an exceptional deformability, a good pressure strength, a high permeability, and a satisfactory permselectivity.

Its interesting specific aniticoagulant activity is a contribution to the realization of a "new bioartificial pancreas," which is able to be performant more than three days, implanted in a vascular system.

In our preliminary experimental conditions, the in vitro perfusion stimulations produce kinetics of insulin more satisfactory than those obtained with our previous hollow fiber device.[8] By reducing the volume of the islet compartment and maintaining a good surface of exchange, we obtain a reduction of functional inertia and an interesting release of insulin by the device when it is submitted to an increasing glucose concentration.

---

# References


1. Chick WL, Like AA, Lauris V. (1975). Beta cell culture on synthetic capillaries: An artificial endocrine pancreas. *Science* 187:847.
2. Chick WL, Perna JJ, Louis W, Law D, Galletti PM, Panol G, Wittemore AB, Like AA, Colton CK, Lysaght MJ. (1977). Artificial pancreas using live beta cells. Effects on glucose homeostasis in diabetic rats. *Science* 97:780.
3. Tze WJ, Wong FC, Chen IM, O'Young S. (1976). Implantable artificial endocrine pancreas unit used to restore normoglycemia in diabetic rat. *Nature* 264:466.
4. Sun AM, Parisius W, Healy GM, Vacek L, McMorine HG. (1977). The use in diabetic rats and monkeys of artificial capillary units containing cultured islets of Langerhans. *Diabetes* 26:1136.
5. Orsetti A, Zouari N, Guy C, Hagelsteen C, Puech AM (1977). Mise en place d'un distributeur bio artificiel d'insuline chez le chien totalement dépancréaté. *XIV Congrés International de Thérapeutique* Montpellier 1977 (Ed) Expansion Scientifique Française Paris.
6. Orsetti A, Guy C, Zouari N, Deffay R. (1978). Implantation du distributeur bio artificiel d'insuline chez le chien utilisant des ilots de Langerhans d'espèces animales différentes. *CR Soc Biol* 172:144.
7. Reach G, Poussier Ph, Sausse A, Assan R, Mitsuyau Itah, Jerich JE. (1981). Functional evaluation of a bio artificial pancreas using isolated islets perifused with blood ultrafiltrate. *Diabetes* 30:296.
8. Orsetti A, Bouhaddioui N, Zouari N, Jacquemin JL. (1982). Etude expérimentale d'un pancréas bio artificiel chez le chien. *Journées de Diabétologie Hôtel Dieu*, 189, Ed. Flammarion Médecine Science.
9. Sparks RE, Mason NS, Finley TC, Scharp DW. (1982). Development, testing and modelling of an islet transplantation chamber. *Trans Am Soc Artif Intern Organs* 28:229.
10. Lacy P, Kostianovsky M. (1967). Method for isolation of intact islets of Langerhans from the rat pancreas. *Diabetes* 16:35.

# Chapter 9

# Encapsulated Islets of Langerhans as a Bioartificial Pancreas

Anthony M. Sun
Geraldine M. O'Shea

Insulin therapy has prolonged the lives of diabetics by controlling hyperglycemia, but it has not cured diabetes nor prevented the development of the secondary complications of the disease. Transplanted pancreatic islets have been shown to reverse diabetes and also to prevent the complications. Islet transplants in humans, however, have been largely unsuccessful due to rapid rejection of the transplanted tissue. To overcome this problem, we have developed a technique for protecting transplanted islets from the recipient's immune system. The islets are encapsulated within biocompatible, semipermeable membranes that allow free diffusion of insulin and glucose while isolating the islet cells from the host's immune system. The membranes are polyelectrolyte, hydrogel complexes of alginate and polylysine with a diameter of 600–800 μm and a membrane thickness of approximately 4μm.[1] The procedure for cell encapsulation is extremely mild and safe and involves extruding a mixture of cells and sodium alginate into calcium chloride. The resultant calcium alginate gels are subsequently coated with polylysine and alginate and the interior liquified. We have successfully

From: Ensminger WD, Selam JL (eds): *Infusion Systems in Medicine*. Mount Kisco, NY, Futura Publishing Co., Inc., ©1987.

encapsulated rat islets in these membranes and demonstrated that allografts and xenografts of microencapsulated islets reversed streptozotocin-induced (SZ) diabetes in rats and mice.[2-4]

Single intraperitoneal transplants of 4.5−5 × 10³ encapsulated islets reversed diabetes in nonimmunosuppressed SZ-diabetic rats within two days.[2,3] The mean fasting plasma glucose dropped from a pretransplant value of 378 (SEM ± 5.4) mg/dL to 85.4 ± 5.4 mg/dL within two days of transplantation. Normoglycemia was restored for up to 21 months (Fig. 1A−H). Five rats received a second transplant of 5 × 10³ encapsulated islets when they regressed to the diabetic state (Fig. 1B,D,F,G). Two of these transplants functioned for the lifespan of recipients (Fig. 1B,D). Capsules recovered from the abdominal cavities of animals one year post-transplant were still intact and contained viable functioning β-cells, as shown by histological and insulin-secretion studies. The pancreas of these animals were essentially devoid of β-cells, indicating that the prolonged reversal of diabetes could be attributed to the transplanted encapsulated cells. Transplant recipients showed a very rapid increase in body weight, and no evidence of eye cataract develop-

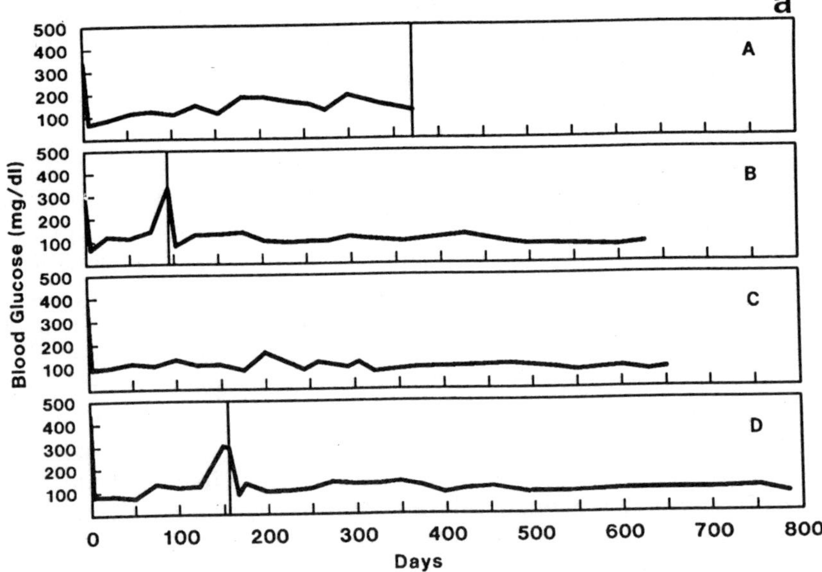


**Figure 1** (*continued*)

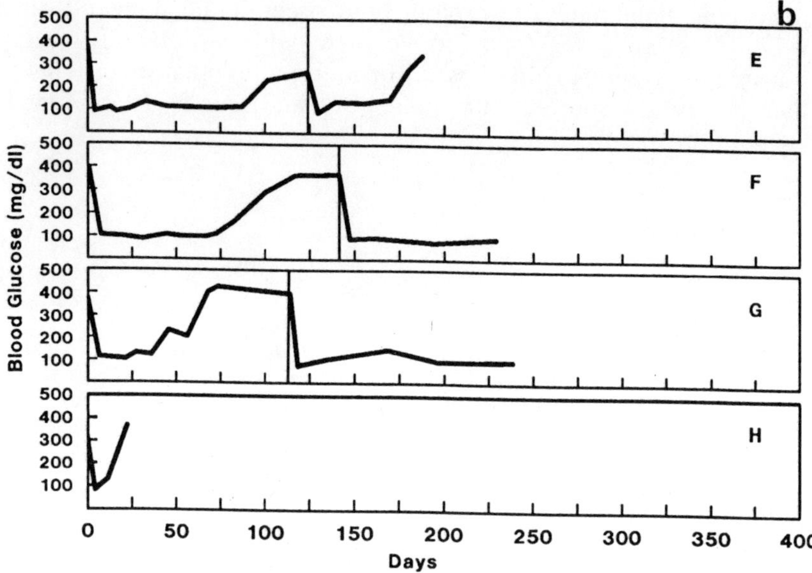



**Figure 1:** Fasting plasma glucose profiles of streptozotocin-induced diabetic rats after transplantation of $4.5-5 \times 10^3$ encapsulated islets. Vertical bars denote time of second transplant. Note different scales in Figures 1a and 1b.

ment was observed. Untreated diabetic controls showed no significant weight increase during the same period and developed eye cataracts within 2 to 3 months.

Xenografts of 1,000 rats islets encapsulated in alginate-polylysine membranes reversed diabetes in nonimmunosuppressed SZ-diabetic mice within three days, and the animals remained normoglycemic for up to 144 days with a mean xenograft survival of 80 days. This was significantly greater than nonencapsulated islets, which functioned for less than 14 days.[4] A second transplant, given after the reappearance of diabetes in 13 animals, again reversed diabetes. Intact capsules with well granulated β-cells were recovered at least two months post-transplantation.

The permeability of these capsules to insulin, glucose, and arginine was demonstrated by Darquy and Reach,[5] who also showed that the membrane protected the encapsulated cells from cytotoxic antibodies in the serum of immunized rabbits and newly diagnosed diabetic patients.

This study demonstrates that pancreatic islets encapsulated in permeable membranes can prolong both allograft and xenograft survival. This technology may prove extremely important for islet transplants in humans in view of the autoimmune nature of type 1 diabetes and the shortage of available human tissue for islet or pancreatic transplants.

## References


1. Goosen MFA, O'Shea GM, Sun AM. (1984). Optimization of microcapsule parameters; semipermeable microcapsules as a bioartificial pancreas. *Biotechnol Bioeng* 27:146−150.
2. O'Shea GM, Sun AM. (1984). Prolonged survival of transplanted islets of Langerhans encapsulated in a biocompatible membrane. *Biochim Biophys Acta* 804:133−136.
3. Sun AM, O'Shea GM. (1985). Microencapsulation of living cells—A long-term delivery system. *J Controlled Release* 2:137−141.
4. O'Shea GM, Sun AM. (1986). Encapsulation of rat islets of Langerhans prolongs xenograft survival in diabetic mice. *Diabetes* (in press).
5. Darquy S, Reach G. (1985). Immunoisolation of pancreatic β-cells by microencapsulation. An in vitro study. *Diabetologia* 28:776−780.

# Chapter 10

# Bionic Closed-Loop Systems for Insulin Administration; Necessity and Reality

P. Abel
U. Fischer

The closed connection between circulating glucose concentration and the amount of insulin provided under all physiological and pathological conditions has led to the concept of a glucose-dependent negative feedback-control between these two parameters. This has also deeply influenced all strategies of diabetes management, because the glucose concentration is still the only variable that is easily accessible and may be measured relatively easily. Thus, the goal of insulin therapy, i.e., permanent normo- or at least euglycemia, can only be achieved if the "loop" between glucose concentration and insulin dose is more or less "closed." There are, of course, fundamental differences among the therapeutic tools in the mechanism, the intervals and the duration of closing the loop. Individually different needs exist to the extent that the loop must be closed to reach optimum metabolic control. But blood glucose stabilization and other variables depending on it are usually better as the loop is "more closed." In many diabetic patients, the so-called "open loop systems," e.g., insulin pumps and possibly "semiclosed loop systems" as pumps in combination with frequent daily blood

From: Ensminger WD, Selam JL (eds): *Infusion Systems in Medicine*. Mount Kisco, NY, Futura Publishing Co., Inc., ©1987.

glucose measurements and with dose calculators are appropriate for daily therapy, but certain patients would obviously require a closed loop system permanently. Much research and technological methods have been devoted to bionic systems, i.e., glucose-controlled insulin infusion pumps. They include the potential advantage that parts of it must be suitable to generate open-loop or semiclosed loop therapeutic strategies. This is important, because—at the moment—none of the systems under development appears ready for human use in routine therapy.

The bionic closed-loop system under development in our laboratories consists of a glucose-measuring system, a computer realizing a mathematical algorithm of the glucose/insulin-relation, and consideration of the patient's individual parameters, and a wearable syringe pump.

The development of the intracorporal glucose sensor is the main problem concerning the long-term function of the system, because all sensing principles being used are dependent on the diffusion qualities of artificial membranes. This problem must be solved in all kinds of artificially closed-loop systems. So far, only one sensing system has really been used in experimental and clinical practice, i.e., the amperometric enzyme electrode, measuring the $H_2O_2$ produced by the glucose oxidation as specifically catalyzed by glucose oxidase (Abel P, et al: *Biomed Biochim Acta* 43:577−584, 1984).

Such sensors have been developed in our laboratory. They have been applied in continuous measurement of whole blood glucose (paracorporal) and of the apparent subcutaneous interstitial glucose concentration after implantation, i.e., they are suitable for glucose measurement without any dilution of the sample due to the usage of a special combination of hydrophobic/hydrophilic material as a covering membrane. A comparison of circulating plasma glucose (PG) and of interstitial glucose concentration (IG) in normal and in diabetic dogs resulted in a linear regression: IG = 0.81 PG − 1.39 (Fig. 1). But there is an influence of the biological system on the diffusion qualities of the covering membrane caused by deposits and limiting the exact sensor function. This is especially true in blood, but it happens in the interstitial tissue also; i.e., the problem of the biocompatible material concerning the enzyme glucose sensor for long-term function has not been solved so far. Using a validated structural model of the glucose−insulin relation for simulating PG and IG after in vivo glucose loads and comparing the calcu-

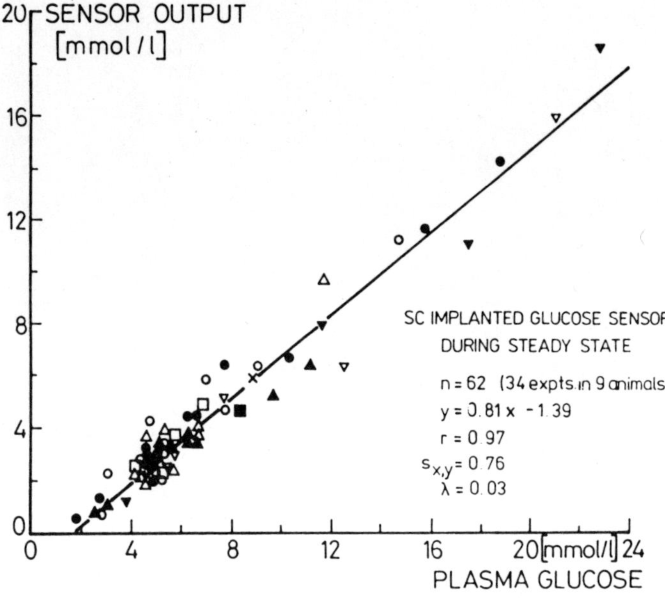


**Figure 1:** Correlation of sensor output (interstitial glucose) and plasma glucose (from steady-state values ≥ 20 min.) in normal and diabetic dogs.

lated results with the measured glucose values in plasma and interstitial fluid, there was an excellent correspondence between the curves as predicted by the model and the measured values.

Also, as a long-term implant for insulin delivery, a basal rate pump of the propellant gas-type has been developed. It will be controllable by a special valve as telemetrically switched. At present, the described system is available for animal experiments at the laboratory stage. Some of its parts, such as the glucose sensor and the microcomputer realizing the mathematical algorithm, are now being prepared for human use to introduce a new developmental stage of semiclosed loop−insulin therapy.

# Chapter 11

# Concanavalin A: Glycosylated-Insulin: Closing the Loop with a Biochemical Pump


Dana E. Wilson
Seo Young Jeong
David L. Holmberg
Sung Wan Kim


A novel approach to coupling circulating glucose concentrations with insulin delivery has been explored in this laboratory. This approach capitalizes on the chemical competition between glucose and glycosylated insulin for binding sites on the lectin, Concanavalin A (ConA). Under properly chosen conditions, the rate of release of glycosylated insulin from the ConA:glycosylated insulin complex should be a function of circulating glucose concentration. If so, the ConA-glycosylated insulin complex could reproduce some of the glucoregulatory functions normally carried out by the endocrine pancreas.

A series of glycosylated insulins was synthesized,[1] differing in their


*From:* Ensminger WD, Selam JL (eds): *Infusion Systems in Medicine.* Mount Kisco, NY, Futura Publishing Co., Inc., ©1987.

carbohydrate moieties, in the spacer molecules connecting them to insulin, and in their affinity for ConA. Several exhibited hypoglycemic potency in a mouse bioassay and showed resistance to aggregation in solution. P-Succinylamidophenyl-$\alpha$-D-mannopyranoside (SAPM) insulin was chosen for further study because of its favorable affinity for the lectin binding site. Glucose in the perfusate bathing an in vitro cell was shown to release glycosylated insulin from ConA-SAPM-insulin at a rate that was proportional to glucose concentration.

The in vivo effects of the SAPM-insulin:ConA complex were then examined in six surgically pancreatectomized diabetic dogs.[2] ConA-SAPM insulin was sealed in a cellophane sac and inserted into the peritoneal cavity. Intravenous glucose tolerance tests were performed prior to pancreatectomy, during insulin treatment of diabetic animals, and 48 hours after insulin withdrawal in the same animals after ConA-SAPM insulin had been implanted. There was marked improvement in glucose tolerance in animals bearing SAPM-insulin sacs (Fig. 1).

Fasting insulin concentrations were supranormal; but despite the normalization of glucose tolerance, there was no secretory peak in immunoassayable peripheral insulin concentrations after intravenous glucose challenge. In other experiments, peripheral insulin concentrations were shown to rise slowly in response to meals.

One of the six implanted animals developed severe symptomatic hypoglycemia. At necropsy the cellophane sac was found to have ruptured, presumably exposing the ConA:SAPM insulin complex to higher ambient glucose concentrations and causing the release of unphysiological amounts of bioeffective glycosylated insulin.

The parallel development of several techniques based on different principles (biomechanical, biological, and chemical) for glucose-coupled insulin replacement might provide clinically useful alternatives for the treatment of insulin-dependent diabetes. The aforementioned results suggest that the chemical pump could eventually find a place in the treatment of insulin-dependent diabetes. Its theoretical limitations include its lack of regulation by endocrine, paracrine or neural stimuli, or by insulin secretagogues other than glucose. Its potential advantages over alternative methods lie in its independence from the availability of biological materials (e.g., pancreatic islets), its low cost, and its simplicity. A great deal of additional work needs to be done to characterize the biological properties of glycosylated insulins more fully and to optimize the insulin delivery system itself.

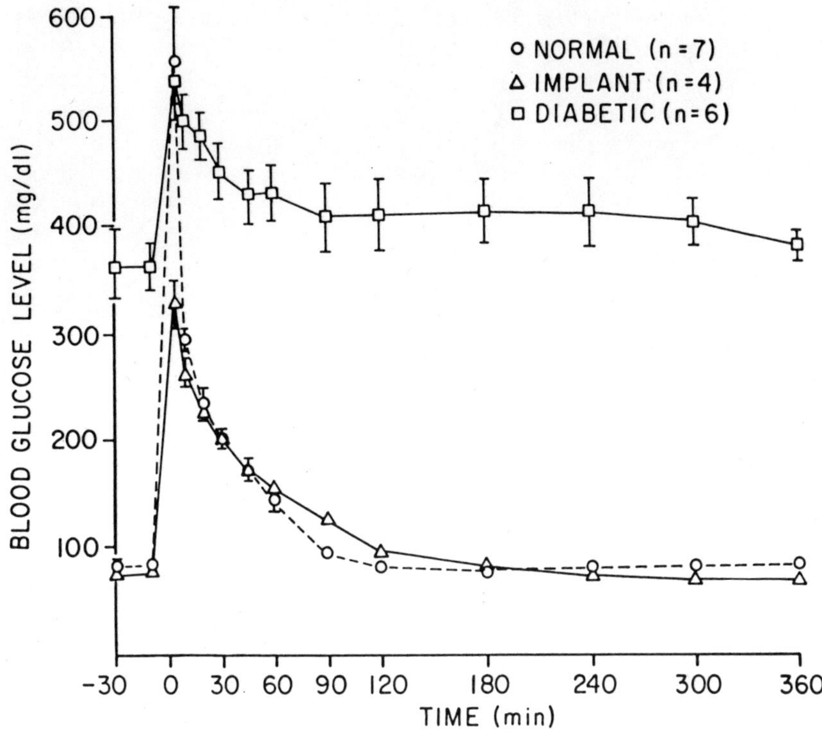


**Figure 1:** IV tolerance test performed before pancreatectomy (○, n=7) during insulin treatment in diabetic animals (□, n=6) and after ConA-SAPM insulin had been implanted (△n=4).

## References


1. Jeong SY, Kim SW, Eenink MJD, Feijen J. (1984). Self-regulating insulin delivery systems. I. Synthesis and characterization of glycosylated insulin. *J Controlled Release* 1:57−66.
2. Jeong SY, Kim SW, Holmberg DL, McRea JC. (1985). Self-regulating insulin delivery systems. III. *In vivo* studies. *J Controlled Release* 2:143−152.

# Chapter 12

# How to Close the Loop in Intraperitoneal Insulin Infusion


K. Piwernetz
J. L. Selam
J. Mirouze
R. Renner
K. D. Hepp


## Introduction

The intraperitoneal route of infusion has proven to be a promising access for insulin delivery by implanted infusion devices. Even if an implantable glucose sensor is not yet available, attempts have been made to look for algorithms for feedback control.[1-3] Insulin absorption kinetics are different compared to the intravenous route. Therefore, the Biostator algorithms cannot be applied without any changes. This has been demonstrated just recently.[3] Problems arise from the delay of the blood glucose lowering effect after the onset of the infusion and the prolonged action thereafter. This paper deals


*From:* Ensminger WD, Selam JL (eds): *Infusion Systems in Medicine.* Mount Kisco, NY, Futura Publishing Co., Inc., ©1987.

with the combination of preprogrammed and feedback control of insulin infusion in insulin dependent diabetic patients (IDDM).

## Patients and Methods

Twelve C-peptide negative patients, who were under long-term treatment with intraperitoneal insulin infusion, received after an overnight fast a standard meal containing 40 g carbohydrates (30 g as white biscuit and 10 g as milk) and 20 g fat; the content of protein was negligible. Two protocols with different infusion regimens were followed, both starting 18 min. before the beginning of the meal:

Protocol A: infusion rate has been increased to the threefold of the basal value; and

Protocol B: infusion rate was set to 10 IU/h for 18 min., to give in total 3 IU in advance of the meal.

With the beginning of the meal under both regimens, the rates have been reset to basal values. The additional postprandial insulin need was administered under strict feedback control with intermittent blood glucose determinations (every 2 to 4 min.); for details, see Reference 1. A control like this is called hybrid because it is a combination of preprogrammed and feedback control.

## Results

The postprandial blood glucose course was markedly different under both protocols. As shown in Figure 1, blood glucose values under protocol A were significantly higher from minute 48 after the beginning of the meal: $p < 0.01$. Not only the maximum under protocol A was much higher $107.9 \pm 27.0$ mg/dl versus $44.2 \pm 38.0$ mg/dl ($p < 0.01$) but also blood glucose returned to values near normal (BG+20 mg/dl) much later $148 \pm 5$ min. versus $79 \pm 38$ min. ($p < 0.001$).

Blood glucose was controlled for three hours from the beginning of the meal. None of the patients under protocol B suffered from hypoglycemia, but two of group A had to receive additional carbohydrates to prevent late postprandial hypoglycemia.

Moreover, though the blood glucose course was much more favorable under protocol B, this result was obtained with less insulin. The difference was statistically significant (protocol A: $12.9 \pm 4.0$ IU versus protocol B: $8.0 \pm 2.3$ IU: $p < 0.025$).

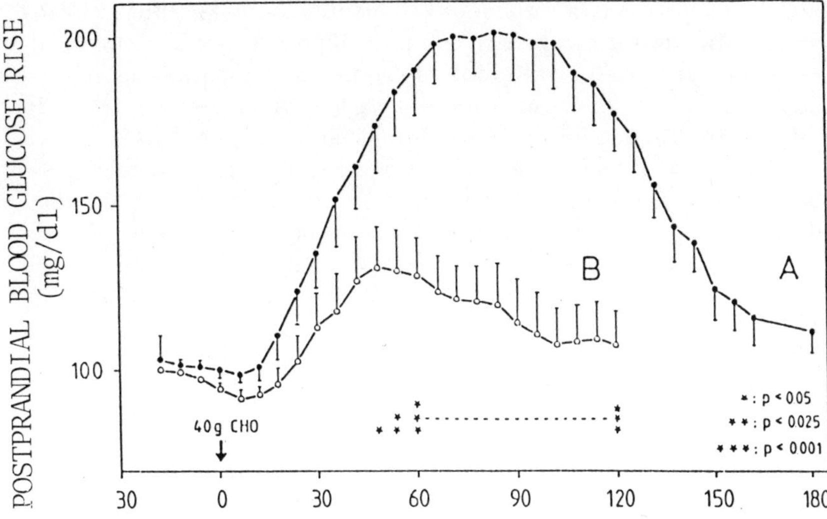


**Figure 1:** Postprandial blood glucose course under hybrid intraperitoneal Insulin infusion. Two different infusion regimens are compared, one with a low (A) and one with a high (B) preprogrammed dose.

## Discussion

Leblanc et al.[3] have demonstrated clearly that the application of the unchanged Biostator algorithms does not provide acceptable control of postprandial blood glucose under intraperitoneal insulin infusion. Not only is the maximum increase exceedingly high but also the risk of late postprandial hypoglycemia is markedly increased. This unfavorable quality of blood glucose control arises from the delay between the beginning of the infusion and the onset of the blood glucose lowering effect of the absorbed insulin. Problems like this are well known from the development of closed-loop control[4]: If not enough insulin is administered in time, a markedly higher dose is needed to bring elevated blood glucose values back to normal.

Even two years ago, a possibility has been shown as to how this problem could be overcome.[2] Part of the insulin has to be administered in advance of the postprandial blood glucose rise. Also, with the intravenous route, this concept improves the quality of pure feedback control.[5] This emphasizes the importance of optimal timing of insulin delivery.

The question is what amount of insulin has to be infused in advance? An answer can be derived from Figure 2. Because the meal-related insulin need is different for each person, the preprogrammed dose of insulin (PP) covers different parts of the total need (MD). In this figure, the maximum postprandial blood glucose rise is drawn over the ratio PP/MD. A statistically significant inverse linear correlation can be calculated, indicating that increasing the preprogrammed dose will tend to normalize the postprandial blood glucose course. From the graph it seems to be optimal to give 50% to 75% of the total insulin need in advance of the meal. The total need has to be estimated from experience according to the planned carbohydrate intake. An error made in the estimation is ruled out within a wide range by the following feedback control.

The introduction of hybrid algorthims for the control of intraperitoneal insulin-infusion may show a possibility of how implantable

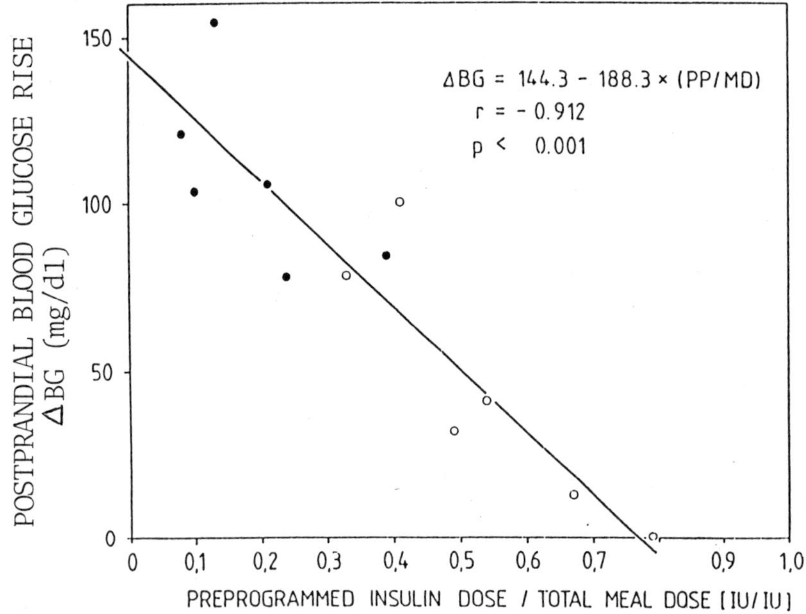


**Figure 2:** Maximum postprandial blood glucose rise correlates with increasing ratio PP/MD. The maximum postprandial blood glucose rise is dependent on the ratio of the insulin dose (PP) administered before the beginning of the meal and the total insulin need (MD). Filled circles: protocol A; open circles: protocol B.

infusion systems could be run as soon as a reliable glucose sensor will have been developed. Regimens such as this render excellent quality of postprandial blood glucose control together with a rather low risk of hypoglycemic reactions in the late postabsorptive phase.

## References


1. Piwernetz K, Renner R, Hepp KD. (1985). Preliminary report: Attempt at glucose-controlled regulation of intraperitoneal insulin infusion. *Proceedings of the Symposium "Continuous Insulin Infusion Therapy."* In: Hepp KD, Renner R, eds, Munich, 1984. Schattauer-Verlag, Stuttgart, New York, 97–104.
2. Piwernetz K, Renner R, Hepp KD. (1985). Is glucose controlled insulin infusion via the intraperitoneal route feasible? *Diabetes* Suppl 1, 34:197A.
3. Leblanc H, Chauvet D, Lombrail P, Robert JJ. (1986). Glycemic control with closed loop intraperitoneal insulin in type I diabetes. *Diabetes Care* 9:124–128.
4. Pfeiffer EF, Thum CH, Clemens AH. (1974). The artificial beta cell. A continuous control of blood sugar by external regulation of insulin infusion (glucose controlled insulin infusion system). *Horm Metab Res* 6:339–342.
5. Piwernetz K, Renner R, Hepp KD. (1981). Approach towards an adequate dosing scheme for continuous insulin infusion in mobile diabetics. *Proceedings of the 2nd Vienna–Lainz Symposium 1980 "New Approaches to Insulin Therapy."* In: Irsigler K, Kunz, KN, Owens DR, Regal H, eds, MTP Press, Lancaster, England, pp 47–54.

# Chapter 13

# Incidence and Severity of Ketoacidosis Due to Technical Problems During Continuous Subcutaneous Insulin Infusion (CSII)

P. Henrivaux
A.J. Scheen
J.C. Daubresse
A.M. Rinaldi
P.J. Lefebvre

## Introduction

One of the goals of the treatment of diabetes is to achieve sufficient metabolic control in the hope of delaying or preventing late complications. Technical facilities are now available to increasing numbers of patients: among them, glucose reflectance meters and insulin pumps. The question is now to assess carefully the risks and benefits of these efforts to obtain (near) normoglycemia.

*From:* Ensminger WD, Selam JL (eds): *Infusion Systems in Medicine.* Mount Kisco, NY, Futura Publishing Co., Inc., ©1987.

In the 1970s, continuous insulin infusion began to be investigated in order to mimic the basal insulin secretion and the meal-related insulin rises observed in normal subjects. Slama et al. in 1974[1] demonstrated the feasibility of improving glucose levels in diabetic subjects during a few days by continuous intravenous insulin administration. In 1977, Pickup and his group achieved good diabetic control by the subcutaneous route for short periods.[2] Subsequently, numerous investigators were rapidly interested by the subcutaneous route considering longer periods of treatment for out-patients.[3-10]

The aim of our report is to analyze the frequency and most common causes of ketoacidosis (KA) episodes during CSII as well as to evaluate the frequency and severity of infusion site infections. Therefore, we have reviewed the follow-up charts of our first 33 patients submitted to CSII since 1980.

## Materials and Methods

### Patients

Our first 33 patients (11 males and 22 females) submitted to CSII were all type-1 C-peptide negative insulin-dependent diabetics. At the start of pump therapy, their mean age was $35 \pm 2$ years (range: $17-53$ years) and the mean duration of diabetes was $16 \pm 2$ years (range: $0.1-36$ years). The mean duration of CSII was $28 \pm 3$ months per patient (range $= 5-57$).

The prevalence of diabetes complications at the time of initiation of CSII in these patients was as follows: (pre-) proliferative and/or ischemic retinopathy in 19 patients (58%), persistent proteinuria and/or GFR below 60 ml/min. in six patients (18%), and electrical and/or clinical polyneuropathy in 17 patients (52%).

The main indications for CSII were insufficient metabolic control under classical insulin therapy for 14 patients (42%) and the occurrence of frequent episodes of hypoglycemic coma for seven patients (21%). Two patients asked CSII for personal conveniences. Ten diabetic women (30%) began CSII in order to achieve adequate prepregnancy diabetic control. Three of these latter preferred to continue with this type of treatment after delivery. Seven among the other patients discontinued insulin infusion therapy after CSII periods ranging from 5 to 57 months. The two youngest female patients (15 and 20 years old) complained of the difficulty of clothing when the summer arrived. Two patients discontinued treatment because of painful subcutaneous lesions. The three last patients were not sufficiently improved regarding the lability and control of their diabetes when compared to the efforts required by CSII treatment and decided to discontinue this type of therapy.

## Materials

Twenty-six patients have been treated with the 1001 HM Mill-Hill infuser (Muirhead Medical Ltd., London, SE25, United Kingdom) because it was the first device available and also the least expensive and easiest to handle. Two patients utilized the AS6C Autosyringe pump (Autosyringe Inc., Hooksett, New Hampshire, United States). Now, the Nordisk infuser (Nordisk Gentofte, Denmark) became our first choice and was used by five patients of this study.

The subcutaneous infusion was performed with 25G needles attached to cannulas of polyvinyl chloride (Butterfly, Abbott Laboratories, Queenborough, Kent, United Kingdom) or polyethylene (Sterilex, Espergaerde, Denmark). The patients were instructed to change the needle in the subcutaneous tissue of the anterior abdominal wall every two to three days. Insulins used included 40 U/mL porcine or human Actrapid (diluted with saline or with the specific diluting medium kindly provided by Novo A.S. Copenhagen, Denmark) and the special prefilled cartridges of 100 U/mL porcine Velosulin (Nordisk, Copenhagen, Denmark).

## Methods

### Home Blood Glucose Monitoring

In most cases, the patients were first instructed to perform home blood glucose monitoring using a reflectance meter. The classical insulin treatment was then optimalized on the basis of the glycemic data recorded in notebooks and discussed with the medical staff at least every two weeks during six to eight weeks. As the diabetic control remained insufficient and/or the patient seemed motivated for pump treatment, he/she was admitted to the metabolic ward for a week in order to learn the handling of the pump and the proper attitude in case of incidents. The basal insulin delivery rate as well as the preprandial insulin supplements were progressively adjusted to achieve the best possible metabolic control. After discharge from the hospital, the patients were seen at our outpatient clinic every six weeks.

The patients were instructed to perform at least four blood glucose controls a day; namely, three determinations before meals and one 2 hours after a meal or before going to bed. Every three weeks, the patients were asked to perform a 6-point-glycemic profile. The values of the home blood glucose monitoring were recorded daily in a notebook and thereafter stored in a computer (Apple II-Basic language). In case of hypoglycemia, metabolic deterioration, or technical incidents, the patients were asked to add a brief comment about the severity of the problem and its possible cause. When they were discharged from the hospital, they received instruction to call our medical staff in case of problems.

## Definition of the Acute Metabolic Deteriorations

We have reviewed the severe ketoacidosis episodes requiring hospitalization as well as the comments of the patients in their notebooks. We have retrospectively considered a 4-step-graduated metabolic alteration scale: (1) Severe ketoacidosis (grade 1) was defined as a marked and prolonged metabolic deterioration with clinical signs of acidosis and/or dehydration and/or a stade-1 coma, situation requiring hospitalization: blood glucose levels were above 600 mg/dL and arterial pH below 7.3; (2) less severe KA (grade 2) was considered when at least three 2-hour-interval blood glucose determinations were over 350 mg/dL with well documented ketonuria or clinical signs of acidosis and without rapid improvement despite multiple insulin supplements; (3) grade 3 metabolic deterioration was considered when at least two glycemic determinations exceeded 300 mg/dL despite insulin supplements; (4) grade 4 was defined as a unique glycemia above 300 mg/dL that was rapidly corrected.

## Results

### Diabetes Control

Improvement of diabetes control during CSII was assessed by the change in $HbA_{1C}$ levels: 7.6 ± 0.2 (mean ± SEM) during CSII versus 8.7 ± 0.3 (2P < 0.10) at the beginning of insulin-pump therapy and 9.0 ± 0.3 (2P < 0.001) during conventional insulin therapy.

### Diabetic Ketoacidosis

During the total period considered (912 patient-months), 35 KA Grade-1 and Grade-2 episodes occurred in 16 of our patients: 5 grade-1 KA occurred in 5 patients and 30 grade-2 KA were presented by 15 patients. Four patients presented both grade-1 and grade-2 KA episodes.

The main causes of grade-1 and grade-2 metabolic deteriorations are summarized in Table 1. Considering the most severe episodes, two were due to needle displacements from the subcutane-

**Table 1**

**Nature of 35 Ketoacidosis Episodes During 912 Patient-Months of CSII Treatment ($N = 33$)**

|  | Grade 1 | Grade 2 | Total | % |
|---|---|---|---|---|
| Number of incidents | 5 | 30 | 35 | |
| Frequency (/patients-year) | 0.06 | 0.4 | 0.46 | |
| Number of patients | 5 | 15 | 16* | |
| Nature of the incidents | | | | |
|   Catheter obstruction | — | 6 | 6 | 17.1 |
|   Battery failure | 1 | 4 | 5 | 14.3 |
|   Needle removed | 2 | 1 | 3 | 8.6 |
|   Empty syringe | — | 1 | 1 | 2.9 |
|   Cannula detachment | — | 1 | 1 | 2.9 |
|   Cutaneous infection | — | 1 | 1 | 2.9 |
|   Intercurrent illness | 1 | 5 | 6 | 17.1 |
|   Not identified or not documented | 1 | 11 | 12 | 34.3 |

*Four patients presented both grades 1 and 2 ketoacidosis.

ous tissue that occurred during the night, and one was attributed to an exhausted battery probably complicated by a catheter obstruction. Another grade-1 ketoacidosis episode was observed in a patient who suffered from a bronchopneumonia and in whom no technical incident could be identified. The fifth case of severe KA occurred in a patient recently discharged from the hospital after initiation of insulin pump therapy; the cause of this incident remained unclear.

It is noteworthy that 22 out of the 35 KA episodes were present in only five patients. Seventeen patients followed during a total of 411 months did not present any KA episode.

As regards grade-3 and grade-4 metabolic deteriorations, 16% of the incidents were clearly related to mechanical obstruction of the infusion set (clotting, catheter kinking, etc. . .) while in 30%, the simple replacement of the infusion set permitted quick restoration of metabolic control. Eleven percent of the incidents were related to infusion-set disruptions (needle displacement, cracked catheter, pump-tube disconnection, etc. . .). The other causes of moderate or minimal blood glucose deteriorations were empty syringe (2.8%), pump failure (0.8%), battery exhaustion (9.0%), and inflammation or infection of the infusion sites (2.3%). In 26% of grade-3 and grade-4 metabolic deteriorations, no specific event was notified by the patient. Furthermore, we have recorded a total of 412 incidents (4.5 /patient-month), which did not result in significant metabolic deterioration.


## Cutaneous Tolerance


### Infectious Complications

"Infections" of the infusion site were defined as the persistence of a tender inflammatory, frequently nodular, area despite removal of the needle and cured by oral antibiotic therapy. The term "abcess" was utilized if surgical drainage or incision was required. Ten such infectious episodes were noted in six patients: nine infections and one abcess (0.011/patient-month considering the entire group of patients). Some patients appeared to have a higher risk, since one patient presented one abcess and two infections and another one exhibited three successive infections. The abcess has been the only infectious incident reported as causing a grade-2 metabolic deterioration. In the other cases, the metabolic deterioration was slight. In all but one case, these infectious incidents always appeared in the first few months of CSII treatment.

## Subcutaneous Nodules

Seven patients complained of frequent subcutaneous nodules at the insulin infusion sites. Usually, these lesions were less accepted by women from an esthetic point of view. These nodosities disappeared 3 to 10 days after changing the infusion site without any specific treatment. Three patients presenting with such nodules requested interruption of CSII.

## Discussion

As reported by others, our experience of CSII confirms the possibility of this mode of treatment to improve diabetes control assessessed by a significant decrease in $HbA_{1C}$ levels. [3−13,16,18,19,22]

The follow-up of our first 33 patients submitted to CSII indicated the occurrence of five severe ketoacidosis episodes over a total period of 912 months (one episode per 182 patient-months or 0.47 per patient-year). These data were compared with those reported in the literature (Table 2). The frequency of ketoacidosis episodes in our patients is comparable to that observed by Lauritzen et al.[11] and Bending et al.[14] Other reports described a higher incidence of KA ranging from one episode every 52 to one episode every 100 patient-months.[15−17] It is noteworthy that the highest incidence of KA episodes was reported by the KROC Collaborative Study Group,[12] which comprised patients treated for an average of eight months only. Indeed, Bending et al.[14] and Knight et al.[17] have already demonstrated that most of the KA episodes occur during the first months of insulin-pump therapy; this finding is also observed in our study. Considering KA incidence, the best results were obtained by Sonnenberg et al.[20] in a center where a major emphasis is put on patient education.[21,22]

While the risk of KA during CSII appears to be slightly higher than that observed with conventional insulin therapy,[12,16] it remains acceptable if the grade-1 KA episodes only are considered. However, in our series, the relatively high incidence of grade-2 KA (where hospitalization was not necessary) emphasizes once more

**Table 2**
**Frequency of Ketoacidosis (KA) Episodes During CSII**

| Studies | Number of Patients | CSII Period Studied (Patient-Months) | Mean Duration of CSII (Months/Patient) | Frequency of KA (/Patient-Month) | Reference |
|---|---|---|---|---|---|
| Lauritzen et al. (1983) | 16 | 186 | 12 | 1/186 | 11 |
| Peden et al. (1984) | 101 | 1,880 | 19 | 1/52 | 15 |
| Mecklenburg et al. (1984) | 161 | 2,978 | 18 | 1/78 | 16 |
| KROC Study (1984) | 34 | 272 | 8 | 1/30 | 12 |
| Sonnenberg et al. (1985) | 114 | 2,291 | 20 | 1/382 | 19 |
| Knight et al. (1985) | 65 | 1,800 | 28 | 1/100 | 17 |
| Bending et al. (1985) | 40 | 1,263 | 10 | 1/180 | 14 |
| Present study (1986) | 33 | 912 | 28 | 1/182 | |

the need for careful education of the patients (who should know to react appropriately) and for responsibility of the medical team (which should be available for giving appropriate advice by phone). In the seven cases who died from diabetic KA during CSII in the Centers for Disease Control survey,[23] five had recognized progressive hyperglycemia and had initially attempted self-treatment, but only three had checked urine samples for ketones. In retrospect, all waited too long to seek medical assistance.

Considering the causes of KA, our study provides results that are quite different from those of other reports (Table 3). In our study, intercurrent illness was not identified as the most frequent cause of KA as it is in other series. In contrast, 46% of KA episodes during CSII were clearly related to technical problems with the insulin infusion devices. Moreover, 20% among the 34% of so-called "not identified incidents" seemed to be related to catheter problems: indeed, in these cases, a glycemic improvement was observed after simply changing the catheter. The reason for this does not appear clearly, but factors such as insulin aggregation or precipitation should certainly be considered.[24-26]

In some cases, the precipitating cause is obscure, and a careful analysis of the incidents is necessary: This may explain the differences between the data of the various studies considered in Table 3. This situation is examplified by the story of one patient reported by Bending et al.[14] in whom metabolic deterioration was first attributed to a viremia, but whose insulin pump syringe was found empty on hospital admission.

Eighteen percent of our patients presented cutaneous infections: All of them used pumps that needed dilution of insulin. It could be hypothesized that such manipulation favors infection. On the basis of the literature,[9,11,16,26] the estimated incidence of infusion-site infections averaged 0.04±0.01 patient-month. As shown in Table 3, this type of incidence is a rare cause of KA.

The relatively high incidence of KA during CSII is secondary to the small amounts of insulin infused continuously. In this situation, insulin deprivation may rapidly occur upon interruption of the subcutaneous infusion. Our group has studied the effects of a nocturnal interruption of CSII. No metabolic deterioration was observed after a one-hour interruption,[28] whereas a two-hour interruption already induced a delayed and sustained increase in blood glucose and plasma $\beta$-hydroxybutyrate levels.[29] A six-hour interruption of CSII resulted, after a two-hour delay, in a marked meta-

**Table 3**
**Causes of Ketoacidosis Episodes During CSII (%)**

| Studies | Intercurrent Illness | Infusion System Leakage | Infected Infusion Site | Not Identified | Reference |
|---|---|---|---|---|---|
| Peden et al. (1984) | 39 | 33 | 8 | 3 | 15 |
| Mecklenburg et al. (1984) | 71 | 8 | 3 | 18 | 16 |
| Knight et al. (1985) | 67 | 11 | 0 | 17 | 17 |
| Bending et al. (1985) | 43 | 14 | 0 | 43 | 14 |
| Present study (1986) | 17 | 46 | 3 | 34 | |

N.B.: Peden et al.: Brittle diabetes = 17% of all causes.
Knight et al.: Noncompliance = 5% of all causes.

bolic deterioration in C-peptide negative diabetic patients: blood glucose levels reached about 17.5 mmol/L and plasma β-hydroxybutyrate levels averaged 1,300 pmol/L. All patients presented marked ketonuria.[30] In all cases, plasma-free insulin levels fell significantly within the first hour after stopping the pump and reached their nadir at the time of reactivating the pump. We have recently shown that the presence of high plasma levels of IgG anti-insulin antibodies gives some protection against such metabolic deterioration occurring during prolonged CSII interruption. [31]

## Conclusion

We confirm the experience of others that significant improvement of diabetes control can be achieved using continuous subcutaneous insulin infusion. Severe ketoacidosis requiring hospitalization occurred in only five instances in 33 patients over a period of 912 months, i.e., 1/182 patient-months. More discrete episodes of ketoacidosis were more frequent (1/30 patient-months) and were mainly due to identified or presumed problems involving the infusion devices. In our series, intercurrent illness is a relatively rare cause of KA. Regular home blood glucose monitoring and frequent urinary checks for ketonuria, together with more attention given to the infusion system whenever a slight metabolic deterioration occurs should reduce the risk of ketoacidosis in the patients submitted to CSII.

## References


1. Slama G, Hautecouverture M, Assan R, Tchobroutsky G. (1974). One to five days of continuous intravenous insulin infusion on seven diabetic patients. *Diabetes* 23:723−728.
2. Pickup JC, Keen H, Parsons JA, and Alberti KGM (1977). The use of continuous subcutaneous insulin to achieve normoglycemia in diabetic patients. *Diabetologia* 13:425 (Abstract).
3. Pickup JC, White MC, Keen H, Parsons JA, Alberti KGM. (1979). Long-term continuous subcutaneous insulin infusion in diabetics at home. *Lancet* 2:870−873.
4. Champion MC, Shepherd GAA, Rodger NW, Dupre J. (1980). Continuous subcutaneous infusion of insulin in the management of diabetes mellitus. *Diabetes* 29:206−212.

5. Schiffrin A, Colle É, Belmonte M. (1980). Improved control in diabetes with continuous subcutaneous insulin infusion. *Diabetes Care* 3:643–649.
6. Schiffrin A, Belmonte MM. (1982). Comparison between continuous subcutaneous insulin infusion and multiple injections of insulin. A one-year prospective study. *Diabetes* 31:255–264.
7. Daubresse JC, Henrivaux Ph, Bailly A, Lemy C, Duchateau A. (1983). Long-term management of insulin-treated diabetic patients with continuous subcutaneous insulin infusion. *Diab Metab* 9:45–52.
8. Nathan DM, Lou P, Avruch J. (1982). Intensive conventional and insulin pump therapies in adult type-1 diabetes. A crossover study. *Ann Intern Med* 97:31–36.
9. Reeves ML, Seigler DE, Ryan EA, Skyler JS. (1982). Glycemic control in insulin-dependent diabetes mellitus. Comparison of outpatient intensified conventional therapy with continuous subcutaneous insulin infusion. *Am J Med* 72:673–680.
10. Mecklenburg RS, Benson JW, Becker NM, Brazel PL, Fredlund PN, Metz RJ, Nielsen RL, Sannar CA, Steenrod WJ. (1982). Clinical use of the insulin infusion pump in 100 patients with type 1 diabetes. *N Engl J Med* 307:513–518.
11. Lauritzen T, Frost–Larsen K, Larsen HW, Deckert T, the Steno Study Group. (1983). Effect of 1 year of near-normal blood glucose levels on retinopathy in insulin-dependent diabetics. *Lancet* 1:200–204.
12. The KROC Collaborative Study Group. (1984). Blood glucose control and the evolution of diabetic retinopathy and albuminuria. A preliminary multicenter trial. *N Engl J Med* 311:365–372.
13. Mecklenburg RS, Benson EA, Benson JW, Blumenstein BA, Fredlung PN, Guinn TS, Metz RJ, Nielsen RL. (1985). Long-term metabolic control with insulin pump therapy: Report of experience with 127 patients. *N Engl J Med* 8:465–468.
14. Bending JJ, Pickup JC, Keen H. (1985). Frequency of diabetic ketoacidosis and hypoglycemic coma during treatment with continuous subcutaneous insulin infusion. *Am J Med* 79:685–691.
15. Peden NR, Braaten JT McKendry JBR. (1984). Diabetic ketoacidosis during long-term treatment with continuous subcutaneous insulin infusion. *Diabetes Care* 7:1–5.
16. Mecklenburg RS, Benson EA, Benson JW, Fredlund PN, Guinn T, Metz RJ, Nielsen RL, Sannar CA. (1984). Acute complications associated with insulin infusion pump therapy. Report of experience with 161 patients. *JAMA* 252:3265–3269.
17. Knight G, Jennings AM, Bailton AJM, Tomlinson S, Ward JD. (1985). Severe hyperkalaemia and ketoacidosis during routine treatment with an insulin pump. *Br Med J* 291:371–372.
18. Berger M, Sonnenberg GE, Chantelau EA. (1982). Insulin pump treatment for diabetes: Some questions can be answered already. *Clin Physiol* 2:351–355.
19. Sonnenberg GE, Spraul M, Chantelau EA, Berger M. (1985). Kontinuierliche subkutane insulin-infusion therapie: Voraussetzungen, Indikationen und Risiken. *Dtsch Med Wschr* 110:1859–1864.

20. Sonnenberg GE, Mulhauser I, Chantelau EA, Berger M. (1985). Incidence of ketoacidosis and severe hypoglycemia in conventionally and CSII treated type-1 diabetic patients (Abstract). *Diabetes* 34 (suppl. 1):117A.
21. Sonnenberg GE, Chantelau E, Berger M. (1982). Routine treatment of insulin-dependent diabetes mellitus with continuous subcutaneous insulin infusion. In: Skyler JS ed, *Insulin Update 1982*, Excerpta Medica, Amsterdam, 223.
22. Sonnenberg GE, Chantelau E, Berger M. (1983). Educational aspects of insulin pump treatment in type-1 diabetic patients. In: Assal JP, Berger M, Canivet J eds, *Handbook of Diabetes Education*, Excerpta Medica, Amsterdam, p 70.
23. Teutsch SM, Herman WH, Dwyer DM, Lane JM. (1984). Mortality among diabetic patients using continuous subcutaneous insulin-infusion pumps. *N Engl J Med* 310:361−367.
24. Lougheed WD, Woulfe−Flanagan H, Clement JR, Albisser AM. (1980). Insulin aggregation in artificial delivery systems. *Diabetologia* 19:1−9.
25. Freeman DJ, Wolfe BM, Mascarenhas M. (1983). Ketoacidosis resulting from precipitation of insulin in syringe used to deliver constant subcutaneous insulin infusion. *Lancet* 1:828.
26. Mecklenburg RS, Guinn TS. (1985). Complications of insulin pump therapy: The effect of insulin preparation. *Diabetes Care* 8:367−370.
27. Pietri A, Raskin P. (1981). Cutaneous complications of chronic continuous subcutaneous insulin infusion therapy. *Diabetes Care* 4:624−626.
28. Scheen A, Henrivaux Ph, Jandrain B, Luyckx AS, Lefebvre PJ. (1985). Lack of systematic metabolic alterations after a one-hour interruption of continuous subcutaneous insulin infusion in type 1 diabetic patients. *Diabetes Care* 8:621−623.
29. Scheen A, Castillo M, Jandrain B, Krzentowski G, Henrivaux Ph, Luyckx AS, Lefebvre PJ. (1984). Metabolic alterations after a two-hour nocturnal interruption of a continuous subcutaneous insulin infusion. *Diabetes Care* 7:338−342.
30. Krzentowski G, Scheen A, Castillo M, Luyckx AS, Lefebvre PJ. (1983). A 6-hour nocturnal interruption of a continuous subcutaneous insulin infusion: 1. Metabolic and hormonal consequences and scheme for a prompt return to adequate control. *Diabetologia* 24:314−318.
31. Scheen AJ, Henrivaux Ph, Jandrain B, Lefebvre PJ. (in press). Anti-insulin antibodies and metabolic deterioration after interruption of continuous subcutaneous insulin infusion. *Diabetes Care*.

# Chapter 14

# Recent Advances in Insulin Stabilization

Ulrich Grau

## Introduction

This is a progress report of our work with the polyethylene-polypropyleneglycol stabilized insulin preparation Hoe 21 PH[1] with two *implantable* programmable pumps, which we have conducted in collaboration with the people from Pacesetter and from Siemens. Those pumps were selected because clinical trials with these implantable pumps are just starting in the United States and Europe. I will not report about our experience with external pumps nor with other implants such as the Medronic or the Infusaid pump.

## Pacesetter Minimed Pump Studies

The pacesetter implantable medication system (PIMS)[2] is a fully programmable, implantable solenoid pump. The drug reservoir and pathway are almost all titanium; the catheter is fabricated from silicone-lined polyethylene. These materials have been demonstrated earlier to be compatible with Hoe 21 PH.[1]

PIMS and Hoe 21 PH of either 100 U/mL or 400 U/mL strength have been evaluated both in vitro and in vivo. The in vivo tests

*From:* Ensminger WD, Selam JL (eds): *Infusion Systems in Medicine.* Mount Kisco, NY, Futura Publishing Co., Inc.,©1987.

have been performed by Dr. Saudek at the Johns Hopkins University. The in vitro test, a summary of which is given in Table 1, was accelerated with regard to insulin stability in that (1) the rate was significantly lower than expected in a human diabetic; (2) the pump was continuously moved; in particular, there was high stress on the catheter since through it the relative movement of pump and collection vial was transmitted; (3) no boli were triggered; and (4) the insulin was collected over one-week periods, which gave rise to certain experimental artifacts (normally the insulin would be distributed in the body immediately).

During the in vitro compatibility tests with U-100 insulin (comprising a total of one device-year) and with U-400 insulin (comprising a total of 1.8 device-years), no insulin precipitate occurred. In the former case, refill cycles lasted four weeks, in the latter up to three months. Insulin quantity and quality have been assessed regularly using high-performance liquid chromatography (HPLC).[3] In PIMS, small proportions of the insulin are being converted slowly to modified insulins. This process, however, is similar to the regular temperature-induced changes seen in a reference glass vial (Table 1). Therefore, refill cycles of about 10 weeks seem

**Table 1**

**Mean insulin quality (% of the total amount of insulin and insulin-like substances) in PIMS eluates under in vitro test condition**

| Residence time (weeks) | Hoe 21 PH U100/ PIMS | | Hoe 21 PH U400/ PIMS | | Hoe 21 PH U100/ glass vial |
|---|---|---|---|---|---|
| | native insulin $\bar{x} \pm SD$ | n | native insulin $\bar{x} \pm SD$ | n | |
| 0 | 97.7 ± 0.8 | 13 | 95.7 ± 0.7 | 9 | 97.5 |
| 1 | 96.7 ± 0.7 | 13 | 93.1 ± 1.9 | 4 | |
| 2 | 96.4 ± 0.8 | 12 | 93.9 ± 1.5 | 9 | 96.6 |
| 3 | 96.5 ± 0.8 | 12 | 93.4 ± 1.0 | 9 | 96.5 |
| 4 | 95.0 ± 1.2 | 10 | 93.4 ± 1.0 | 7 | |
| 5 | | | 92.2 ± 1.6 | 8 | |
| 6 | | | 91.8 ± 2.2 | 8 | 95.0 |
| 7 | | | 91.6 ± 0.8 | 7 | |
| 8 | | | 91.6 ± 1.1 | 7 | |
| 9 | | | 90.2 ± 0.5 | 4 | |
| 10 | | | 89.7 ± 1.7 | 4 | |

feasible, the native insulin content then remaining at about 90% or better.

After six months of in vitro testing, a catheter has been analyzed thoroughly for insulin coating using scanning electron microscopy and x-ray microanalysis. We found slight insulin coating only at a small silicone rubber junction (Figure 1) but very clean surfaces everywhere else (Figure 2). Furthermore, one PIMS device, which had been tested with both Hoe 21 PH U-100 and U-400 in vitro for about one year, was cut apart and inspected along the entire drug pathway at many different locations. One such micrograph is shown in Figure 3. Again, we found only at a few microscopic spots little insulin coating but no major precipitous material anywhere. In fact, the device's interior was remarkably clean, especially in remote corners. These tests, along with results from animal tests performed simultaneously, will be published in greater detail.[4] Clinical trials are to resume shortly in the United States.

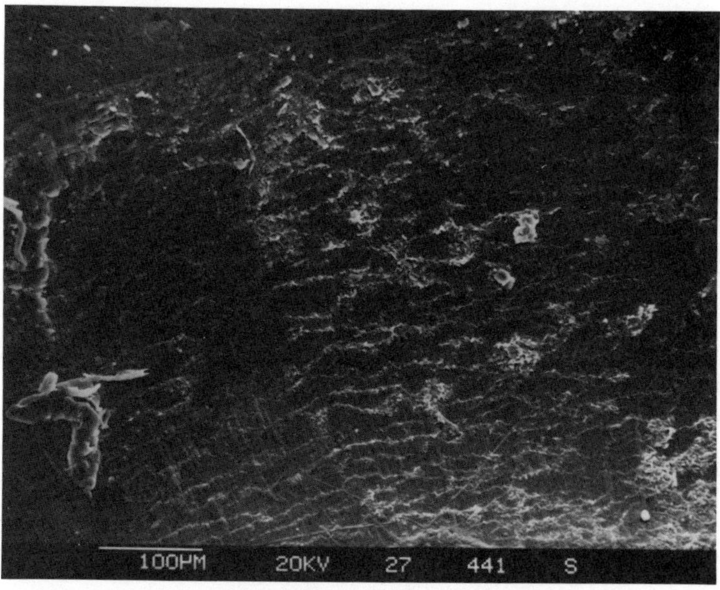


**Figure 1:** Scanning electron micrograph of a portion of a catheter after one year in vitro testing with the PIMS device: insulin coated portion at the silicone junction.

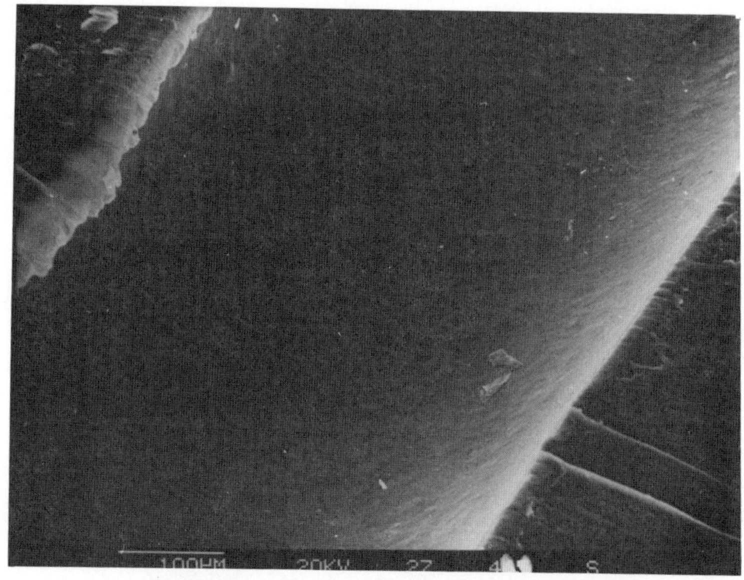

**Figure 2:** as Figure 1, polyethylene portion.

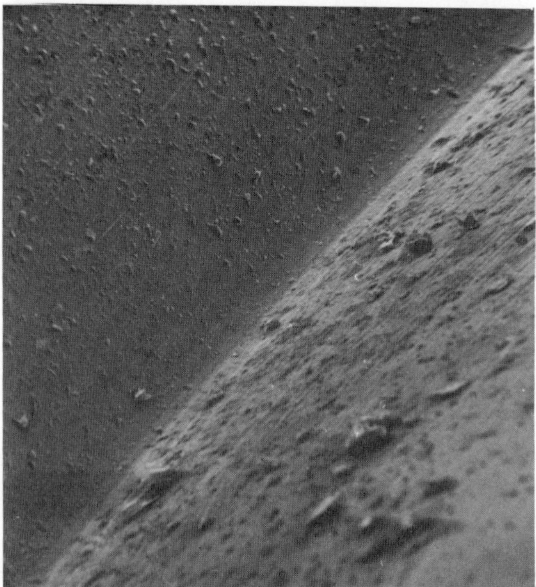

**Figure 3:** Scanning electron micrograph of a portion of the PIMS interior after one year in vitro testing.

## Siemens Pump Studies

The stress on insulin is particularly high in peristaltic pumps. On the other hand, this pump principle is elegant and least prone to handling-related failures, such as the introduction of air into the reservoir. Based on our current data, Hoe 21 PH is not sufficiently stable in the Promedos I1 implantable peristaltic pump. We have, therefore, looked for alternatives that would particularly withstand the peristaltic action inside an elastomer tube.

By the addition of polygeline, which is a gelatin derivative also used as a plasma substitute, the viscosity of the insulin solution has been increased. Thus, Hoe 21 GH combines two stabilizing features, namely the stabilizing effect of the surface active polyethylene-polypropyleneglycol and the increased viscosity. The latter should have the effect of decreasing the tendency for denaturation. Simple rotation-, shaking-, and circular-pumping-experiments have, in fact, shown similarly high stability between Hoe 21 PH and Hoe 21 GH, except that Hoe 21 PH is superior with respect to a circular pumping test (Table 2).

Hoe 21 GH U-100 has been tested successfully in the Promedos I1 pump in vitro for a total period of more than five device years. Part of this work has been conducted by P. Jährling at Siemens. Figure 4 shows the summary of the HPLC results. Panel A shows the time of operation of the individual pumps, some of these still in operation. Panel B shows the quantity of insulin at the catheter tip and panel C the proportion of native, unmodified insulin in the pump eluate.

**Table 2**
**Physical stability of Hoe 21 PH and Hoe 21 GH**

| Preparation | Stability in the rotation test | Stability in the shaking test | Stability in the circular pumping test |
|---|---|---|---|
| Conventional insulin preparation | < 2 days | < 2 days | ~28 hours |
| Hoe 21 PH U-100 | > 60 days | > 40 days | ~20 hours |
| Hoe 21 GH U-100 | > 50 days | > 14 days | ~ 5 days |

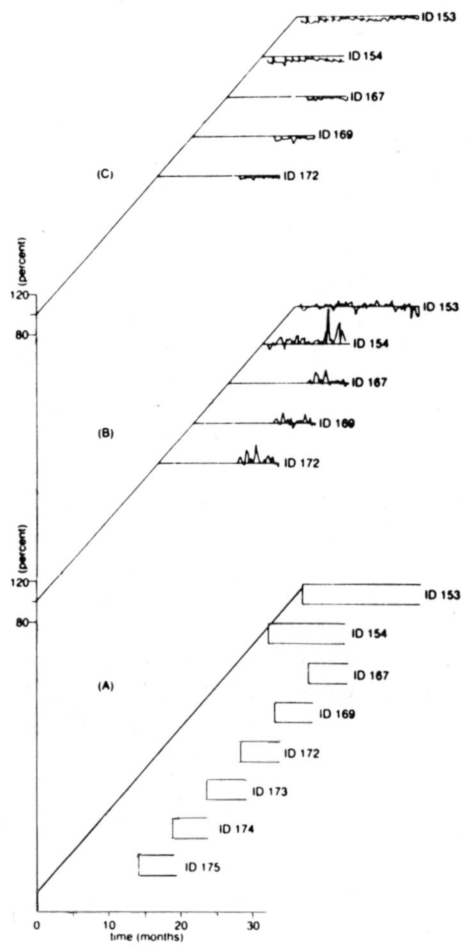



**Figure 4:** Summary of the in vitro tests of Hoe 21 GH with the Promedos I1 pump. Panel A: time of operation. Panel B: insulin quantity in the eluate. Panel C: native, unmodified insulin content in the eluate, as measured by HPLC.

It is evident that both the quantity and the quality of the insulin were almost always near 100%. Device 154 had some elevated insulin contents toward the end due to malfunction: The rate had dropped drastically so that evaporation took place in the collection vial.

The overall mean insulin quantity out of 180 eluate samples has been determined to be 101.9% ± 58% (standard deviation). Our requirements for clinical trials—six devices for six months—have well been exceeded in these tests without insulin precipitation.

In vivo tests of Hoe 21 GH and Promedos I1, which are being done by Dr. K. Geisen, are now in excess of 7.5 device years (Fig. 5). These data, along with the in vitro data, were such that clinical trials could be started earlier this year.

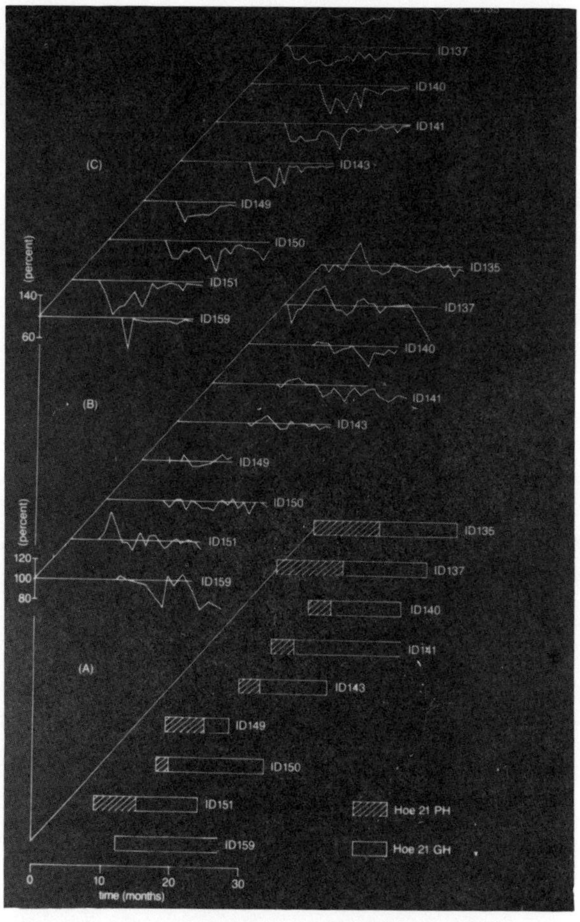


**Figure 5:** Summary of the in vivo tests of Hoe 21 PH and Hoe 21 GH with the Promedos I1 pump. Panels A, B, and C as in *Figure 4*.

In conclusion, the project of diabetes therapy with programmable pumps has now reached the clinical stage. While in the past device reliability and insulin stability have been limiting steps toward the clinical use of implantable insulin infusion devices, we may see more and more other factors arising, such as the catheter access. It will probably, again, need some ingenuity and subtle refinements to lead this project to a success eventually.

## References


1. Grau U. (1985). In: Hepp KD, Renner R, eds, *Continuous Insulin Infusion Therapy. Experience from One Decade*, Schattauer, Stuttgart, New York, pp 33–46.
2. Taylor G, Lebisch H, Weinmann P, Champion J.R. (1983). In: K. Irsigler, H. Kritz, R. Lovett, eds, *Diabetes Treatment with Implantable Insulin Infusion Systems*. Urban & Schwarzenberg, Munich, Vienna, pp 29–39.
3. Grau U, (1985). Chemical stability of insulin in a delivery system environment. *Diabetologia* 28:458–463.
4. Grau U, Saudek C.D., (1986). *Diabetes*, (submitted.)

# Chapter 15

# Computer-Assisted Insulin Therapy

J. Beyer
G. Schulz
J. Schrezenmeir
T. Strack
H. Achterberg
G. Klausmann
F. Hohleweg

Diabetes therapy provided an exact knowledge of the action of the single therapeutic components on the blood glucose, such as the food intake required, the insulin preparations, the body weight, and the physical activity.[1,3,4,8,24,25] It is difficult to coordinate this for numerous diabetics. Blood glucose levels are usually measured for self-control, but the corresponding steps of regulation are not performed with sufficient reliability. In most cases, only single components in insulin dosage are altered in such a way that the full spectrum of the therapeutical possibilities are not completely dealt with. For this reason, we developed various programs for the Sharp pocket computer PC 1500 A for continuous adaption of the insulin doses for different therapeutic strategies on the basis of blood glu-

From: Ensminger WD, Selam JL (eds): *Infusion Systems in Medicine.* Mount Kisco, NY, Futura Publishing Co., Inc., © 1987.

cose self-control and 2 to 4 daily injections of rapid- and long-acting insulin. This computer was able to store blood glucose values, injected insulin doses, and hypoglycemias over three months. A connection to a personal computer or a small printer allows a rapid analysis of the stored data. We developed and tested computer programs for the following different therapeutic strategies.[3,4,6,11−27]

1. Conventional insulin therapy, which is based on NPH and regular insulin injections given 2 to 3 times daily.[3,4,21−23,26,27]

2. Meal-dependent insulin therapy, where meal-dependent regular insulin is injected in addition to a basal insulin.[11−20]

3. Insulin therapy with insulin infusion pumps, where the meal-dependent insulin requirement is calculated based on a pre-prandial blood glucose measurement and the amount of food given, and further calculations will cause a corresponding change of the basal insulin requirement need.

## Study 1

In our first studies carried out years ago, simple regulation principles were used.[21−23] Blood glucose increases were convert-ed directly to insulin units with the help of a regulation matrix. In this way, it is possible to raise or to lower the insulin doses by a nomogram depending on the current blood glucose level for a given glucose target level of 100−120 mg/dL.

The simple principle first used already provided good thera-peutic results (Fig. 1). The blood glucose values of poorly regu-lated diabetics returned to therapeutic blood glucose ranges in a period of about seven days with the use of this program. We tested this with 10 badly regulated hospitalized type I diabetics. Regula-tion of blood glucose values improved during the first seven days mainly by an increase of the NPH insulin dose in the evening, less of the doses of normal insulin in the morning and in the evening [21−23] (Fig. 2).

## Study 2

In a second study with nine outpatient diabetics (Fig. 3), we used a more complex model of regulation. The effect of computer-regulated conventional therapy was studied over 6 to 8 periods of

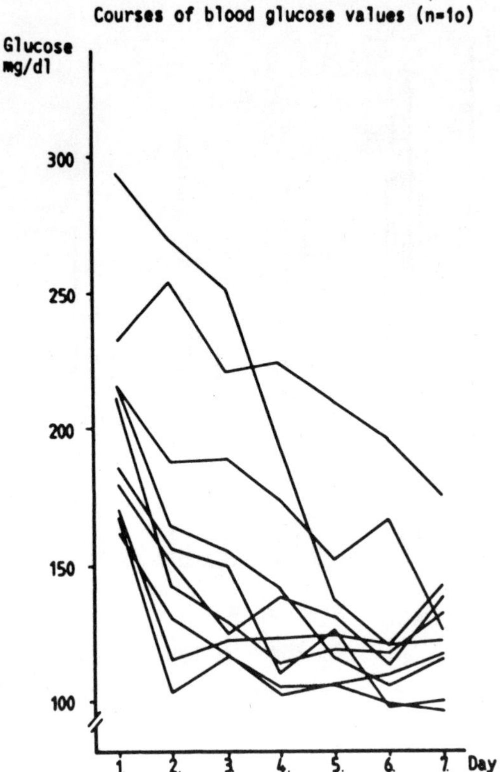


**Figure 1:** Study 1: Courses of blood glucose values (n=10). From Reference 22, with permission.

one week. After a control period without a computer, a phase of computer-aided insulin therapy followed, which in turn was followed by an eight-week control phase of conventional therapy. In this study, computer-aided conventional therapy led to a significant decrease of the HbA1 values in the formerly poorly regulated patient.[26,27] The control phase led to a deterioration of the diabetics who were regulated better before. This agrees with the results published by other investigators.[2,5,7,9,10,28]

## Study 3

In the third group of nine diabetics, whose diabetes was well regulated, and who had performed self-control for a consider-

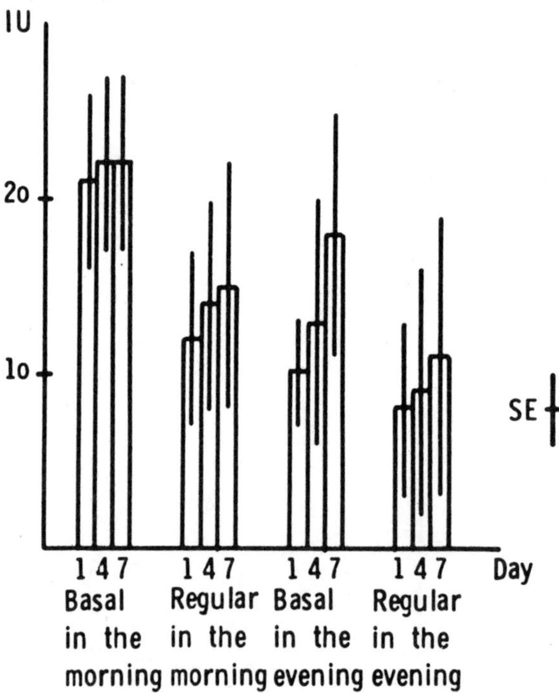


**Figure 2:** Study 1: Alteration and distribution of the daily insulin requirement. From Reference 22, with permission.

able period of time and who where trained in dose adaptation, computer-aided conventional insulin therapy had no significant effect on the metabolic state, except for weak stabilization of the daily blood glucose profile and a reduction of the elevated fasting blood glucose. The total insulin dose for the morning and evening insulin injection did not change significantly, as compared with the earlier period of conventional insulin therapy. No significant changes were observed in the distribution between the regular and NPH insulins in the morning and in the evening.

## Study 4

In a further study, we tested computer use in a cross-over study in the meal-dependent insulin therapy (CAMIT). Twelve type

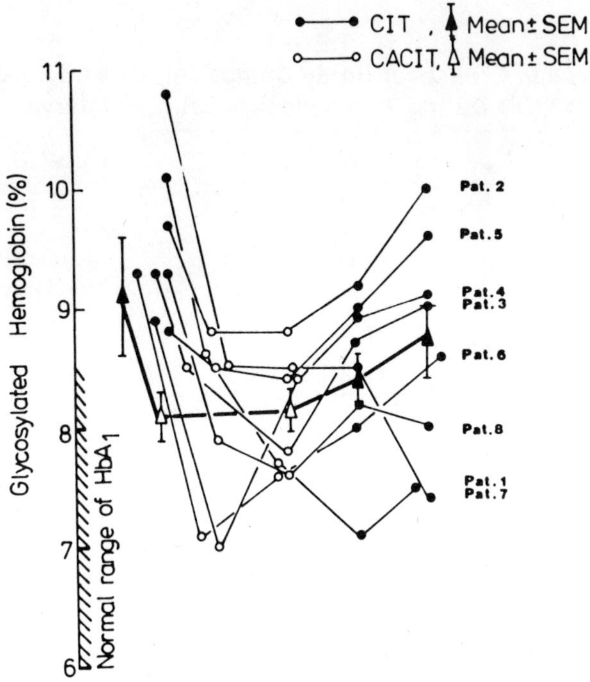


**Figure 3.** Study 2: HbAl changes

I diabetics were observed for 12 weeks. Each patient underwent a six-week period of conventional therapy and a period of CAMIT of the same duration. According to a controlled crossover study design, the order of regimes was randomized (Table 1). Following the conventional therapy regimen, patients injected insulin two to three times daily and ingested six to seven meals of fixed carbohydrate content at defined times of the day. With CAMIT, the patients had one to two insulin injections more and were allowed to vary meal size and time. At the beginning and at the end of each treatment period, HbA1 values were determined. Preprandial blood glucose values were measured by the patients at least four times daily during the whole observation period. Comparison of both treatment periods showed a significant difference between their regimes.[11−20] Although the number of meals was reduced from 6 to 7 small to 3 to 5 larger meals and carbohydrate intake was allowed to vary from day to day, parameters of metabolic control

**Table 1**
**Controlled Crossover Study Comparing CT and CAMIT**
**In 12 IDD During Two 6-week Treatment Intervals**

|  | CT | CAMIT |
|---|---|---|
| Number of meals per day | 6−7 | 3−5 |
| COH intake | fixed | variable |
| Preprondial glucose levels (mmol/L) | 8.86 ± 1.83 to 6.91 ± 0.90 | 9.10 ± 2.96 to 6.22 ± 0.65 |
|  | $p < 0.05$ | |
| $HbA_1$(%) | 9.8 ± 1.3 to 9.1 ± 1.0 | 10.2 ± 1.5 to 8.6 ± 0.8 |
|  | $p < 0.05$ | |

were significantly improved by CAMIT compared to conventional therapy. The average daily insulin requirements in the treatment interval were reduced significantly as well.

## Conclusion

The results of our studies show that a good diabetes regulation can be achieved in a short time with the aid of our computer algorithms on the basis of a diabetes self-control. The therapeutic effect is the more impressive the worse the earlier metabolic state. The limit of therapy is at the well-regulated diabetic who learned to carry out blood glucose self-control and to vary insulin dosages. To summarize, the computer, together with our various programs, was safe and therapeutically effective and found good acceptance in our patients.

## References


1. Albisser M J. (1986). First International Symposium on Computer Systems for Insulin Adjustment Diabetes Mellitus. *Diabetes Care* pp 208−209.
2. Albisser A M, Schiffrin A, Mihic M, Leibel B S, Schulz M. (1984). The insulin dosage computer: A new approach to optimizing conventional insulin therapy. *Diabetologia* 27:250A.

3. Beyer J, Alabisser M, Schrezenmeir J, Lehmann L. (1985). Computer systems for insulin adjustment in diabetes mellitus. Proceedings of the First International Symposium on Computer Systems for Insulin Adjustment in Diabetes mellitus. Mainz, May 15/17th, 1985, ISBN 3-907994-01-9.
4. Beyer J, Becker G, Schulz G, Gaberle E, Wolf E, Hassinger W, Cordes U. (1981). Blood glucose controlled insulin insufion systems for rapid adjustment of insulin dependant diabetics. *Deutsche Medizinische Wochenschrift* 106:1644−1649.
5. Furler S M, Kraegen E W, Smallwood R H, Chrisholm D J. (1985). Blood glucose control by intermittent loop closure in the basal mode: Computer simulation studies with a diabetic model. *Diabetes Care* 8:553.
6. Küstner E, Schrezenmeir J, Strack T, Schulz G, Scholl G, Zwiener K, Rothhaar I, Beyer J (1985). Der Insulindosis-Computer: Hilfsmittel oder Konkurrenz zur Diabetikerschulung? *Akt Endokrin Stoff* 6:118.
7. Pernick N L, Rodbard D. (1986). Personal computer programs to assist with self-monitoring of blood glucose and self-adjustment of insulin dosage. *Diabetes Care* 9:61.
8. Schade D S, Santiago J V, Skyler J S, Rizza R A. *Intensive Insulin Therapy*. Excerpta Medica, Amsterdam, p 341.
9. Schiffrin A, Albisser A M, Mihic M. (1984). Optimizing conventional insulin therapy using an insulin dosage computer. *Diabetes* 33:(Suppl. 1):39A.
10. Schiffrin A, Mihic M, Leibel B S, Albisser A M. (1985). Computer-assisted insulin dosage adjustment. *Diabetes Care* 8:545.
11. Schrezenmeir J, Achterberg H, Bergeler J, Küstner E, Hutten DH. Beyer J (1985). Development of an insulin dosage computer enabling conversion to and optimizing of meal-related insulin injection regimes. Artificial Insulin Delivery Systems, Pancreas and Islet Transplantation. Fourth Workshop, February 3−5, 1985, Igls/Austria.
12. Schrezenmeir J, Achterberg H, Küstner E, Bergeler J, Hutten H, Beyer J. (1985). Computer-assisted meal-related insulin therapy (CAMIT)—New approach to multiple subcutaneous injections and continuous subcutaneous insulin infusion (CSII) regimes. XII Congress of the International Diabetes Federation, Diabetes Research and Clinical Practice, Elsevier Science Publishers, Suppl. 1, p 503.
13. Schrezenmeir J, Achterberg H, Bergeler J, Küstner E, Stürmer W, Hutten H, Beyer J. (1986). Controlled study on the use of hand-held insulin dosage computers enabling conversion to and optimizing of meal-related insulin therapy regimens. Artificial Insulin Delivery Systems, Pancreas and Islet Transplantation. Third Workshop, February 5−7, 1984, Igls/Austria, Life Support Systems 1986, in press.
14. Schrezenmeir J, Achterberg H, Bergeler J, Küstner E, Stürmer W, Hutten H, Beyer J. (1985). Computer-assisted meal-related insulin therapy (CAMIT). In: Beyer J, Albisser M, Shcrezenmeir J. (eds). Proceedings of the First International Symposium on Computer Systems for Insulin Adjustment in Diabetes Mellitus. ISBN 3-907994-01-9.
15. Schrezenmeir J, Achterberg H, Bergeler J, Küstner E, Hutten H, Beyer J.

(1985). Computerassistierte mahlzeitenbezogene Insulintherapie (CAMIT), neuer therapeutischer Ansatz für multiple subkutane Injektions (MSI) and CSII-Regime. *Akt Endokrin Stoff* 6:109.

16. Schrezenmeir J, von Aerssen M, Kasper H. (1984). Use of formula in the management of intensified insulin therapy. Third Workshop of the Study Group of the EASD on Artificial Insulin Delivery Systems, Pancreas and Islet Transplantation. Igls/Austria p 45.

17. Schrezenmeir J, von Aerssen J, Küstner E, Kasper H, Beyer J. (1985). Eine Formel zur Einstellung und Anpassung insulinpflichtiger Diabetiker mit mahlzeitenbezogenen Insulininjektionen. *Klin Wschr* Suppl. IV, 63:263.

18. Schrezenmeir J, von Aerssen M, Tato F, Tato S, Strack T, Kasper H, Beyer J. (1985). Unterschiedlicher Insulinbedarf bei verschieden artigem Frühstück: Der Kohlenhydratgehalt ist nicht das alleinige Maß in der diätetischen Therapie des Diabetes. *Akt Endokrin Stoff* 6:109.

19. Schrezenmeir J, Küstner E, Beyer J. (1985). Die Vermittlung von Regeln zur quantifizierten Selbstanpassung der Insulindosis. *Akt Endokrin Stoff* 6:119.

20. Schrezenmeir J, Tato F, Tato S, Achterberg H, Schulz G, Strack T, von Aerssen M, Kasper M, Beyer J. (1985). Food-dependent insulin consumption. In: Beyer J, Albisser M, Schrezenmeir J. Proceedings of the First International Symposium on Computer Systems for Insulin Adjustment in Diabetes Mellitus. ISBN 3-907994-01-9.

21. Schulz G, Beyer J. Fortschritte in der Therapie insulinpflichtiger Diabetiker. *Krankenhauspharmazie* 5:104.

22. Schulz G, Beyer J, Hohleweg H, Bergeler J, Hutten H. (1985). Die rechnergestützte Diabeteseinstellung. *Klin Wschr* 63:1098−1101.

23. Schulz G, Beyer J, Hohleweg F, Bergeler J, Küstner E, Hutten H. (1985). A computerized program for intentified subcutaneous insulin therapy by diabetes self-adjustment. *Diabetologia* 27:330A.

24. Skyler J S, Seigler D E, Reevers M L. (1982). Optimizing pumped insulin delivery. *Diabetes Care* 5:135−147.

25. Skyler J S, Skyler D L, Seigler D E, O'Sullivan M J. (1981). Algorithms for adjustment of insulin dosage by patients who monitor blood glucose. *Diabetes Care* 4:311.

26. Strack T, Bergeler J, Hutten H, Beyer H. (1985). Rechnergestütze Diabetesbehandlung mit konventioneller Insulintherapie und tragbaren Insulininfusionspumpen. *Akt Endokrin Stoff* 6:109.

27. Strack T, Beyer J, Schrezenmeir J, Bergeler J, Schulz G, Krause U, Hutten H. (1986). Computer assisted conventional insulin therapy in the treatment of insulin-dependent diabetics. (in press).

28. Wilson D, Clarke D H. (1983). Profiling self-monitored blood glucose results with the personal microcomputer. *Diabetes Care* 6:604.

# Chapter 16

# Insulin Delivery Devices: The Vienna–Lainz Pump Experience (1978–1986)

Karl Irsigler

## Introduction

With ongoing solutions of some of the problems encountered with pump treatment and new types of pumps, an optimistic outlook can be given for the future for improvement of pump treatment strategy. The intravenous (IV) and/or intraperitoneal (IP) route of insulin delivery is feasible for long-term treatment. This paper reports the Vienna–Lainz pump experience.

Work was begun in 1978 with a closed-loop system (Biostator) and the first prototypes of the externally worn Siemens pump. First, implantations were done in April 1981 with two Infusaid (constant basal infusion, CBI) pumps and one programmable Siemens implant. The Vienna–Lainz pump experience is based on results of 223 treatment years in 97 patients (one year programmable pump, 146 years CBI intraperitoneal, 76 years CBI intravenous). The IP route was used for 57 patients, and the IV route for 39 pa-

From: Ensminger WD, Selam JL (eds): *Infusion Systems in Medicine.* Mount Kisco, NY, Futura Publishing Co., Inc., ©1987.

tients. For the newer generation of externally worn pumps with subcutaneous insulin infusion (Nordisk-Infuser, Lilly CPI-pump, Autosyringe, Medix, Millhill, Hoechst Dise-tronic), we now have an observation period of 117 years. Therefore, a comparison is possible between 92 patients with externally worn devices and 69 patients with implanted devices with ongoing function for long-term treatment (38 IP, 31 IV).

## Metabolic Control

Three categories of $HbA_{1c}$ were established (below 6%, 6−8%, and above 8%, normal range ending at 5.6%). A comparison of metabolic control achieved with external versus implanted pumps could be made with all three delivery routes (IV, IP, SC). Programmable pumps gave a slightly superior metabolic control than constant basal rate pumps. The IV route proved to be superior to the IP or SC route. Only 24% of patients with externally worn IV pumps had $Hb_{A1c}$ values above 8%, whereas 33% of CSII treated patients were in this unsatisfactory stage of metabolic control.

With eleven ketoacidosis per 100 patient years with CSII treatment, there was an unacceptably high rate of metabolic derangement with this type of pump treatment (similar to rates reported in the literature). With implanted pumps and IP or IV insulin delivery, the rate was only of one and two ketoacidosis per 100 patient years, respectively. The single experienced case of ketoacidosis with IP was due to noncompliance of the patient to come to refills.

## Causes of Explantations (n = 39)

In addition to a few cases of pumpbed infections postsurgically or from pump refill manipulation, the major cause of explantation was slowdown of the pump flow (p = 13). Rinsing procedures were developed with acidic or alkaline solutions to dissolve insulin aggregates but proved not to be very successful.

No single technical failure occurred in CBI pumps (Infusaid). The first programmable pump (Siemens-Erlangen), also implanted in April 1981, lasted for eight months and the second pump for four months.

## Catheters

For the CBI Infusaid pump, a silicone rubber catheter was used while a polyethylene catheter was used with externally worn IV or IP pumps. The catheter tip proved to be the most critical part of the pump catheter unit. Pump slowdowns were mainly caused by obstruction of the catheter tip. These obstructions were previously explained as being insulin aggregates, but could be shown now as being mainly fibrin clots. Therefore, new rinsing procedures were developed, and plasmin and/or urokinase were able to dissolve obstructions in IV and also in IP pumps.

## Insulin

Acidic insulin (Hoechst Ag, Frankfurt, FRG) proved to be stable enough for externally worn pumps. Infusaid pumps were used with insulin-glycerol-bicarbonate mixtures. Filtration of glycerol instead of autoclaving has minimized deterioration of insulin. Stability of Genapol insulin (Hoechst AG, Frankfurt) has proven to be satisfactory in dog experiments and also when used in externally worn pumps in diabetic patients.

## Quality of Life

There is evidence now, that compared to the prepump phase in our patient group, a considerable reduction of days in hospital and also of sick leave days per year was achieved. According to a psychological evaluation, depression was considerably reduced especially in patients with implanted pumps. The major drawback up to now has been short refill intervals of only three weeks, which could be prolonged with higher concentrated insulins.

## The Future: Insulin Delivery Route

In spite of the long experience with the IV and the IP route, a definite conclusion cannot be drawn. An actuarial analysis of catheter-pump lifetime in our implanted patient group gives a slight superiority for the IV route. According to this analysis, the probability of a long-term function for more than three years is 70%

for the IV and 60% for the IP insulin delivery with an implanted pump (Infusaid). The IV route has a good chance for further improvement since most of the catheters that were occluded were those which did not stay in optimal position within the superior vena cava.

## The Future: Pumps

The closed-loop system is not in sight for the future, because the long-term function of sensors has not been achieved. The sensor will be used for intermittent blood glucose measurements in tissue or blood and possibly will substitute for fingerpricking and paperstrips.

During the second half of 1986, new programmable devices will be introduced into clinical trials with insulin. The Siemens device has been improved and will function with a three-year battery. The Pacesetter Minimed device (solenoid-pump) with a titanium chamber inside will soon go into clinical trials. Several other new developments of programmable insulin pumps are now used with pain-killing drugs or with chemotherapeutic agents. Though a continuous basal-rate insulin infusion alone is able to stabilize unstable diabetes with additional injections, in the long run, the CBI insulin infusion will not be used in large patient groups until a programmable device is available. For the future, a three-year uninterrupted function of implanted pumps seems satisfactory and economically feasible as well.

# Chapter 17

# Drug Delivery Devices in Oncology

William D. Ensminger

The history of drug delivery devices in oncology is intimately associated with hepatic arterial chemotherapy. In fact, as a treatment modality, hepatic arterial chemotherapy can be divided into the time period before the implanted pump and the time period after the implanted pump. Prior to the introduction of the implanted pump, hepatic arterial chemotherapy frequently utilized angiographically placed, percutaneous catheters with external pumps for protracted drug infusions. The level of difficulty in dealing with such catheters and drug infusion systems limited the number of physicians practicing such therapy. However, the response rates claimed (Table 1) tended to be much higher than those associated with the use of intravenous chemotherapy regimens for the treatment of colorectal cancer metastatic to the liver.

Several developments during the late 1970s provided impetus to interest in hepatic arterial chemotherapy. Pharmacologic studies carried out with 5-fluoro-2'-deoxyuridine (FUDR) and 5-fluoro-uracil (FU) demonstrated how high hepatic extraction could lead to reduced systemic drug levels and potentially generate increased drug levels within the hepatic artery when hepatic arterial chemotherapy was used.[7] The results of these pharmacological studies indicated that hepatic tumor exposure to FUDR might be increased

**Table 1**
**Intraarterial Therapy of Hepatic Metastases Using External Pumps**
**in Patients with Colorectal Cancer**

| Reference | Drugs Used | No. of Evaluable Patients | Response Rate Claimed (%) |
|---|---|---|---|
| Sullivan and Zurek[1] | Multiple regimens | 39 | 62 |
| Watkins et al.[2] | FUDR | 82 | 73 |
| Cady et al.[3] | FUDR | 51 | 57 |
| Oberfield et al.[4] | FU/FUDR | 48 | 75 |
| Patt et al.[5] | Mitomycin/FUDR | 12 | 83 |
| Reed et al.[6] | FUDR | 77 | 76 |

as much as several hundred-fold by direct hepatic arterial administration.[8,9] In light of these pharmacologic studies, the earlier reports of high response rates with hepatic arterial chemotherapy could be seen as a logical extrapolation of dose response effects for the fluorinated pyrimidines.

During the late 1970s, nuclide angiography was introduced as a technique to define and mimic drug flow distribution patterns during low flow rates as used in hepatic arterial chemotherapy. Radioactively-labeled, gamma-emitting particles (Tc99m-macroaggregated albumin, TcMAA) were injected at slow flow rates into hepatic arterial catheters. The pattern of flow distribution as seen by the entrapment of these microparticulates within (the first capillary bed of) the liver was found to correlate with the pattern of regression of tumor.[10] Nuclide flow to a particular region of the liver was correlated with a high probability of response for tumors in that region, whereas a lack of direct drug flow was found to correlate with a lack of response. This pointed out the necessity that catheters should always be positioned within the hepatic artery such that there is direct drug infusion to the entire tumor-bearing liver.

In 1980, Buchwald and associates reported on the treatment of five patients with hepatic arterial chemotherapy using an implantable infusion pump, which they had invented at the University of Minnesota.[11] Unfortunately, their results were not impressive due to lack of definition of complete hepatic coverage by drug (see above) and to the toxicity generated by continuous infusion, without break periods, of FUDR for from 13 to 29 weeks. In 1979, investigators at the University of Michigan obtained this implantable pump from the Infusaid Division of the Metal Bellows Corporation (Sharon, Massachusetts). The model 400 Infusaid® pump, as obtained from the manufacturer, had a sideport® that bypassed the pumping mechanism and allowed direct catheter injection for nuclide angiography, bolus drug administration, and for clearing of blocked catheters. The initial clinical experience with the first 13 patients having this pump implanted at the University of Michigan was published in 1981.[12] This study defined the utility of the pump sideport® to clear catheter occlusions and to define drug flow distribution using nuclide angiography (see above) with TcMAA injection into the sideport®. The limiting toxic effects of continuous hepatic arterial infusion of FUDR in this study were gastrointestinal and hepatic; most patients developed elevations in serum bilirubin and of liver enzymes after 6 to 8 weeks of continuous FUDR infusion. Resolution of gastrointestinal symptoms and signs of chemical hepatitis were noted to occur when drug was withheld for periods of 1 to 4 weeks. The application of a drug-free "break" using alternate pump refills with saline only was described as a way to decrease toxicity. Most remarkably, however, 11 of the 13 patients (85%) in the study were stated to have achieved partial response of their hepatic tumor by physical examination or liver scan criteria. In 1982, Ensminger and associates described therapeutic results in 60 evaluable patients with colorectal cancer receiving FUDR at 0.3 mg/kg/d for two weeks alternating with normal saline for two weeks using the implanted pump.[13] Short infusions of Mitomycin (over 15 to 30 minutes) were administered through the pump sideport® when FUDR failed to induce a response. Fifty of the sixty evaluable patients were found to have partial responses of hepatic tumor ascertained by physical examination and/or nuclide liver scans. Approximately half of these patients were noted to have symptoms of gastritis, and half were felt to have developed "chemical hepatitis" by serum enzyme determinations. The variety of catheter placement techniques necessary to achieve total hepatic drug infusional patterns (by TcMAA nuclide angiography) in these patients was described.[14]

There have been multiple phase II studies reported in the last three years utilizing primarily the Infusaid® implanted pump for hepatic arterial chemotherapy (Table 2). All of these studies have utilized FUDR, and many of them have added other drugs to the treatment regimen, including primarily mitomycin C (Mito) administered

**Table 2**
**Phase II Studies Utilizing an Implanted Drug Delivery System**

| Investigators | No. of Patients | Drugs Utilized | Response Rate Claimed | Comment |
|---|---|---|---|---|
| Balch et al.[15] | 81 | FUDR/Mito | 88% | Response by drop in CEA |
| Niederhuber et al.[16] | 93 | FUDR/Mito | 78% | |
| N. Kemeny et al.[17] | 41 | FUDR/Mito | 44% | 52% response in previously untreated patients |
| M. Kemeny et al.[18] | 24 | FUDR | 73% | |
| M. Kemeny et al.[19] | 24 | FUDR | 52% | |
| Patt et al.[20] | 29 | FUDR/Mito/Cisplatin | 52% | Infusaid and Medtronics Pumps |
| Cohen et al.[21] | 36 | FUDR/Mito/BCNU | 70% | |

as a short infusion through the pump sideport®. A variety of response criteria have been applied ranging from use solely of a fall in CEA to strict use of measurable reductions in lesions by CT scanning. The majority of response rates claimed have exceeded 50% (Table 2).

There are two randomized studies from which preliminary information is available as to the comparison of hepatic arterial venous intravenous FUDR administration. Unfortunately, neither of these studies has been published as yet. Both of these studies have a similar design and basically compare the response rate of colorectal liver metastases to treatment with FUDR administered by the hepatic artery route versus the intravenous route on a 14-day on, 14-day off drug cycle.

The study conducted at Memorial Sloan Kettering Cancer Center used previously untreated patients with colorectal cancer confined to the liver.[22] All patients underwent an exploratory laparotomy to evaluate the extent of liver involvement and to determine eligibility with an absence of extrahepatic disease. At the time of surgery, catheters were placed into the hepatic artery and a central vein. Patients were then randomized to receive either hepatic arterial infusion or intravenous infusion with the Infusaid® pump connected to the appropriate catheter. Of note, patients who subsequently failed treatment on the intravenous arm were crossed over to hepatic arterial chemotherapy although crossover in the other direction was not performed. Patients on the two arms were matched for all pertinent variables. The toxicities in the hepatic arm were similar to those previously reported for hepatic arterial chemotherapy. The dose-limiting toxicity for the intravenous group was diarrhea in two-thirds of the patients. As reported by Dr. Nancy Kemeny at the Fifth NCI/EORTC Symposium on New Drugs in Cancer Therapy in Amsterdam, the response to intrahepatic therapy was significantly higher than that obtained with systemic infusion, 50% versus 19.6%. Of the 31 systemically treated patients who underwent crossover into intrahepatic therapy, 58% were stated to have a documented response or stable remission on intrahepatic infusion.

The Northern California Oncology Group randomized trial of intravenous versus hepatic arterial FUDR for colorectal cancer enrolled 110 evaluable patients.[23] FUDR dosages were adjusted according to toxicity. Major hepatic responses (greater than 50% reduction in tumor volume by CT scan) occurred in 10% of patients receiving intravenous therapy and 37% of patients receiving intraarterial therapy. Measurable responses (any reduction in tumor volume) occurred in 25% of intravenous patients and 59% of intraarterial patients. These differences in response rate are highly significant statistically. Stable disease was seen in 39% of intravenous patients versus 27% of intraarterial patients, with disease progression occurring in 36% of intravenous and 14% of intraarterially treated patients. Median times to hepatic tumor progression were 203 days for the intravenously treated patients and 658 days for intraarterially treated patients (statistically significant with P≤ 0.0003). Differences in times to extrahepatic progression were insignificant.

The commerical approval by the U.S. Food and Drug Administration in early 1982 of the implantable Infusaid® pump for hepatic arterial chemotherapy led to the implantation of some 15,000 pumps in subsequent years at 1,400 centers in the United States and other countries. The widespread introduction of the Infusaid® pump demonstrated the capability of a multitude of surgeons and medical oncologists to implant and refill an implanted pump. Although hepatic arterial chemotherapy remains controversial and the Infusaid® pump may have been applied to some inappropriate patients,[24] the device itself proved to be highly reliable in delivering a constant infusion. Demonstration of the marketability of the Infusaid® pump has provided impetus to the development of other implanted pumps and of the implantable injection ports, which were a direct offshoot of the sideport® of the Model 400 Infusaid® pump.[25] Due to the nature of the disease in question, the risk−benefit ratio is likely to continue to make oncology applications important in the development and introduction of new drug delivery devices.

In a real sense, at this juncture, infusion technology is not the sole limitation to the applicability of drug delivery devices to the treatment of cancer. Instead, the demonstration that there are suitable drugs that would display more activity or an improved therapeutic index on a protracted infusion schedule remains a major problem to expansion of the role of implanted pumps and, to a lesser degree, to greater use of external pumps in an outpatient setting (see below). The restrictions on an agent that would be appropriately used in a constant infusion transcend those applicable to standard drugs given by bolus or short-term infusion.

The first criterion in choosing an agent of constant infusion is a need to have demonstrated therapeutic superiority of a protracted, sustained drug level for the agent in question. It is noteworthy that only recently has it been possible, and then with considerable cost/effort, to use protracted drug infusions for testing in animal models, further restricting our knowledge as to useful agents for infusions. A second criterion is that the drug possess a high total body clearance and short plasma drug half-life, making constant infusion necessary. A recent review of continuous infusion chemotherapy has defined a number of antineoplastic agents for which infusional therapies may be reasonable in certain treatment regimens.[26] These include 5-FU and FUDR, cytosine arabinoside, vinca alkaloids, doxorubicin, and cisplatin. Clearly, without FU and FUDR there would be no viable market for portable external pumps (FU) or implanted pumps (FUDR) in oncology.

Implanted pumps bring further constraints to bear. Due to a limited reservoir size and the desire not to refill the devices more frequently than every week, the drug used must be both potent and sufficiently soluble. FUDR is very potent (daily dose by constant infusion being about 20 mg) and soluble (over 100 mg/mL) so that 1 mL holds five day's worth of drug. FU, on the other hand, is less potent (daily dose by constant infusion being 1,000−2,000 mg) and less soluble (50 mg/mL) so that one day's worth of drug requires 20 mL or 100 times more volume than required for an equitoxic dose of FUDR. Thus, although the Infusaid® pump and FU are compatible, the 50 mL pump reservoir would require refills every two days. Solubility can sometimes be improved upon by pH or solvent changes. For example, our investigations with 5-bromo-2'-deoxyuridine (BUDR) using the Infusaid® pump have been conducted using a pH 9.5 buffer which improves the solubility by some 25-fold so that the daily dose can be contained in 3−4 mL of solution. The use of implanted pumps also raises the problem of drug stability at 37°C and compatibility with the device for the days to weeks involved between refills. Pharmaceutical firms generally have little information on drug stability at 37°C making it incumbent upon pump manufacturers or individual investigators to carry out stability as well as compatibility studies.

Although "second generation" programmable pumps such as the Medtronic Drug Administration Device have become available for investigations in oncology,[27] apart from their use in chronobiology[28,29] (see Chapter 18), one can see little advantage to applying these more sophisticated devices to chronic, steady-rate drug infusions such as are common in oncology. The more complex the device, the less reliable and more costly it will be, intrinsically. Unfortunately, apart from some leads from Dr. Hrushesky's group in the chronobiology of several oncolytic agents, little is known as to whether varying drug levels with time make any significant difference. Certainly, rate variable programmable external pumps are probably best used to define the role of unique schedules prior to implanting a programmable subcutaneous pump.

As noted earlier, implantable injection ports attached to intravenous or intraarterial catheters were a direct offshoot of the sideport® of the Infusaid® pump.[25] This device appears to be reliable, safe, and easy to use, leading to many thousands being sold. It is this writer's opinion that there is a proliferation of such ports on the market, most representing clones of the initial design. There has been a notable lack of creativity in the design and use of such ports. Many improvements in port design and means of access/use seem possible, which should expand port use throughout medicine and surgery where repeated protracted access to a vascular tree or body space is required. The expansion of port use has, in turn, facilitated application of external pumps (of which there are now a wide variety). To date, however, none of the external systems approaches the implanted pumps for patient convenience, and all external pumps present some impediment to normal function.

In conclusion, oncology and, in particular, hepatic arterial chemotherapy has played a major role in the widespread acceptance of implanted devices in the medical community. Expansion of the utility/applicability of implanted pumps depends largely on new drugs and new indications (for example, the use of carotid arterial 5-bromo-2'-deoxyuridine (BUDR) for gliomas; see Chapter 21). In this regard, the constant drug levels achievable with protracted constant infusions should facilitate (on the basis of drug concentration and exposure) correlations between in vitro cell culture studies and in vivo effects on tumor and host tissues in patients. Finally, offshoots of implanted pump technology, such as injection ports for vascular access and improved catheter materials, may impact more broadly on all of medicine. The severe nature of cancer has and will continue to provide the seedbed for the germination of innovative and daring approaches often involving drug delivery technology.

# References


1. Sullivan RD, Zurek WZ (1965). Chemotherapy for liver cancer by protracted ambulatory infusion. *JAMA* 194:481.
2. Watkins E, Khazei AM, Nahra KS (1970). Surgical basis for arterial infusion chemotherapy of disseminated carcinoma of the liver. *Surg Gynecol Obstet* 130:581.
3. Cady B, Oberfield RA (1974). Regional infusion chemotherapy of hepatic metastases from carcinoma of the colon. *Am J Surg* 127:220.
4. Oberfield RA, McCaffrey JA, Polio J, et al (1979). Prolonged and continuous percutaneous intraarterial hepatic infusion chemotherapy in advanced metastatic liver adenocarcinoma from colorectal primary. *Cancer* 44:414.
5. Patt YZ, Mavligit GM, Chuang VP, et al (1979). Percutaneous hepatic arterial infusion (HA) of mitomycin C and floxuridine (FUDR): An effective treatment for metastatic colorectal carcinoma in the liver. *Cancer* 46:261.
6. Reed ML, Vaitkevicius VK, Al-Sarraf M, et al (1981). The practicality of chronic hepatic artery infusion therapy of primary and metastatic hepatic malignancies. *Cancer* 47:402.
7. Ensminger WD, Rosowsky A, Raso V, et al (1978). A clinical–pharmacological evaluation of hepatic arterial infusions of 5-fluoro-2′-deoxyuridine and 5-fluorouracil. *Cancer Res* 38:3784.
8. Collins JM (1984). Pharmacologic rationale for regional drug delivery. *J Clin Oncol* 2:498.
9. Ensminger WD, Gyves JW (1984). Regional cancer chemotherapy. *Cancer Treat Rep* 68:101.
10. Kaplan WD, Ensminger WD, Come SE, et al (1980). Radionuclide angiography to predict patient response to hepatic artery chemotherapy. *Cancer Treat Rep* 64:1217.
11. Buchwald H, Grage TB, Vassilopoulos PP, et al (1980). Intraarterial infusion chemotherapy for hepatic carcinoma using a totally implantable infusion pump. *Cancer* 45:866.
12. Ensminger W, Niederhuber J, Dakhil S, et al (1981). Totally implanted drug delivery system for hepatic arterial chemotherapy. *Cancer Treat Rep* 65:393.
13. Ensminger W, Niederhuber J, Gyves J, et al (1982). Effective control of liver metastases from colon cancer with an implanted system for hepatic arterial chemotherapy. *Proc ASCO* 1:94.
14. Niederhuber JE, Ensminger WD (1983). Surgical considerations in the management of hepatic neoplasia. *Sem Onc* 10(2):135.
15. Balch CM, Urist MM, Soong S-J, et al (1983). A prospective phase II clinical trial of continuous FUDR regional chemotherapy for colorectal metastases to the liver using a totally implanted drug infusion pump. *Ann Surg* 198:567.
16. Niederhuber JE, Ensminger W, Gyves J, et al (1984). Regional chemotherapy of colorectal cancer metastatic to the liver. *Cancer* 53:1336.

17. Kemeny N, Daly J, Oderman P, et al (1984). Hepatic artery pump infusion: Toxicity and results in patients with metastatic colorectal carcinoma. *J Clin Oncol* 2:595.
18. Kemeny MM, Goldberg DA, Browning S, et al (1985). Experience with continuous regional chemotherapy and hepatic resection as treatment of hepatic metastases from colorectal primaries. *Cancer* 55:1265.
19. Kemeny MM, Goldberg D, Beatty JD, et al (1986). Results of a prospective randomized trial of continuous regional chemotherapy and hepatic resection as treatment of hepatic metastases from colorectal primaries. *Cancer* 57:492.
20. Patt YZ, Boddie AW Jr, Charnsangavej C, et al (1986). Hepatic arterial infusion with floxuridine and cisplatin: Overriding importance of anti-tumor effect versus degree of tumor burden as determinants of survival among patients with colorectal cancer. *J Clin Oncol* 4:1356.
21. Cohen AM, Schaeffer N, Higgins J (1986). Treatment of metastatic colorectal cancer with hepatic artery combination chemotherapy. *Cancer* 57:1115.
22. Kemeny N (1986). Personal communication and, as quoted in "Intrahepatic administration of FUDR yields more responses than systemic." *The Clinical Cancer Letter* 9:1.
23. Hohn D, Stagg R, Friedman M, et al (1987). The NCOG randomized trial of intravenous (IV) vs hepatic arterial (IA) FUDR for colorectal cancer metastatic to the liver *Proc ASCO.* (in press)
24. Ensminger WD (1987). Intraarterial chemotherapy for the treatment of hepatic metastases. *Updates for Cancer Principles and Practice of Oncology* 1(3).
25. Gyves JW, Ensminger WD, Niederhuber JE, et al (1984). A totally implanted injection port system for blood sampling and chemotherapy administration. *JAMA* 251:2538.
26. Vogelzang NJ (1984). Continuous infusion chemotherapy: A critical review. *J Clin Oncol* 2(11):1289.
27. Vogelzang NJ, Ruane M, DeMeester TR (1985). Phase 1 trial of an implanted battery-powered, programmable drug delivery system for continuous doxorubisin administration. *J Clin Oncol* 3(3):407.
28. von Roemeling RW, Hrushesky WJM, Kennedy BJ, et al (1986). Programmed automatic FUDR chronotherapy improves therapeutic index. *Surg Forum* 37:401.
29. von Roemeling R, Hrushesky W (1987). Circadian shaping of FUDR infusion reduces toxicity even at high-dose intensity. *Proc ASCO.* (in press)

# Chapter 18

# Programmable Automatic Drug Delivery: New Perspectives for Cancer Therapy

William J. M. Hrushesky
Reinhard V. Roemeling
Jeffrey T. Rabatin

## Introduction

Although spectacularly effective in a few malignancies, chemotherapy cannot cure most metastatic solid tumors. These cancers are often primarily and/or will eventually become drug resistant. Many attempts have been made to overcome this resistance. In the previous decade, it was assured that optimal doses and schedules of anticancer treatment would emanate from knowledge of the cytokinetics of cancer cells. These efforts have been disappointing.[1] Recently, limited host treatment tolerance has been emphasized as a major cause of treatment failure by Chabner[2] and Devita.[3] Most chemotherapeutic agents kill malignant cells only when the cells are actively cycling. Prolonged and continuous exposure of tumor cells to antineoplastic drugs can result in regression of malignant

*From:* Ensminger WD, Selam JL (eds): *Infusion Systems in Medicine.* Mount Kisco, NY, Futura Publishing Co., Inc., ©1987.

cells of low-growth fraction tumors, even if they are refractory to conventional therapy. Frequent high-dose administration of cytotoxic agents or continuous infusion is theoretically necessary to increase tumor cell kill and to minimize the probability of the development of drug-resistant clones. The amount of drug delivered per unit of time (dose intensity) clearly determines the quality and longevity of tumor control in a variety of malignancies.[4]

Biological rhythms along daily, monthly, annual, or other time spans characterize processes that may be involved in the malignant transformation of cells, cellular proliferation of both normal and tumor tissues as well as their susceptibilities to cytotoxic agents, and the pharmacokinetics of chemotherapeutic agents used. Variations result from interaction of many component rhythms, like cell cycles and endocrine and immunological changes.[5,6] In the hypothetical example (Fig. 1), the circadian times of best and worst drug tolerance differ between host and tumor, whereas the quantitative differences between peak and trough and the rhythm frequency are

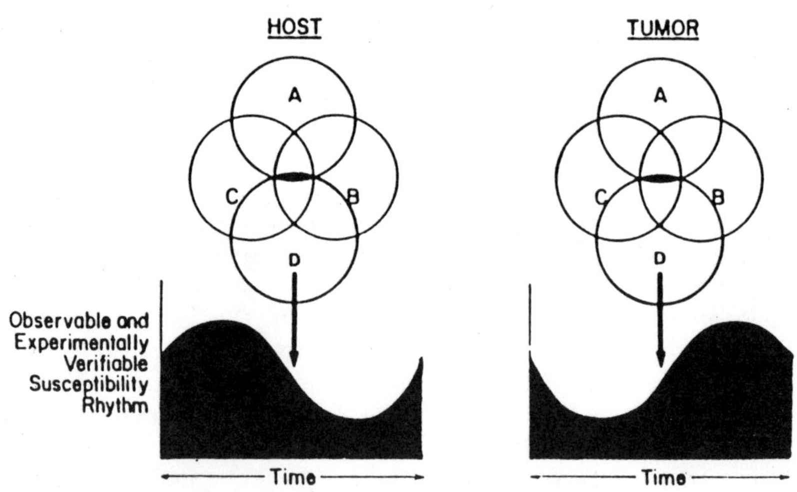


**Figure 1:** Host and tumor susceptibility rhythms. Results from the interaction of many component rhythms.

the same. These differences theoretically can be used to increase the differential cell kill by drug timing. Optimal circadian drug timing may maximize therapeutic effect and minimize toxicity. The timing, sequence, and interval between agents may also be relevant if multiple agents are given.

The toxicity of at least 15 of the most commonly used anticancer drugs has been shown to be circadian stage-dependent in murine systems.[7] The anticancer effects of many of these agents have also been shown to be time-dependent in mice and rats. Clinical studies have documented that anticancer drug pharmacokinetics are circardian stage-dependent in human beings.[8-10] Most clinicians do not specify the time of day when a drug is to be given. Patients usually receive drugs at times most convenient for clinical or hospital staff. Until recently, prolonged continuous infusion could be accomplished only with great difficulty and in a hospital. The development of programmable implantable or external, wearable pumps allows treatment in the outpatient setting with minimal impact on lifestyle. The development of programmable drug administration devices makes time-qualified drug delivery practical, safe, and cost effective. Two such devices are discussed below.

## Programmable Drug Administration Devices

The Medtronic Drug Administration System (DAS; Medtronic Inc., Minneapolis, MN) is an implantable, programmable drug infusion system (Fig. 2). It consists of (1) an infusion pump that can be noninvasively programmed to a specific infusion pattern; (2) a programmer for setting or changing the pump's infusion pattern (instructions are noninvasively transmitted via coded radiofrequency signals); (3) a sideport for injections bypassing the pumping mechanism; and (4) various size catheters.

The pump contains a collapsible 20 cc drug reservoir. A peristaltic roller pump, driven by a lithium thionyl battery module, delivers the drug. The rate of delivery is controlled by an inbuilt microcomputer. The infusion rate can be programmed to vary between 0.009 cc/h and 0.9 cc/h. Program options allow time-qualified bolus injections, continuous infusion at a constant flow rate, or a combination of both modes so that virtually any temporal infusion pattern can be achieved. For example, a complex delivery cycle can be created that consists of continuous infusion with multiple increases

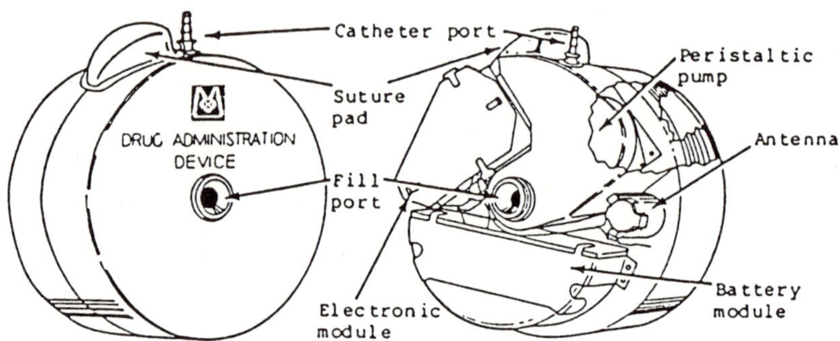


**Figure 2:** Medtronic drug administration device.

and decreases of the flow rate over time, resembling a sinus curve (10 steps per cycle; maximum cycle length = 100 h).[11] The accuracy of the Medtronic pump has been calculated to be within an error margin of 2.2%. This has been demonstrated in 799 refills of 122 pumps.

An implantable drug administration device is superior for arterial (e.g., intrahepatic) drug infusion. If the metastatic disease is confined to the liver, as is frequently the case in colon cancer patients, a laparotomy may be performed to place a pump and catheter for hepatic arterial drug infusion. During such an operative procedure, the abdomen is explored to search for and quantify extrahepatic cancer deposits, which are resected if possible. Prophylactic gallbladder removal is recommended because cholecystitis is a frequent side effect of hepatic arterial FUDR infusion.[12] During this operation, the liver is inspected and palpated in order to assess the degree of tumor involvement. This estimation of the tumor mass is the single most important prognostic factor for determining subsequent survival in patients whose disease is limited to that organ.[13] Chemotherapy is usually begun within a week of pump implantation and is conducted entirely on an outpatient basis.

If chemotherapy is to be given systemically, the pump is placed in a subcutaneous pocket in the right or left subclavian fossa. The catheter tip is placed in the superior vena cava. This implantation procedure can be performed under local anesthesia in an outpatient surgery clinic. Chemotherapy can usually be initiated on the same day as surgery and is conducted on an outpatient basis.

Whereas the Medtronic pump can deliver only one drug at a time, treatment schedules may be desirable that include a combination of various drugs. The Intelliject system (Intelligent Medicine, Inc., Englewood, CO) offers an external pump capable of administering four drugs simultaneously. This system consists of three major elements: (1) the pump itself, which contains four disposable 30 mL syringes connected through a manifold; (2) the programming software to be written on an IBM-AT computer; and (3) a control cartridge inserted into the back of the pump, which contains the program information. This information is stored permanently in the cartridge. The pump may be programmed for cycle lengths of up to 31 days or as short as one minute, and can deliver fluids at a flow rate between 0.015 mL/h to 40.5 mL/h per syringe; it is battery powered and weighs 1.5 kg.

Our current experience with the pump used in patients and small animals (275 complete treatment courses) indicates extremely precise drug delivery according to preprogrammed time schedules. Accuracy was greater than 95%.

## Clinical Studies at the University of Minnesota Illustrating the Importance of Drug Timing

### Intrahepatic Infusional 2'-Deoxy-5-Fluorouridine (FUDR)

Hepatic-arterial FUDR is effective in controlling malignancies confined to the liver,[14] but liver toxicity is very frequent ($> 60\%$) and often severe (in 5% of the cases irreversible and occasionally fatal).[15] In a series of murine experiments, we determined that both FUDR toxicity and efficacy are circadian-stage dependent.[16] Forty patients with metastatic malignancies confined to the liver (28 with colon primaries and 12 with other primary adenocarcinomas) received either Infusaid (24) or Medtronic (16) pumps for hepatic-arterial FUDR at 0.25 mg/kg/day $\times$ 14 days every month. All Infusaid pump patients had constant-rate infusions. With programmable Medtronic pumps, the infusion shape was sinusoidal with 68% of the daily dose given during a presumed "safe" time of day: 3−9 P.M. Both treatment groups had comparable risk factors. Toxicity was more frequent ($p < 0.01$), more severe, and occurred earlier with the flat infusion shape, in spite of lower dose intensity (Table 1). Objective response rates observed in patients with colon

**Table 1**
**Toxicity of Intrahepatic FUDR Infusion**

| Infusion Shape | Cholangitis* | Hepatitis* | Jaundice* | DI (mg/kg/wk) |
|---|---|---|---|---|
| Flat | 64%/3.8 | 38%/2.2 | 24%/2.8 | 0.529 |
| Sinusoidal | 29%/6.0 | 13%/3.0 | 0%/0 | 0.761 |

*Rate per patient group/time to toxicity in months.

primaries were 50% for both flat and sinusoidal infusion. Quality of life was significantly better for those receiving the time-modified infusion shape. Chronobiological modification of FUDR infusion shape in hepatic-arterial infusion reduced toxicity without any loss of antitumor efficacy and allowed greater dose intensity and longer uninterrupted treatment duration.

## Systemic FUDR Infusion for Progressive Metastatic Renal Cell Carcinoma

Intravenous infusion of FUDR is accompanied by substantial toxicity. In a frequently used schedule, monthly courses of constant rate infusion over 14 days at a low dose (equal or higher than 0.125 mg/kg/day) are associated with debilitating diarrhea in the majority of cases.[17,18] To test whether long-term exposure of usually chemotherapy-refractory renal cell cancer (RCC) to FUDR can improve the response rate, we treated 19 patients with proven-progressive, measurable metastatic RCC (3 female, 16 male; ages 36−73), 52% of whom had received previous chemotherapy. All received Medtronic pumps for automatic drug delivery. Sixteen patients had intravenous infusion. Because disease was limited to the liver in three cases, they were given hepatic arterial therapy. FUDR was continuously infused for 14 days at monthly intervals at starting doses of 0.15 mg/kg/day systemically or 0.25 mg/kg/day via the hepatic artery. These starting doses were escalated and de-escalated in increments of 0.025 mg/kg/day, as permitted by toxicity. Abdominal pain, diarrhea, and mucositis limited the systemic continuous infusion tolerance, whereas malaise, anorexia, and hepatic function abnormalities were limiting for hepatic-arterial continuous infusion. Time modification of the infusion shape (68% of the daily dose given during a presumed "safe" time of day: 3−9

P.M.) virtually eliminated toxicity of systemic continuous infusion. Maximum-tolerated dose intensity of time-modified systemic infusion was 0.55 /± 0.02 mg/kg/week, which is twice that of constant-rate infusion as found in a previous study[19] and described by others.[20] In 18 patients evaluable for response who had at least two courses, we observed one complete response, four partial responses, and two minor responses. During a median follow-up span of 7.5 months (range 2–21 months), only 4 of the 18 patients had objective tumor progression (none of the responders). Objective responses have been durable; one complete response has lasted longer than one year (six months off therapy). Overall survival of the 19 patients at 7.5 months was 84%. Continuous infusion of time-qualified, high-dose intensity FUDR is a safe and effective outpatient treatment for progressive renal cell carcinoma.

## Doxorubicin and Cisplatin in Metastatic Ovarian Cancer

The time of day at which cytotoxic drugs are given, their sequence, the span between them, and the dose intensity of drugs are of critical importance for optimal control of epithelial ovarian cancer. Sixty-three consecutively diagnosed women (median age 60, range 29–87) with FIGO stage III (46) and IV (17) epithelial ovarian cancer were treated using the same drugs in one of four temporal schedules to test whether drug timing affected tumor control. Fifteen of these 63 women had optimal debulking operations; 48 had bulky disease with residual masses (massive disease of >10 cm masses in 40 patients) at the start of chemotherapy. Each of the four treatment groups was comparable with regard to patient age, FIGO stage, histological grade of cancer, and quality of debulking surgery. Sixteen women had received prior chemotherapy, and nine had abdominal pelvic irradiation. In each case, induction treatment consisted of monthly doxorubicin and cisplatin (each 60 mg/m$^2$) for nine months. Four different schedules were compared: *U*: Treatment with doxorubicin and cisplatin at unspecified times of the day with no consistent sequence or interval between drugs. *A*: Women were randomized to receive doxorubicin at 6 A.M. followed 12 hours later by cisplatin. *B*: Patients randomly received doxorubicin at 6 P.M., followed 12 hours later by cisplatin. *A/B* : Patients were alternated monthly on A and B. Toxicity was lowest with schedule A.[21] Circadian scheduling significantly increased

**Table 2**
**Response Rate and Survival in Metastatic Ovarian Cancer**

| Schedule* | N | %CR | %CR+PR | Med. Survival (mo.) | % Survival at 60 mo. |
|:---:|:---:|:---:|:---:|:---:|:---:|
| U | 15 | 13 | 40 | 8 | 0 |
| A | 17 | 85 | 100 | 23 | 50 |
| B | 20 | 82 | 100 | 25 | 25 |
| A/B | 11 | 91 | 100 | 80 | 78 |

*U = doxorubicin and cisplatin at unspecified time of day, A = doxorubicin at 6 A.M. followed 12 hours later by cisplatin; B = doxorubicin at 6 P.M. followed 12 hours later by cisplatin; A/B = patients were alternated monthly on A and B.

response rates ($X^2 = 38.8$, $p < 0.001$) and survival (Table 2). Median follow-up of all patients is now 57 months (6–95 months).

## Doxorubicin and Cisplatin for Transitional Cell Bladder Cancer

Locally advanced (stage C and $D_1$) transitional cell carcinoma of the urinary bladder (TCCB) usually causes death within two years. Metastatic disease (stage $D_2$) kills patients within a few months. We have treated 43 patients with stage $D_2$ TCCB. Of 35 patients evaluable for response, 1/3 failed prior radiation therapy and half underwent prior cystectomy. Nine monthly cycles of doxorubicin 60 mg/m$^2$ followed 12 hours later by cisplatin at 60 mg/m$^2$ were given. This schedule was randomly begun at either 6 A.M. or 6 P.M. Fifty-seven percent of the patients with metastatic disease responded objectively for at least three months. Eight of the 20 responders had complete disappearance of cancer (CR, 20%). Median survival for patients with CR was 27 months (range 11–39+ months) compared to 10 months (range 4–25) for partial responders ($p < 0.05$). Three of the complete responders are alive and well without evidence of disease at 29, 48, and 93 months after the initiation of chemotherapy, off all chemotherapy for 17 months to 7 years.

Full doses of this two-drug combination given over a relatively long span and using chronobiological schedules have yielded good treatment results. The fact that three patients with biopsy-proven metastatic TCCB have been taken off all chemotherapy without disease recurrence may portend its chronochemotherapeutic curability.

Adjuvant chemotherapy is indicated in patients with locally advanced TCCB because of their high risk for postoperative recurrence or dissemination and a five-year survival rate smaller than 15%. Adjuvant therapy in 16 consecutive patients with stage C (5) and $D_1$ (11) TCCB was initiated within one month following radical cystectomy and lymphadenectomy. This therapy consisted of nine monthly cycles of doxorubicin followed 12 hours later by cisplatin, both at 60 mg/m$^2$. Treatment was randomly begun at either 6 A.M. or 6 P.M. Eleven of these 16 patients showed no recurrence after a median follow-up period of 3.5 years (range 1−>5.5 years); these patients have not received chemotherapy for a median duration of three years (range 2−5 years). Circadian scheduling allowed us to administer 93% and 96% of the planned dose intensity for doxorubicin and cisplatin, respectively, as calculated by the method of Hryniuk.[4] Toxicity was mild in all but one patient who developed severe anemia and neurotoxicity; cardiomyopathy was not observed. This time-qualified adjuvant chemotherapy delays and may prevent local and distant recurrence of stage C and $D_1$ bladder cancer when given in full doses for nine courses.

The Intelliject pump is currently being utilized to administer automatically doxorubicin and cisplatin according to the time-qualified schedules described above.

While it has been adequately demonstrated that the therapeutic ratio of toxicity to anticancer drugs is dependent, to a large extent, upon the timing of drug delivery (relative to circadian time, time between doses, and drug sequence), these variables are likely to be more relevant to the effective use of biological response modifiers.[5] The time of day when these biological response modifiers (interferons, leukotrienes, tumor necrosis factors IL-2, or LAK cells) are given may, to an even larger extent, determine how effective they are.[22,23]

The standard phase I and phase II approaches to the study of these agents will not work in defining the activity or even the relevant toxicities without specification of temporal variables. Giving milligram quantities of biologicals without regard to the complexity of the relationship between host and tumor will only result in great expense, great toxicity, and finally, great frustration. The availability of instruments able to stipulate sequence, interval, circadian stage, and infradian pattern of immune modulation is a sine qua non to optimal biotherapy.

## Perspectives in Automatic Drug Delivery

### Economic Pressures of Governmental Origin

The latest and highly effective governmental attempt to decrease the costs of medical care mitigates strongly against inpatient medical evaluation and therapy. Whereas two years ago most cancer therapy was given in the hospital, currently very few patients are admitted for inpatient treatment. While the outpatient clinic is the major site of cancer therapy, these clinics are not optimally configured to give complex, time-oriented, multiday, multidose, or even multidrug therapy. On the other hand, the most effective anticancer regimens are becoming much more complex, not simpler. If patients are to receive the benefit, economically, of the latest and most effective multidrug, multiday, multidose, and time-specified treatments, a way must be devised. Programmed automatic drug delivery devices obviously provide the method, both in principle and in practice. Many complex protocols for the treatment of a variety of cancers could be moved from the inpatient to the outpatient setting by the intelligent use of these kinds of devices.

### Industrial-Based Economic Pressure

The scientific drought, reflected by the lack of promising new anticancer drugs combined with the length of time required to gain FDA approval for a new drug, has resulted in tremendous pressure on large pharmaceutical firms producing anticancer drugs. At the same time, the lack of exciting, new, even tarnished "silver bullets," has many physicians and cooperative clinical research groups thinking about new ways to give old drugs. These "old drugs" are not proprietary.

If new therapies and new drugs are ever to develop, the huge costs of research, development, marketing, and jumping through the required regulatory hoops must be paid. One approach to this is a natural tripartite alliance among drug makers, device manufacturers, and clinical research laboratories to develop regimens that can be protected by meaningful method patents. Optimal complex therapeutic regimens developed at universities, using research funds supplied by both device and drug manufacturers, may be protected by method patents and patents upon hardware, software, and single-device-compatible drug packaging. This would result in nonproprietary drugs regaining a proprietary advantage. This approach will result in the most advanced and complex protocols being available to patients largely in the outpatient setting. It will also result in the cost accounting of clinical research and in appropriate return to device and drug manufacturers for funding the research that develops these regimens.

The medical community will insist on the availability of such devices, because their proper use will allow the simpler, easier administration of the optimal, disease-related complex protocols, protocols that are more effective than current ones. No physician will adopt the use of a device that will complicate and increase the cost of his/her practice by requiring more of the physician's or the nurse's time. However, these devices will ultimately be put together in such a way as to require less time and less attention than standard methods of giving therapy. Shell programs and premixed, prepackaged hardware and/or software-specific drug regimens,combined with long-term parenteral access catheters, will ultimately make delivery of complex regimens simpler.

Pharmacy-related costs are also a sizeable component of inpatient and outpatient treatment costs. The use of automatic drug delivery systems and prepacked drug regimens can markedly reduce these costs as well.

## Medical Consumer (Patient) Pressure

The "patient as consumer" will exert substantial pressure. The oversupply of physicians of all varieties has resulted in a profound and increasing competition for patients. This has put physicians in a position of needing to deliver the highest quality and most current protocols, in order to maintain their patient base and income. When patients become aware of the advantages of automatic drug delivery systems, they will demand them, and the physician will supply this demand.

## Treatment Accuracy

Errors of dosage and errors of drug timing and sequence can be eliminated by the employment of simple-to-use, smart devices. The frequency of inpatient and outpatient therapeutic errors is not something discussed frequently, but something about which each physician, nurse, and pharmacist is acutely aware. Errors do occur. Sometimes they result in insignificant and sometimes grave consequences. In our own University hospital, we have traced 11 steps between the writing of an intravenous medication order and its actual delivery. At each juncture, an error of several varieties is possible. New hardware, software, and premixed drug modules can result in elimination of nearly all of these errors.

## Scientific Pressures

For clinical trials, use of such delivery systems may also allow improved compliance in national cooperative study group protocols. Clinical research trial sponsors, whether federal or industrial, can more easily assure that common research done in several centers is truly common. The use of these systems will improve comparability across institutions.

## Summary

Increased dose intensity, long-term infusion of certain drugs, and the use of combinations of noncrossresistant anticancer agents can improve therapeutic index. Optimal circadian drug timing, interval between drugs, and the sequence of drugs reduce toxicity and improve cancer control. Without automatic drug delivery systems, complex therapy schedules are impractical and expensive because of the high demand on support personnel. Programmable pumps allow complex treatment schedules to be given with higher accuracy and lower cost. The circadian timing of bolus drug delivery or the circadian shape of continuous drug infusion profoundly affects the therapeutic index of some anticancer drugs. The systems described make the delivery of temporally specific therapy no more difficult than single-rate, pump-based, continuous infusion treatment.

## References

1. Tannock I. (1978). Cell kinetics and chemotherapy: A critical review. *Cancer Treat Rep* 62:1117−1133.

2. Chabner B. (1985). The oncologic end game. 16th Annual D. A. Karnofsky Memorial Lecture, 21st Annual Meeting of ASCO, May 20, 1985. (See also, Chabner B, Curt GA, Fine RL. (1985). Implications of drug resistance for cancer drug development. *Proc AACR* 25:390–391.)
3. DeVita VT Jr. (1986). Chemotherapy of the lymphomas: Looking back—moving forward. 10th R. and H. Rosenthal Foundation Award Lecture, 77th Annual AACR Los Angeles, May 7th, 1986. (See also, Longo DL, Young RC, Wesley M, Hubbard SM, Duffey PL, Jaffe ES, Devita VT Jr. (1986). Twenty years of MOPP therapy for Hodgkin's disease. *J Clin Oncol* 4(9):1295–1306.
4. Hryniuk W, Levine MN. (1986). Analysis of dose intensity for adjuvant chemotherapy trials in stage II breast cancer. *J Clin Oncol* 4:1162–1170.
5. Levi F, Canon C, Blum JP, et al. (in press). Circadian and/or circahemidian rhythms in nine lymphocyte-related variables from human peripheral blood. *J Immunol*(in press).
6. Haus E, Lakatua DJ, Swoyer J, et al. (1983). Chronobiology in hematology and immunology. *Am J Anatomy* 168:467–517.
7. Levi F: (forthcoming). Chronopharmacology of anticancer agents and cancer chronotherapy. In: Kuemmerle H, ed, *International Handbook of Clinical Pharmacology*. Ecomed, Landsberg am Lech, (FRG).
8. Hrushesky WJM, Borch R, Levi F. (1982). Circadian time dependence of cisplatin urinary kinetics. *Clin Pharmacol Ther* 32:330–339.
9. Hecquet B, Meynadier J, Bonneterre J, et al. (1985). Time dependency in plasmatic protein binding of cisplatin. *Cancer Treat Rep* 69:79–83.
10. Sinkule J, Choi K, Roemeling R, et al. (1986). Preliminary investigations into the circadian variation of doxorubicin (adriamycin) plasma concentrations and systemic clearance when administered as a prolonged IV infusion. In: Reinberg A, Smolensky M, Labrecque G, eds., *Annual Review of Chronopharmacology Vol 3*, Pergamon Press, New York, pp 215–216.
11. Medtronic Model 8800M Physician Programmer, Technical Manual. Medtronic, Inc. Minneapolis, Minnesota 55440.
12. Kemeny M, Goldberg D, Browning S, et al. (1985). Experience with continuous regional chemotherapy and hepatic resection as treatment of hepatic metastases from colorectal primaries. *Cancer* 55(6):1265–1270.
13. Kemeny N, Daly J, Oderman P, et al. (1985). Prognostic variables in patients with hepatic metastases from colorectal cancer: Importance of medical assessment of liver involvement. *Proc Am Soc Clin Oncol* 4:88 (Abstr).
14. Vogelzang NJ. (1984). Continuous infusion chemotherapy: A critical review. *J Clin Oncol* 2:1289–1304.
15. Hohn DC, Rayner AA, Economou JS, et al. (1986). Toxicities and complications of implanted pump hepatic arterial and intravenous floxuridine infusion. *Cancer* 57:465–470.
16. Roemeling R, Mormont M-C, Walker K, et al. (1987). Cancer control depends upon the circadian shape of continuous FUDR infusion. *Proc AACR* 28: (Abstr. #1293).
17. Kemeny N, Daly J. (1985). Randomized study of intrahepatic vs sys-

temic infusion of FUDR in patients with liver metastases from colorectal carcinoma. ICRCT 85 Giessen, Italy, August 26–28, 1985, p 25 (Abstr).

18. Lokich JJ, Sonneborn H, Paul S, et al. (1983). Phase I study of continuous venous infusion of floxuridine (5-FUDR) chemotherapy. *Cancer Treat Rep* 67:791–793.

19. Roemeling RV, Hrushesky WJM, Kennedy BJK, et al. (1986). Programmed automatic FUDR chronotherapy improves therapeutic indes. In: Pannell M ed, Surgical Forum (Proc for 42nd Annual Sessions of the Forum on Fundamental Surgical Problems; 72nd Annual Clinical Congress, New Orleans, October 1986) Chicago: American College of Surgeons, Publ. XXXVII:400–402.

20. Ensminger WD, Rosowsky A, Raso V, et al. (1978). A clinical-pharmacological evaluation of hepatic arterial infusions of 5-fluoro-2'-deoxyuridine and 5-fluorouracil. *Cancer Res* 38:3784–3792.

21. Hrushesky WJM. (1985). Circadian timing of cancer chemotherapy. *Science* 228:73–75.

22. Abrams PF, McClamrock E, Foon KA. (1985). Letter to the Editor. Evening administration of alpha interferon. *N Engl J Med* 312(7): 443–444.

23. Langevin T, Young J, Walker R, et al. (1987). The toxicity of tumor necrosis factor (TNF) is reproducibly different at specific times of the day. *Proc AACR* 28: (Abstr. #1580).

# Chapter 19

# Arterial Therapy: Percutaneous Catheters or Implantable Infusion Devices (Medtronics DADS, Infusaid® Pump)

Yehuda Z. Patt
Arthur Boddie
Marilyn Soski
Laura Claghorn

## Introduction

The feasibility of delivering single and multiple drug combinations by the hepatic arterial route to patients with liver metastases from colon cancer has been reported by various investigators. The advantage of this route has been demonstrated in terms of a high response rate.[1-4] Although a survival advantage was recently suggested for patients treated arterially over those given intravenous therapy,[5] studies confirming such an advantage are still lacking.

We have previously delivered chemotherapy intraarterially with percutaneously placed catheters.[1,2] With the introduction of im-

From: Ensminger WD, Selam JL (eds): *Infusion Systems in Medicine*. Mount Kisco, NY, Futura Publishing Co., Inc., ©1987.

plantable infusion devices, we decided to study the benefits of delivering arterial chemotherapy using implantable pumps as opposed to percutaneously placed catheters in terms of accuracy of regimen delivery, cost-effectiveness, patient convenience, and complication rate. The regimen used in the study contained cisplatin and fluorodeoxyuridine (FUDR) alternating with mitomycin and FUDR given by the hepatic arterial route.

## Materials and Methods

Forty-four patients with colorectal cancer metastatic to the liver were treated with a hepatic arterial infusion of cisplatin, 100 mg/m$^2$ given as a two-hour infusion on day 1, followed by FUDR, 100 mg/m$^2$/day continuously infused daily for five days as described in Table 1. This combination was alternated with hepatic arterial infusion of mitomycin C and FUDR when response to cisplatin-FUDR had peaked or did not occur, as previously described.[1] All patients had an initial hepatic arteriography by the Seldinger technique to determine their anatomy and in some cases to deliver chemotherapy into the liver. In all 13 patients treated percutaneously, catheters were left in place following angiography.[6] Ten of the 20 patients treated via Infusaid pumps were initially given chemotherapy with percutaneous catheters; an Infusaid pump was placed subcutaneously when response occurred. In the other 10 patients,

**Table 1**
**Treatment Plan***

| Arterial infusion device | Cisplatin | | FUDR | |
|---|---|---|---|---|
| | Dose mg/m$^2$ | Duration hours | Dose | Duration (days) |
| Percutaneous | 100 on day 1 | 2 | 100 mg/m$^2$ | 5 |
| Medtronic DADS | 100 on day 1 | 2 | 100 mg/m$^2$ | 5 |
| Infusaid Pump | 100 on day 1 | 2 | 50 mg/mL of fluid in chamber (2–3 mL/day) | 5 |

*Cisplatin plus FUDR was switched to mitomycin C plus FUDR after response had peaked. Treatment cycles were repeated every 5–6 weeks.

hepatic arterial therapy was delivered throughout treatment with an Infusaid pump. Similarly, all patients treated with the Medtronic drug administration delivery system (DADS) had only diagnostic angiography, which was followed by a laparotomy and placement of the device and a catheter access port.[1] Patients treated exclusively with percutaneous catheters were those who had only a brief response (four of 13, 31%), or a minimal response (two of 13).

## Accuracy of Delivery

Accuracy of delivery was measured by subtracting the volume actually delivered from the desired delivery and dividing it by the desired volume according to the formula described by Boddie et al.[7]:

$$\frac{\text{Desired flow rate} - \text{Actual flow}}{\text{Desired flow}} = \text{Variance of delivery}$$

## Cost Effectiveness

Cost involved in percutaneous arterial chemotherapy included a hospital stay, a clinic visit, angiography, infusion catheter placement, flow study, abdominal x-rays, laboratory work-up, etc. All of these costs were calculated from typical statements submitted to the patients by the hospital billing department. Median cost for pump implantation was calculated by analyzing patients' billing statements. The cost included a median hospital stay of 12 days, operating room charges, anesthesia, medications, hydration, supplies, laboratory expenses, pathology, blood replacement, postoperative care, angiography, cost of the pump, a clinic visit, and a flow study.

The typical cost of chemotherapy delivery with a Medtronic DADS was calculated in a similar fasion. A hospital stay charge was required only when cisplatin was added to the therapy. When FUDR alone or FUDR and mitomycin were given, there was no need for hospitalization. Medication and hydration (required for cisplatin therapy), supplies, a flow study, laboratory, and clinic visit charges were all added into the calculation of each treatment.

The inconvenience associated with percutaneous therapy or

implantable device therapy with either Medtronic or Infusaid pump was assessed from a review of the chart and listed in a separate table. All complications associated with the drug delivery systems were reviewed and listed.

## Results

### Accuracy of Delivery

There was no variance between the desired flow rate and the actual flow rate in patients treated with percutaneously placed catheters. Since these patients were treated with bedside pumps, the desired volume was actually delivered to the patient. Among patients treated with Medtronic pumps, the variance from the desired flow rate was 11.5 ± 8.5%, and among patients treated with Infusaid pumps variance from the desired flow was 38 ± 5.0% (Table 2).

### Cost-Effectiveness

Cost comparison of drug delivery with percutaneous therapy or with implantable infusion devices is shown in Table 3 for FUDR and FUDR and mitomycin C. The cost of percutaneous therapy exceeded that of implantable infusion pump therapy when the number of treatment courses was greater than four. A similar observation was made for cisplatin and FUDR therapy; the breakeven-point for both modes of therapy was at about four therapy cycles[8] (Table 4).

**Table 2**
**Accuracy of Delivery**

| Delivery System | No. of Patients | Variance from Desired Flow Rate (%) |
|---|---|---|
| Percutaneous catheter | 13 | 0 |
| Medtronic DADS | 11 | 11.5 ± 8.5% |
| Infusaid pump | 20 | 38 ± 5.0% |

---

**Table 3**

**Cost Comparison: Implantable Pumps Versus Percutaneous Catheters for Delivery of FUDR or FUDR plus Mitomycin-C**

| Treatment Cycles No. | Cost | |
|---|---|---|
| | Percutaneous Therapy | Implantable Pump |
| Surgery | 0 | $14,155.60 |
| I | $4,456.65 | 429.30 |
| II | 4,456.65 | 429.30 |
| III | 4,456.65 | 429.30 |
| IV | 4,456.65 | 429.30 |
| Total | $17,826.60 | $15,872.00 |

---

**Table 4**

**Cost Comparison: Implantable Pumps Versus Percutaneous Catheters for Delivery of Cisplatin plus FUDR**

| Treatment Cycles No. | Cost | |
|---|---|---|
| | Percutaneous Therapy | Implantable Pump |
| Surgery | 0 | $14,155.60 |
| I | $4,605.68 | 1,229.46 |
| II | 4,605.68 | 1,229.46 |
| III | 4,605.68 | 1,229.46 |
| IV | 4,605.68 | 1,229.46 |
| Total | $18,422.72 | $19,073.44 |

## Patient Convenience

Table 5 compares the various drug delivery systems in terms of patient convenience. Percutaneous therapy requires hospital stay and confinement to bed (Table 5). Patients treated with an implantable infusion device, however, could be gainfully employed during

**Table 5**
**Patient Convenience**

| Event | Percutaneous Catheter | Medtronic DADS | Infusaid Pump |
|---|---|---|---|
| Hospitalization | + | — | — |
| Confinement to bed | + | — | — |
| Continued employment during treatment | — | + | + |
| Catheter and pump maintenance between treatments | — | —* | +** |

*Patients require pump evacuation at the end of the five-day FUDR infusion.
**Patients require pump evacuation at the end of the five-day FUDR infusion and pump refills between treatment courses every two weeks.

treatment. When off therapy, patients treated with percutaneous catheters did not require a visit to the doctor's office unless an unexpected complication occurred. Since the flow rate of the Medtronic pump could be slowed to a very low rate, patients treated with the Medtronic pump did not require a doctor's office visit between treatments; intervals of up to 35 days between treatments were achieved by slowing the pump flow to 0.5 mL per day. Patients treated via an Infusaid pump required an office visit every two weeks to refill the nonprogrammable device to avoid the possibility of the pump emptying and not infusing any fluid into the catheter, which could result in its occlusion.

## Complication Rate

Table 6 shows the complications observed with the various infusion devices. Uncontrolled rapid flow occurred in a febrile patient treated via an Infusaid pump. Leakage around the catheter tip (after "whistle tip"-type catheter placement in a replaced right hepatic artery) occurred in one patient treated with the Infusaid

**Table 6**
**Comparison of Delivery System-Associated Problems**

| | No. of Problems | | |
| | Percutaneous Catheters | Medtronic | Infusaid |
| Problem | N = 13 patients | N = 11 patients | N = 20 patients |
|---|---|---|---|
| Uncontrolled rapid flow rate | 0 | 0 | 1 |
| Leakage at spliced catheter ("whistle tip" leak) | 0 | 0 | 1 |
| Catheter puncture in pump pocket | 0 | 1 | 1 |
| Catheter occlusion | 0 | 2 | 2 |
| Hepatic artery occlusion | 3* | 1 | 0 |
| Iliac artery occlusion | 1 | 0 | 0 |
| Sideport occlusion | 0 | 2 | 0 |
| Infection | | 0 | 0 |
|   Catheter tip | 2 | | |
|   Blood | 1 | | |
|   Perforation site | 1 | | |
|   Urinary | 2 | | |
|   Pulmonary | 3 | | |

*Two additional patients had a portal vein pump placed after hepatic artery occlusion on percutaneous catheter treatment.

pump. Catheter puncture during refill occurred once in a patient with an Infusaid pump. Catheter occlusion occurred in two patients treated through the Medtronic pump and in two patients treated with the Infusaid. Hepatic artery occlusion occurred in a total of five patients, three who were not subsequently treated and two who were subsequently treated with an Infusaid pump placed in the portal vein. An iliac artery occlusion occurred in one patient treated with a percutaneous catheter. Occlusion of the sideport occurred in two patients treated with a Medtronic pump. Infectious complications occurred only in patients with percutaneous catheters and included catheter tip infection (two patients), septicemia (one patient), and perforation site infection (one patient). Two patients had a urinary tract infection and three patients had a pulmonary infection. The latter two types of infection occurred among patients with percutaneous catheters.

## Discussion

We have compared the accuracy of regimen delivery, cost-effectiveness, patient convenience, and complication rate using percutaneous catheters, Medtronic pumps, or Infusaid implantable infusion pumps. Chemotherapy delivery was most accurate through a percutaneous catheter and second most accurate through the programmable Medtronic DADS. The Infusaid pump flow rate was temperature- and altitude-dependent and so varied with the patient's body temperature and residence altitude. Since the chemotherapy regimen was adjusted according to the pump used (Table 1), no major complication resulted from inaccuracy in drug delivery. However, one febrile patient treated with FUDR developed stomatitis because of rapid emptying of an Infusaid pump. This situation is potentially dangerous: patients' compliance with the need to report temperature elevations that could induce an accelerated emptying of the pump should be stressed. Such a complication would not affect patients with a Medtronic DADS since it is body temperature- and altitude-independent. Although possible, it is unlikely that the variations in flow of both Infusaid and Medtronic pumps were related to human error. Decreased DADS emptying could be related to partial obstruction of the catheter resulting in an increased residual volume compared to the expected. Variance with the Infusaid was usually accelerated emptying, which could be related to temperature elevation or change in altitude.

A cost analysis (Tables 3 and 4) indicates that patients who were candidates for four or more cycles of hepatic arterial therapy could benefit from early pump implantation in terms of a decrease in cost of therapy and increased comfort. Additionally, patients who were treated with implantable infusion devices could spend more time at home or could be gainfully employed during treatment, resulting in further financial benefit. Pump implant surgery was associated with a median hospital stay of 12 days and obvious laparotomy-related morbidity. The procedure was not associated with mortality. For maximal benefit, it would seem advisable to try and detect patients who are likely to respond to hepatic arterial therapy and select those for early pump implantation. One such indicator is the serum level of lactate dehydrogenase (LDH). Kemeny et al.,[9] have observed that patients with an LDH of less than 300 mL had significantly longer survival times than those with a higher value. We have made a similar observation among 29 patients treated with hepatic arterial infusion of cisplatin and FUDR alternating with mitomycin C and FUDR. Sixteen patients with an LDH level of less than 400 $\mu$/mL had a median survival time of 16 months versus 13 patients with an LDH level greater than 400 $\mu$/mL who had a median survival of 6 months ($p$ = 0.004, Wilcoxon sign rank). Additionally, the response rate among patients with an LDH level less than 400 $\mu$/mL was 75% as opposed to only 23% among those with an LDH level greater than 400 $\mu$/mL ($p$ < 0.05, chi-square).[1]

The latter observation, together with the cost-effectiveness of long-term therapy with implantable infusion devices, their convenience, the possibility of the patient's continued gainful employment, and the low infection rate among patients treated with them suggests the advisability of early use of implantable infusion devices in patients who are candidates for long-term hepatic arterial therapy for the treatment of metastatic colorectal cancer in the liver.

Circadian timing of chemotherapy delivery may be associated with decreased toxicity, as proposed by Hrushesky et al.[10] It was suggested by the same investigators that delivering the bulk of FUDR (68%) over a six-hour period from 15:00 to 21:00 hours may be associated with decreased hepatic and gastrointestinal toxicity. Such circadian timing can be accomplished only with a programmable pump like the Medtronic DADS. A randomized trial comparing flat to timed FUDR delivery is currently being implemented. Attempts should also be made to identify new chemotherapeutic regimens to achieve better control of metastatic colorectal cancer in the liver.

## Summary

Forty-four patients with colorectal cancer metastatic to the liver were treated with hepatic arterial infusion of cisplatin and fluorodeoxyuridine (FUDR) alternating with mitomycin C and FUDR. Thirteen were treated with percutaneous catheters placed by the Seldinger technique, 11 were treated with an implantable Medtronic Drug Administration Delivery System (DADS), and 20 were treated with an Infusaid pump. We compared the three delivery systems in terms of accuracy of regimen delivery, cost-effectiveness, patient convenience, and complication rate. Hepatic arterial therapy with percutaneous catheters was accurate, and no variance from desired flow rate was observed. Among patients treated with the Medtronic DADS variance from the desired flow rate was 11.5 ± 8.5%, and among patients treated with the Infusaid pump it was 38 ± 50%. Percutaneous therapy with angiographically placed catheters cost a total of $4,456.65 for each treatment; when cisplatin was added, the therapy cost an additional $140.00. A median cost for Medtronic pump implantation was $14,155.80. Each treatment cost was $429.30 when FUDR was used alone and $1,249.46 when cisplatin (which involved a two-day hospital admission) was added. Thus, the initial cost for pump implantation was higher, but the increment for each treatment cycle smaller than the cost of percutaneously placed catheters. The cost curves crossed at about four cycles.

Treatment with Medtronic and Infusaid pumps did not require hospitalization or confinement to bed. In addition, patients treated with implantable infusion devices could be gainfully employed. Patients treated with percutaneous catheters, however, required no physician or clinic visits between treatment cycles. Patients with Infusaid pumps required a clinic visit once every two weeks to replenish the pump with fluid and avoid catheter occlusion. The Medtronic pump could be programmed to deliver fluid into the artery at a very low flow rate and thus maintain patency without requiring an additional clinic visit between treatment cycles. Infectious complications were more frequent with percutaneous catheters. Catheter occlusion occurred in two of 11 patients with Medtronic pumps and in two of 20 patients with the Infusaid. Sideport occlusion occurred in two of 11 Medtronic DADS.

We conclude that patients who are candidates for more than three or four hepatic arterial therapy cycles would benefit from early placement of an implantable infusion device. Early identification of patients likely to respond to arterial therapy would further enhance the cost-effectiveness of implantable pumps and help prevent unnecessary surgery.

---

## References

1. Patt YZ, Boddie AW, Charnsangavej C, et al. (1986). Hepatic arterial infusion with 5-FUDR and CDDP: Overriding importance of antitumor

effect versus degree of tumor burden as determinants of survival among patients with colorectal cancer. *J Clin Oncol* 4:1356.
2. Patt YZ, Peters RE, Chuang VP, et al. (1983). Effective retreatment of colorectal cancer patients. *Am J Med* 75:237.
3. Niederguber JE, Ensminger W, Gyves J, et al. (1984). Regional chemotherapy of colorectal cancer metastatic to the liver. *Cancer* 53:1336.
4. Balch CM, Urist MM, McGreogor ML. (1983). Continuous regional chemotherapy for metastatic colorectal cancer using a totally implantable infusion pump. *Am J Surg* 145:285.
5. Kemeny N. (1986). Innovative cancer chemotherapy for tomorrow. Presented at Chemotherapy Foundation Symposium VII, New York, New York, November 12–14, 1986.
6. Patt YZ, Wallace S, Hersh EM, et al. (1978). Hepatic arterial infusion of Corynebacterium parvum and chemotherapy. *Surg Gynecol Obstet* 147:897.
7. Boddie AW, Patt YZ, McBride CH, et al. (1986). MDAH surgical experience with implantable Infusaid Pump and Medtronic drug administrations devices. In: Proceedings of the II International Conference on Advances in Regional Cancer Therapy, Giessen, West Germany, 1986, forthcoming.
8. Patt YZ, Claghorn L, Soski M, et al. (1987). Hepatic arterial therapy for liver neoplasms: Treatment cost analysis of percutaneous angiographically placed catheters versus programmable implantable Medtronic Drug Administration System. *Proceedings ASCO* 6:321.
9. Kemeny N, Daly J, Oderman P, et al. (1984). Hepatic artery pump infusion: Toxicity and results in patients with metastatic colorectal carcinoma. *J Clin Oncol* 2:595.
10. Hrushesky WJM. (1985). Circadian timing of cancer chemotherapy. *Science* 228:73.

# Chapter 20

# Regional Intraarterial Chemotherapy for Colorectal Cancer Hepatic Metastasis: Implanted Pumps Versus Ports for Direct Access


J.P. Fraioli
L. Schwarzenberg
S. Crepin
N. Avetyan
M. Castot
F. Fraioli


## Introduction

The prognosis with hepatic metastases of colorectal origin is poor. Natural survival of patients with such metastases is on average 6 to 10 months.[1-3] Survival depends upon numerous prognosis factors: the degree of hepatic involvement of solitary versus multiple metastases, the degree of alteration of hepatic enzyme functions (especially the alkaline phosphatases, the bilirubin, and the transaminases)


From: Ensminger WD, Selam JL (eds): *Infusion Systems in Medicine.* Mount Kisco, NY, Futura Publishing Co., Inc.,©1987.

and, finally, whether there is confinement to the liver or coexistence with extrahepatic disease.

Average survival is quite different for a solitary small metastasis as opposed to multiple, bilateral metastases. Thus, survival is five years for 35% of cases with a small, solitary metastasis that is resected, but only a few months for multiple bilateral metastasis with alteration of the hepatic function. Survival is usually between three and four months when diffuse hepatic as well as extrahepatic metastasis coexist.[4,5]

Therapeutically speaking, if one excludes surgical resection that can, in a few patients, lead to cure, the other therapeutic possibilities are limited when metastases are multiple and bilateral. Systemic chemotherapy for the treatment of hepatic metastasis produces few responses. For this reason, loco-regional intraarterial chemotherapy has been developed. Presently, two techniques are used: continuous intraarterial chemotherapy by totally implantable pumps and continuous or sequential intraarterial chemotherapy using implanted catheters attached to subcutaneous ports.

We have implanted 56 intraarterial pumps, 44 of which were for hepatic metastasis from colorectal cancers; 241 direct access ports of which 107 were intravenous and 95 intraarterial (of which 37 were for hepatic metastasis from colorectal cancers). An additional 36 ports were for intraperitoneal access and three were for miscellaneous uses.

We shall compare the pump versus the port method of delivering chemotherapy.

## Methods

Between April 1982 and December 1985, 44 patients underwent implantation of an Infusaid® Model Pump 400 (Figs. 1 and 2). There were 27 men and 17 women aged between 31 and 75 years (average 52.4 yrs.).

Between April 1983 and February 1986, 37 cases of hepatic metastases from colorectal cancer received a direct access device, either an Infuse-a-Port® (Figs. 3 and 4) or another similar vascular access port. In this group, there were 23 men and 14 women aged 36 to 75 years with an average of 58.8 years.

Criteria of selection for implantation of an Infusaid® Model 400 Pump included involvement of less than 50% of the hepatic mass,

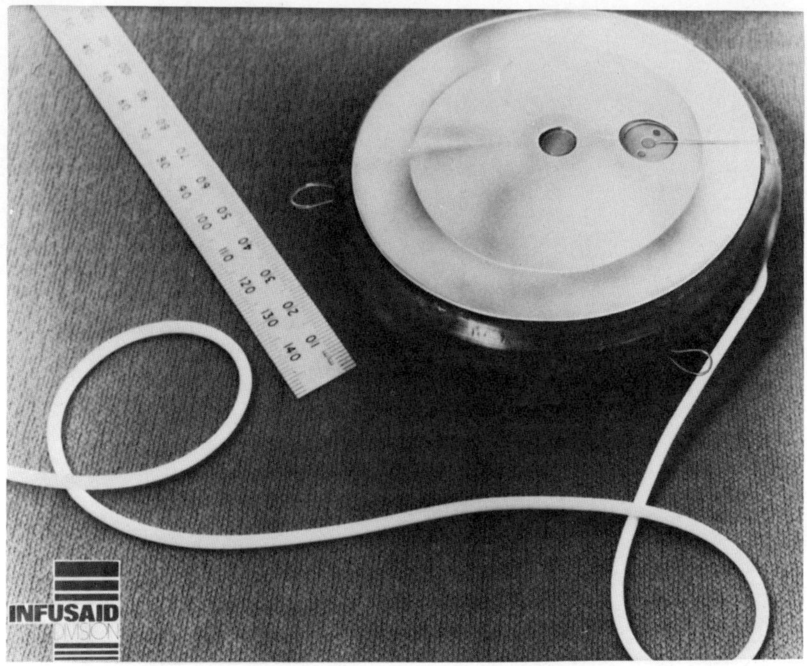


**Figure 1:** Totally implantable pump - Infusaid® 400.

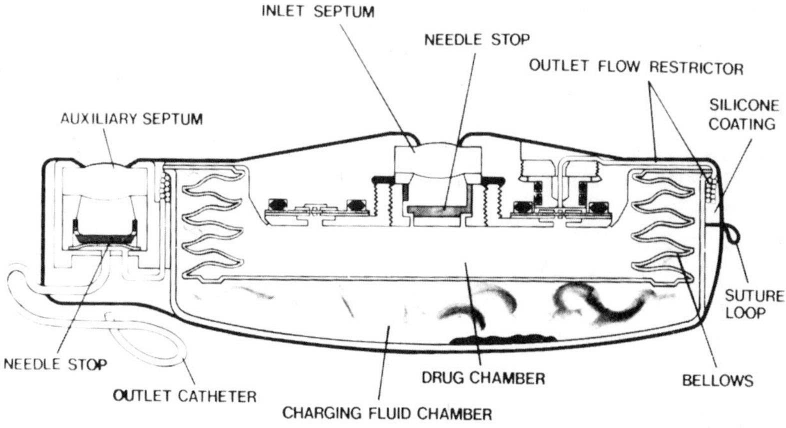


**Figure 2:** Totally implantable pump - Infusaid® 400.

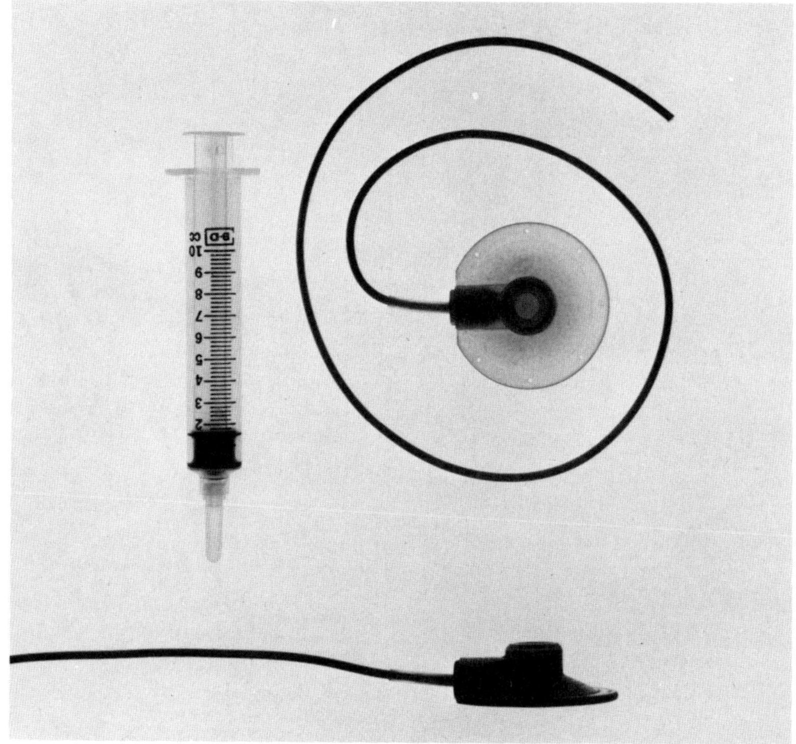

**Figure 3:** Access direct arterial implantable model Infuse-a-Port.

absence of extrahepatic metastases, and a bilirubin lower than 30 mg%. For direct access, we did not use hepatic arterial catheter implantation in the case of peritoneal carcinosis, abundant ascites, and portal hypertension.

In the case of Infusaid® Model 400 Pumps, the localization of the original tumor was found in 4.5% of cases at the level of the right colon, 9% at the level of the transverse colon, 72.7% at the level of the left colon, and 13.6% at the level of the rectum. Using implanted ports, primary tumors were located as follows: 13.5% at the level of the right colon, none at the level of the transverse colon, 72.9% at the level of the left colon, and 13.5% at the level of the rectum. As these figures show, the most frequent tumors leading to hepatic metastasis are cancers of the left colon and of the rectum. The metastases were synchronous in 72.7% of cases for the pumps and in 48.6%

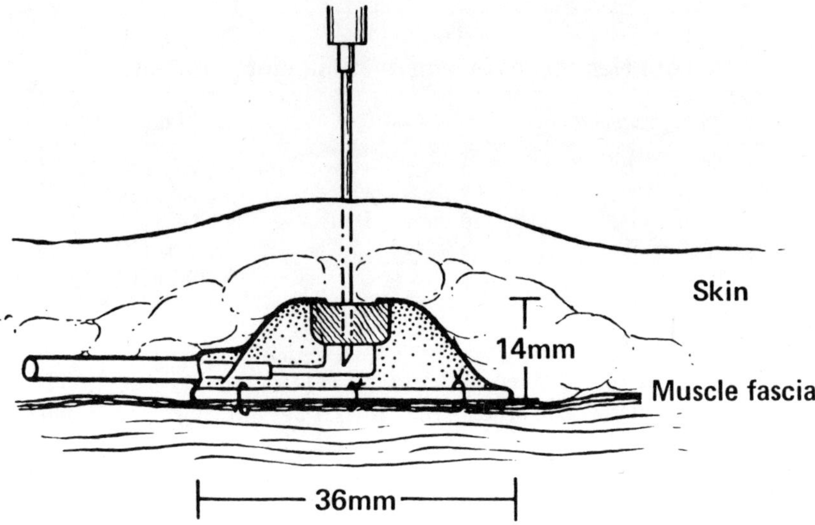



**Figure 4:** Access direct arterial implantable model Infuse-a-Port.

for ports. They were metachronous in 27.3% of cases for the pump and 38% for direct access ports.

One must note that in five cases, or 13% of total cases, chemotherapy by direct access ports was used as adjuvant or preventive therapy. These were five patients carrying a colic tumor, Dukes C, for whom we decided to apply adjuvant intraarterial chemotherapy by direct access ports for a period of six months post primary resection. These five patients are still living, but the experience is too recent and numbers of patients too small to decide whether the therapy has modified the natural relapse rate.

It must also be stated that in one case of implantation, the hepatic resection was "macroscopically radical." This patient presented with two hepatic nodules, which we were able to totally resect; unfortunately, the patient died 16 months later with widespread metastases. In three cases of direct access by ports, we were able to make a macroscopically satisfactory hepatic resection: These three patients are still alive.

Among the prognostic factors, the importance of hepatic damage plays a determining role. The majority of cases having had implantation of a pump had hepatic involvement averaging between 25% and 50% (20 cases). Most direct access (port) cases had hepatic in-

**Table 1**
**Percent Hepatic Involvement in Implanted Patients**

| % Hepatic Involvement | Pump | Ports |
|---|---|---|
| 0 | 0 | 5 cases (10.9%) |
| < 25% | 21 cases (47.7%) | 9 cases (24.3%) |
| 25–50% | 20 cases (45.4%) | 4 cases (10.8%) |
| 50–75% | 3 cases ( 6.8%) | 15 cases (40.5%) |
| > 75% | 0 | 4 cases (19.9%) |

volvement ranging between 50% and 75% (15 cases) (Table 1). This difference is related to the fact that in the beginning of our experience, we selected the most favorable cases in whom to install the totally implantable Infusaid® Model 400 Pumps, while reserving the least favorable cases for direct access ports.

The implantation technique is similar for both systems. The objective is to achieve total perfusion of the liver by direct arterial catheterization. The most frequently used artery is the gastroduodenal. The only technical difference between pump and port implantation is the making of a smaller pocket in the case of ports, this pocket being often made in the prethoracic area, which provides the support of a hard surface for injections. In the case of the implantable pump, the pocket is generally made in the right lower quadrant of the abdomen because of the size of the pump.

During laparotomy, other surgical interventions conducted include (as indicated): colectomy, rectal resection, cholecystectomy, and partial hepatectomy (Table 2).

## Postsurgical Mortality/Morbidity

Mortality was nil in the case of pump implantations. Two patients, or 5.4%, died in the case of port implantations. Morbidity remains relatively low. In the case of the pumps, we had to reexplore one patient for a biliary leak (which stopped spontaneously). One patient developed a colic fistula, and six patients had seromas of the pocket, which stopped after several evacuations. Three patients had an extended ileus lasting longer than eight days. In the use of ports, we had to reexplore two cases of colic fistulas, of which one resulted in death by hemorrhage. There were seven instances of postsurgical icterus (which took several days to weeks to resolve).

**Table 2**
**Concurrent Surgical Procedures with Pump and**
**Port Implantation**

|  | Pump | Ports |
|---|---|---|
| **Colon** | | |
| Left or right colectomy | 4 | 6 |
| Rectal resection | 1 | 4 |
| Reanastomosis | 0 | 1 |
| **Biliary Tract** | | |
| Cholecystectomy | 24 | 37 |
| Biliary stone extraction | 1 | 0 |
| **Foie** | | |
| Metastasectomy | 1 | 1 |
| Segmentectomy | 5 | 12 |
| L. lobectomy | 4 | 3 |
| R. lobectomy | 0 | 2 |
| Macroscopic resection of metastases | 1 | 3 |

Since the modification of our anesthetic technique, we no longer have such incidents. For 18 months, all patients with hepatic metastasis from colorectal cancers have had peridural thoracic anesthesia, which causes less disturbance of the hepatic function.

## Long-term Morbidity

For chemotherapeutic pumps, the main complication that subsequently developed was chemical hepatitis, encountered in 12 cases (27%) of our patient population. Some patients had repetitive attacks of hepatitis that led to interruption of the therapy for 6 to 8 weeks (Table 3).

Three cases of chemical cholecystitis also occurred in the beginning of our experience when we did not take out the gallbladder. These three cases of chemical cholecystitis led to secondary cholecystectomy. None of these complications occurred in the case of port implantation/use. Eleven percent of the cases led to removal of the pumps, in two cases because of infection, and in three cases because of chronic inflammation caused by the pump itself. Removal of ports was necessitated in 2.7% of the cases, one case because of infection.

**Table 3**
**Long-term Morbidity Associated with Therapy**

|  | Pump | Ports |
|---|---|---|
| **Treatment Complications** | | |
| *Toxic hepatitis | 12 cases (27.2%) | 0 |
| *Chemical cholecystitis | 3 cases | 0 |
| *Liver pain | 2 cases | 0 |
| *Hemorrhagic gastritis | 1 case | 0 |
| **Technical Complications** | | |
| *Device removal due to | (11%) | (2.7%) |
| Infection | 2 cases | 1 case |
| Irritation | 3 cases | 0 |
| *Blood collection | 6 cases | 0 |
| *Catheter thrombosis | 3 cases | 3 |
| *Transformation IA IV | | |
| Persistent hepatitis | 2 cases | 0 |
| Artery/AL thrombosis | 1 case | 1 case |
| Septicemia | 0 | 1 case |

Among the other main complications, thrombosis of the catheter occurred three times with pumps. In one case, thrombosis was irreversible and led to thrombosis of the hepatic artery. The catheter became clotted three times in the case of ports.

Finally, we transformed intraarterial pumps into venous pumps in three cases: twice for repetitive toxic hepatitis and once for thrombosis of the catheter with thrombosis of the hepatic artery. In one case involving a port, we transformed an intraarterial catheter into an intravenous catheter.

An interesting complication occurred in one case: colonic/bacillus septicemia with infection carried from outside to inside, which confirms the necessity of strict asepsis while filling the pumps and using ports.

## Long-term Mortality and Survival

Presently, 41 patients out of 44 have died after implantation of a pump, with an average survival of 17 months (ranging from 1 to 56 months). Three patients are alive at 44, 18, and 21 months. Unfortunately, all three patients show an increase of CEA, indicating an escape from therapy. We have had no case of a complete response.

In the use of ports, 17 out of 37 patients are still alive, with an average survival of 15 months (ranging between 6 and 40 months). Twenty of the 37 patients lived beyond eight months.

It is difficult to speak of recovery in the five cases of adjuvant chemotherapy, as all the patients have been treated recently.

In the pump method, the death of patients occurs generally either due to terminal cachexia or with irreversible jaundice caused by progression of the hepatic metastases. It must be noted that while the hepatic disease was improving and the hepatic metastases were regressing, extrahepatic disease frequently developed: pulmonary metastases (4 cases), bone metastases (3 cases), cerebral metastases (2 cases), intraperitoneal and nodal extensions (5 cases). There were no secondary colonic primaries noted.

In the use of ports, death occurred due to terminal cachexia (10 cases), irreversible jaundice (4 cases), cerebral metastases (2 cases), secondary colonic metastases (1 case).

Thus, it appears that continuous regional chemotherapy has a real efficiency at the hepatic level, but does not prevent the progression of extrahepatic cancer using the drugs in question (see below).

The chemotherapy utilized was different for the pump method and the direct access port method. For the pumps we used 5-fluoro-2′-deoxyuridine (FUDR) in the reservoir with a dosage of 0.2 to 0.3 mg/kg/day with complimentary chemotherapy by the sideport® with ametycine. FUDR was used continuously for 15 days. With ports, we used a protocol of bolus and continuous infusion chemotherapy: day 1, Adriblastine; day 2, ametycine; days 1 to 5, 5-fluorouracil and leucovorin either continuously by means of a transportable pump, or discontinuously by means of a peristaltic pump.

## Conclusion

The implantable pumps enable better comfort for the patients and easy continuous chemotherapy, but unfortunately represent a hepatic only chemotherapy or, the administration of adjuvant chemotherapy, which does not treat systemic cancer. The devices are very expensive. They cause few complications, which are mostly local but very disconcerting: mainly FUDR hepatitis (30% of our patients). This requires a 6- to 8-week break in the treatment, which impedes the therapy. Treatment may lead to sclerosing cholangitis and may also produce gastroduodenal ulceration and hemorrhagic gastritis.

With the direct access port method, we observed no hepatitis and less distant metastatic dissemination. The ports are less expensive. On the other hand, there are more therapeutic constraints, including a need for more work to use the device and for rigorous asepsis. With ports, other complications are scarce, mainly being catheter thrombosis.

Regional intraarterial chemotherapy appears superior to systematic chemotherapy. For the moment we have abandoned the totally implantable pumps in favor of ports. The only way to compare the efficiency between pumps and ports would be to carry out a randomized prospective study.

In the future, it would be valuable to manufacture totally implantable pumps that would include at least two chambers, the first one for continuous intraarterial chemotherapy and the other one for systematic chemotherapy.

It may be illusory to believe that hepatic metastases are strictly localized in the liver and have not spread to other places. We feel that intraarterial chemotherapy plus systematic chemotherapy is necessary.

---

## References


1. Martin C. (1976). Surgical treatment of hepatic metastases. *Arch Surg* 111:330.
2. Martin C. (1979). Hepatic metastasis symposium. *Dis Colon Rect* 22:653.
3. Bengmark S, Hafstrom L. (1978). The natural course for liver cancer. *Prog Clin Cancer* 7:195.
4. Audigier JE, Lambert R. (1979). Epidemiologie des cancers du colon. *Rev Prat* 29:1055.
5. Jaffe BM, et al. (1968). Factors influencing survival in patients with untreated hepatic metastases. *Surg Gynecol Obstet* 127:1.
6. Collins JM. (1984). Pharmacological rationale for regional drug delivery. *J Clin Oncol* 2:498.
7. Ensminger WD, Gyves JW. (1984). Regional cancer chemotherapy. *Cancer Treat Rep* 68:101.
8. World Health Statistics Annual. Année, 1979–1980.
9. Blackshear, Dermon FD, Blackshear PJ Jr. (1972). The design and initial testing of an implantable infusion pump. *Surg Gynecol Obstet* 184:51.
10. Ensminger WD, Niederhuber JE, Dakhil S, Thrall J, Wheeler R. (1981). Totally implanted drug delivery system for hepatic arterial chemotherapy. *Cancer Treat Rep* 65:393.

11. Niederhuber JE, Ensminger WD. (1983). Surgical considerations in the management of hepatic neoplasia. *Sem Oncol* 10(2):135.
12. Niederhuber JE, Ensminger WD, Gyves JG, Thrall J, Walker S, Cozzi E. (1984). Regional chemotherapy of colorectal cancer metastatic to the liver. *Cancer* 53:1336.
13. Sullivan RD, Norcross JW, Watkins E Jr. (1964). Chemotherapy of metastatic liver cancer by prolonged hepatic artery infusion. *N Engl J Med* 270:321.
14. Weiss GR, Garnick MB, Osteen RT, Steele GD, Wilson RE, Shade D, Kaplan WD, Boxt LM, Kandarpa K, Mayer R, Frei E. (1983). Long-term hepatic arterial infusion of 5-fluorodeoxyuridine for liver metastases using an implantable infusion pump. *J Clin Oncol* 1:337.
15. Balch CM, Urist MM, Soong SJ, McGregor M. (1983). A prospective phase II clinical trial of continuous FUDR regional chemotherapy for colorectal metastatic to the liver using a totally implantable drug infusion pump. *Ann Surg* 198:567.
16. Cohen AM, Schaeffer N, Higgins J. (1986). Treatment of metastatic colorectal cancer with hepatic artery combination chemotherapy. *Cancer* 57:1115.

*(Appendix follows)*

# Outline Listing Technical Complications with Drug Delivery Systems for Chemotherapy Except Direct and Side Effects of Drugs: Experience on 341 Patients and 4,000 Perfusions Over Four Years


N. Avetyan
S. Crepin
M. Castot
J.P. Fraioli
F. Fraioli
L. Schwartzenberg



From: Ensminger WD, Selam JL (eds): *Infusion Systems in Medicine*. Mount Kisco, NY, Futura Publishing Co., Inc.,©1987.

## 341 Drug Delivery Systems

Most of the patients were implanted in our center. A few of them came for treatment of complications with an already implanted system.

Intraarterial: 139 cases

        Infusaid® 400 (46 cases)

  Hepatic

        Other (85 cases)

  Carotid (6 cases)
  Other (2 cases)

Intravenous (153 cases)
  Portal vein: 3 cases
  Umbilical vein: 1 case
  Cephalic or axillary or collateral veins: 149 cases

Intraperitoneal (47 cases)

Other (2 cases)

---

P. A., the percentage per implanted patients.
P. U., the percentage per puncture.

## Introduction

With a four-year study and experience of chemotherapy with implantable materials either intraarterial, or intravenous, or intraperitoneal, we can conclude the following:

1. 70% of the patients prefer chemotherapy by the system known as: Infuse-a-Port, e.g., pump through the veins.

2. 62% of the patients find the second effects are less stressing with this system.

3. 83% of the patients prefer the treatment of chemotherapy by continuous perfusion of the portable infusion pump.

4. Following certain necessary precautions, we can diminish different complications, which could deteriorate this system of treatment.

## Surgical Complications

Peri-Operative Complications

### *Wrong Positioning of the Catheter*

(1) Bad Direction: Drug Runs Out Against Blood Flow

The tip of the catheter proceeds up the common hepatic artery in the case of hepatic implantation.

> Treatment:  good surgical exposure
> fluoroscopic x-ray system

(2) Partial Irrigation of the Organ

Manifold or unusual irrigation of organs with terminal type arteries. Liver irrigation from different main blood vessels: left hepatic artery born of coeliac artery.
Right hepatic artery born of superior mesenteric artery.

> Treatment:  good surgical exposure
> hepatic arteriography before surgery
> fluorescein angiography
> ligature of one of these arteries
> implantation of two systems

(3) Ejection in Collaterals or Outside of the Vessel

Blood vessels shaken by heartbeats and expelled catheters.
Catheters can jump from superior vena cava to internal jugular.

> Treatment:  gentle curves of catheter
> keep clear of heart proximity
> right length of catheter
> proof against blood and stability checked by gentle traction of catheter.

(4) Endovascular or In-The-Pocket Bended Catheters

Hindrance during the insertion and tiny pocket are the main causes.

> Treatment:  use of collaterals of main vessels
> fluoroscopic x-ray system control
> good appreciation of injection pressure
> right length of catheter in a comfortable pocket

(5) Injury of Catheter

The danger of surgical diathermy or sharp instruments (scalpels, scissors, or needles) is well known.

Treatment: delivery system must be picked up only after perfect exposure and hemostasis of vessels and pocket

(6) Insertion Above Thrombosis

The bad diffusion of drug can induce toxicity on the walls of vessel.

Treatment: arteriography or phlebography before surgery radiopaque medium injection

## Excessive Tied Knot

Thin ligature or excessive tied knot injures the catheter and obstructs lumen of vessels.

One case: 0.2% P.A.
Treatment: thick and steady wall catheters
large linen thread (0/0) or (0)
ligature must compound with stability and permeability appreciated by injection

## Errors in Creation of the Pocket

(1) Insufficient Excision of Fat Tissue

Makes localization of the site of injection difficult.
Four cases: 0.8% P.A.
Treatment: tissues facing the pump must not exceed 5 millimeters.
(2) Unsteady Implantation of the Lower Part of the Pump creates difficulties for introduction of the needle.

Treatment: large flat-based pumps
implantation against rib cage (fat patients)
(3) Bad Suture of the Pump

One ligature allows several sites of injection whereas two ligatures, prevent pump from turning upside down.

Two cases: 0.4% P.A.
(4) Wrong Site of the Pocket

One must avoid sites of belts and straps.

Two cases: 0.4% P.A.
(5) Nonoperative Pump (Infusaid 400)

One case: 2.17% Infusaid 400

## Postoperative Complications

### Bulging of the Pocket

Before any perfusion, hematoma, ascite diffusion, or edema can occur.
In hepatic or peritoneal pump, ascite shoots out in the pocket.

Hematoma:  Six cases: 13% Infusaid 400
Two cases: 0.5% other patients

Treatment:  perfect hemostasis or surgical drainage avoids a blind entry
medical therapy may be considered (diuretic, non-steroid anti-inflammatories

### Exteriorization of Catheter or Pump is a Pure Mechanical Complication by Cachectic Patients.

### Thrombosis of Catheter or Blood Vessels

Is a rare early post-operative complication.

Treatment: catheter:  permeability checked by the surgeon
heparin flush during implantation early perfusion

vessels:  if possible, the tip of catheter must stay out of blood flow in arteries (use of collaterals)
medical therapy may be considered (anti-coagulant, antiaggregation of platelets).

### Ejection of the Catheter Out of Blood Vessel

Internal hemorrhage has never occurred.

However, pain, bulging or fibrosis of the pocket, ineffective drug treatment, sound the alarm.

>Three cases: 0.6% P.A.
>Treatment: radiopaque or isotopic medium injection.

### *Necrosis of the Gallbladder in Liver Chemotherapy and Liver Cholangiosclerosis*

Must be taken into account as possible direct or side effect of drug. Cholecystectomy is one part of the treatment.

## Perfusion Complications

### *Leakage of Chemotherapy Drugs*

Is the serious complication.
Aggravating circumstances are
>type of drug:  cisplatine (cisplatyl)
>>doxorubicine (Adriblastine)
>>mitomycine (Ametycine)
>
>Volume or concentration of drug
>Continuous drug delivery systems: three cases: 0.08% P.U.
>Site of the pocket: belly

Main causes are:
>Incorrect injection
>Pump or catheter failure
>Catheter injury
>>Twelve cases: 0.3% P.U.
>>Seven cases explantation: 1.4% P.A. 0.18% P.U.

>Preventive treatment:  the choice of "the right" drug delivery system
>no catheter winding in the pocket
>no injection without being sure of the position of the tip of the needle: if in doubt radiopaque medium injection
>cold water injection sensed by the patient taste of heparin after injection

Curative treatment:  early needle or surgical drainage
                     sclerosis generally precedes necrosis
                     osmogel
                     early explantation
                     pocket washing increases septic risks

## *Thrombosis of Catheter*

Physical impossibility of injection is an incurable complication.
Injection with high pressure, leads to bursting of catheter.
Injection against pressure gradient ending in a slight flowback
marks progressive occlusion.
It can be crystals or red blood clotted.

Thirteen cases: 2.6% P.A. 0.32% P.U.
Thirteen second operations

Treatment:  early and frequent heparin flush
            rinsing with physiological serum after each perfusion
            highly resistant catheter wall
            thrombolitic treatments through the catheter after
            making sure of arterial permeability
            one must not take any blood sample or do any
            transfusion through the pump and catheter

## *Thrombosis of Blood Vessels*

Its late detection leads again to surgery.

Two cases: 0.4% P.A. 0.05% P.U.

Treatment:  tip of catheter must stay out of blood flow in ar-
            teries (use of collaterals).
            use of heavy flow veins
            anticoagulant therapy?
            surgery
            internal saphenous vein must be avoided for im-
            plantation

### *Septic Injection or Fixation on Endovascular Prosthesis*

Is a very severe complication

> Seven cases: 1.2% P.A. 0.20% P.U.
> Seven explantations

> Treatment: percutaneous puncture must be avoided for implantation
> strictly aseptic handlings (injections, punctures, drainage)
> systematic prophylactic antibiotic therapy in septic risk circumstances
> explantation and antibiotic therapy
> one must not take any blood sample or do any transfusion through the pump and catheter

### *Blood Vessel Injury During the Puncture*

Leads to bulging of the pocket
The frequency and the recurrence in the same patients must lead to consideration of other etiological causes.

> Six cases: 13% P.A. Infusaid 400
> Treatment: puncture or surgical drainage

## Conclusion

The complications of implanted pump chemotherapy must be correctly known, to be able to utilize this system.

The following four points are necessary to succeed in a totally implanted system chemotherapy.

1. One must find a reliable system.

2. The technique concerning the surgery of implanting the pump is very important for the functioning of a chemotherapy system.

3. The aseptic conditions before, after, and during each perfusion must be seriously respected.

4. The presence of a highly qualified medical team seems indispensable in putting chemotherapy into practice.

# Chapter 21

# Radiosensitization With Constant Intraarterial Infusion of Bromodeoxyuridine (BUdR) and Focal External Beam Radiation in the Treatment of Malignant Astrocytomas

Harry S. Greenberg, William F. Chandler
Richard F. Diaz, William D. Ensminger
Larry Junch, Michaelyn A. Page
Stephen S. Gebarski, Terry W. Hood
Philip L. Stetson, Allen S. Lichter

## Introduction

Malignant glioma of the brain (anaplastic astrocytoma, malignant astrocytoma, glioblastoma multiforme) treated with "conventional" therapy of maximal surgical resection followed by radiation therapy, with or without intravenous (IV) nitrosourea chemother-

From: Ensminger WD, Selam JL (eds): *Infusion Systems in Medicine.* Mount Kisco, NY, Futura Publishing Co., Inc.,©1987.

apy has a poor prognosis. Surgery followed by radiation therapy has resulted in a median survival of 36 weeks and a 24-month survival of only 10%. The addition of IV BCNU or oral procarbazine chemotherapy has only extended the median survival to 51 weeks and increased the 24-month survival rate to 15%.[5]

Unique characteristics distinguish malignant gliomas from malignant neoplasms of other organs. Malignant gliomas do not metastasize except in rare instances. Local tumor progression in a confined inelastic space is the cause of death in virtually all cases. Total surgical excision of malignant gliomas is rarely feasible because of the tumor's infiltrative nature. Additionally, malignant gliomas are heterogeneous tumors. In vitro cloning studies have shown multiple morphological cell types within a single tumor or region of a tumor with varying karyotypic numbers and differential chemosensitivity.[6]

Radiation therapy is beneficial in the treatment of malignant gliomas of the brain, and its effects are dose related.[7,8] Dose limitations relate to normal brain tissue tolerance to external beam radiation.[8] This limitation has led many investigators to explore the interaction of external beam radiation and drugs that selectively increase tumor kill without increasing normal tissue toxicity. In theory, BUdR is an ideal drug to produce a clinically useful radiation sensitizing effect. BUdR is a halogenated pyrimidine analogue (bromine in BUdR replaces the methyl group in thymidine)[9] that is incorporated into the DNA of dividing cells in place of thymidine. BUdR has been shown to sensitize both bacterial and mammalian dividing cells to ultraviolet light and radiation.[3,9-12] A definite BUdR dose-radiation effect relationship has been demonstrated in both in vitro and in vivo experiments.[3,13]

Several clinical trials have been undertaken to investigate the efficacy of radiation sensitization with halogenated pyrimidines. In the late 1960s and early 1970s, Hoshino and coworkers in a series of reports presented a clinical trial of IA BUdR radiosensitization in 107 patients with malignant brain tumors.[14-16] Their infusion began 7 to 14 days prior to radiation therapy and was continued throughout the radiation therapy. Of 48 malignant gliomas in their study, 50% survived more than 18 months. This trial was ultimately discontinued due to difficulties with percutaneous IA BUdR delivery. A second trial evaluating IA BUdR radiosensitization in the treatment of head and neck tumors showed no advantage in local tumor control with significant normal tissue toxicities.[17,18] Normal tissue toxicity was due to the high mitotic index of the oral mucosa in comparison to tumor.

The optimal route of delivery of BUdR has been controversial. Initial studies indicated that BUdR has its maximum effect when given IA by constant infusion for a prolonged period of time.[19,20] A low tumor mitotic rate requires prolonged continuous infusion for BUdR incorporation into all dividing cells. Metabolism of BUdR was previously thought to be primarily by dehalogenation in the liver; however, plasma clearance of BUdR is three times hepatic plasma flow, suggesting that extrahepatic metabolism may be important. This high rate of metabolism may necessitate IA infusion. Russo et al.[2] conclude that common carotid IA infusion could yield a regional BUdR concentration 11- to 16-fold (1 log) higher than with IV infusion, resulting in optimum delivery of BUdR to tumor with minimal systemic toxicity.

Malignant gliomas have several characteristics that make them ideally suited for IA radiosensitization with BUdR. They are surrounded by supporting glial fibrillary network and brain neurons, which have virtually no ongoing mitosis. This tissue will not incorporate BUdR, and a therapeutic advantage will develop between radiosensitized tumor and nonradiosensitized normal tissue. Approximately 75% of malignant gliomas are unilateral and are supplied by a single internal carotid artery, allowing IA delivery of BUdR. In order to deliver a prolonged, continuous, high regional concentration of BUdR to brain tumors, a totally implantable Infusaid pump system has been developed.[1]

Because of the theoretical advantage of IA BUdR,[2,21] we initiated a primate toxicity study comparing carotid IA BUdR infusion to IA buffer infusion in control animals with both groups receiving external beam radiation to the brain. The study demonstrated no increase in pathology in the BUdR-infused hemisphere (Greenberg et al., submitted for publication). A clinical phase I protocol was developed utilizing IA infusion of BUdR prior to and concurrent with focal external beam radiation treatment.

## IA BUdR Radiosensitization and Radiotherapy

Patients with histologically confirmed unilateral malignant gliomas (grade III, grade IV, anaplastic astrocytoma, malignant astrocytoma, glioblastoma multiforme) with blood supply from one internal carotid artery were eligible for this phase I trial. Patients were required to have a Karnofsky rating of 30 or better and be capable of giving informed consent. Other eligibility criteria included normal peripheral blood count (WBC > 4,000 cells/$\mu$L; platelets > 200,000/$\mu$L), normal renal function (creatinine < 1.5; BUN < 30 mg%) normal liver function studies (bilirubin < 2.0; SGOT < 2 × normal; alkaline phosphatase < 2 × normal), and a life expectancy of at least three months.

Nine patients were entered and treated on this study through September 1986 (Table 1). Six patients had grade IV astrocytomas or glioblastoma multiforme, and three patients had grade III anaplastic astrocytomas. The average age of this group was 46.5 years (range 20-71).

BUdR was infused IA into the carotid system continuously using an Infusaid pump system. This system was surgically implanted subcutaneously in a pocket overlying the clavicle, and the outlet catheter of the pump was passed retrograde down the external carotid artery to the carotid bifurcation. The distal external carotid artery and superior thyroid artery were ligated (Fig. 1). This resulted in the infused drug flowing exclusively into the internal carotid artery. Patients received the BUdR infusion for eight weeks, beginning two weeks prior to focal external beam radiation treatment and continuing concurrently with radiation. Patients received

**Table 1**
**Patient Characteristics (Intraarterial BUdR + Concurrent XRT)**

| Patient (Age) | Grade | BUdR Infusion Rate (mg/m²/day) | Status (Months F/U) |
|---|---|---|---|
| 1. JB  (39) | IV | 400 | NED (14) |
| 2. LB  (44) | IV | 400 | Progressed @ 12 months |
| 3. DD  (20) | III | 400 | NED (13) |
| 4. PS  (36) | IV | 500 | Progressed @ 8 months |
| 5. PR  (71) | III | 450 | Progressed @ 8.5 months |
| 6. JK  (67) | IV | 450 | Stable (7.5) |
| 7. GD  (59) | IV | 500 | Stable (5.5) |
| 8. KW  (29) | III | 500 | Stable (4.5) |
| 9. MY  (55) | IV | 600 | Stable (3.5) |

Median follow-up = 8.5 months.
Average age = 46.5 years.

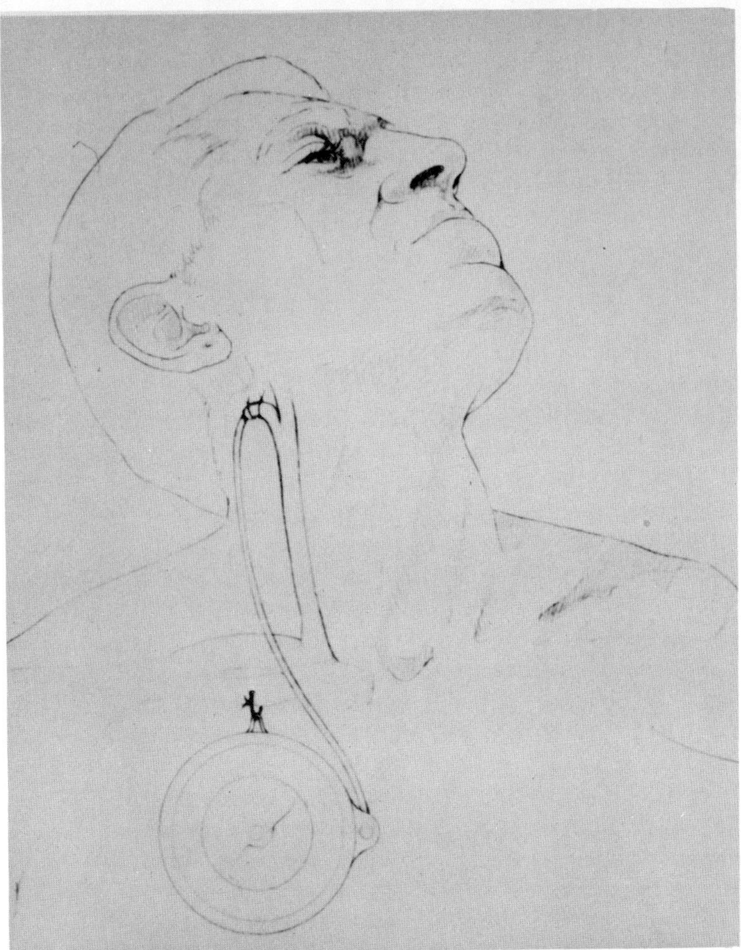

**Figure 1:** Schematic drawing of the Infusaid pump in the infraclavicular sub-cutaneous pocket with the outlet catheter placed retrograde down the external carotid artery to the carotid bifurcation. The external carotid artery has been ligated distally. The small circle in the center represents the inlet septum for refilling the drug chamber with BUdR, and the small circle at the periphery represents the auxiliary septum for direct bolus injection of BCNU into the carotid artery. (Drawn by Lewis L. Sadler.)

BUdR at doses ranging from 400 to 600 mg/m$^2$/day. After the eight-week BUdR infusion, the pump was filled with buffer solution for two weeks followed by water, then 17% glycerol, and finally 22% glycerol solution.

Systemic venous plasma steady-state levels were measured in all patients using HPLC with UV-absorption peak detection.[22] An estimated $R_d$ was calculated utilizing the definition of the ratio of tumor exposure following IA and IV administration, where exposure is the concentration-time integral.[21] Assuming linear kinetics of drug distribution and metabolism with negligible clearance by the lungs, the following equation is appropriate:

$$R_d = 1 + \frac{CL}{F}$$

where F is flow in the artery infused (L/min), and CL is the rate of metabolic clearance of the drug (L/min).[21]

One patient (no. 7) underwent emergency surgical resection of his malignant glioma after initiating BUdR infusion. A DNA assay of BUdR incorporation in the resected tumor tissue was performed using gas chromatography/mass spectrometry with selected-ion monitoring.[23]

Radiation therapy was begun two weeks after the initiation of BUdR infusion. Patients received focal partial brain radiation to the tumor volume measured by contrast-enhanced CT scan with an additional 3 to 4 cm margin around this tumor volume. A custom cerrobend block was utilized in shielding the scalp region as well as the nasopharynx and orbital regions. Treatment was administered with 6 to 10 MV photons on the linear accelerator. Daily dose was 180 cGy/fraction to a total dose of 5940 cGy over 6.5 weeks of treatment. Patients were followed by neurological exams as well as by general physical exams weekly. Complete blood and platelet counts were performed weekly, and liver function studies were obtained prior to and following completion of radiation therapy. CT brain scans were performed six weeks following radiation and every three months thereafter. PET scans using [18]F-fluorodeoxyglucose were obtained in selected cases in an effort to correlate CT scan findings with disease status.

## Results

The nine patients treated on this study through September 1986 (Table 1) have all completed their external beam radiation treatment and full BUdR infusion course. The initial three patients were treated with 400 mg/m$^2$/day of BUdR during their eight-week infusion. Patients nos. 4 and 5 were treated at 450 mg/m$^2$/day of BUdR, and patients nos. 6, 7, and 8 at 500 mg/m$^2$/day. The ninth patient received 600 mg/m$^2$/day of BUdR.

Two patients have no evident disease at 13 and 14 months, respectively. Four patients are stable between 3.5 and 7.5 months postdiagnosis. Three of the nine patients have had progression of their tumor with a median follow-up of 8.5 months and a maximum follow-up of 14 months postdiagnosis. The progression of their tumor occurred at 8, 8.5, and 12 months postdiagnosis, and all patients are alive. These patients had development of CT scan-enhancing lesions consistent with progressive tumor in addition to progressive clinical symptoms. In one patient, PET scan images showed increased $^{18}$F-fluorodeoxyglucose metabolism in the area of the CT scan abnormality consistent with recurrent tumor.

In three patients, early post treatment CT scans have identified new areas of abnormal increased contrast enhancement within the radiation field (Fig. 2). These abnormalities were initially noted on the CT scans at 4 to 6 weeks post treatment and thought to be consistent with tumor progression. PET scan images were obtained in two of these patients and showed no hypermetabolic foci suggestive of tumor. These patients were followed clinically and are doing

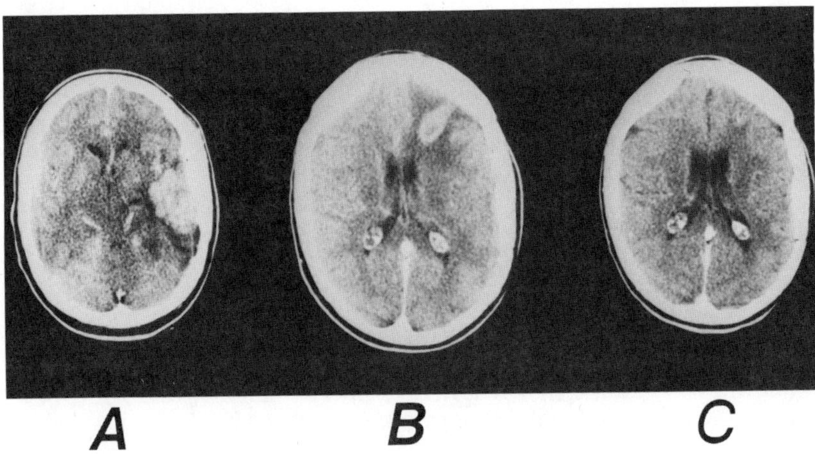


**Figure 2:** Patient no. 1 with Grade IV left temporal lobe astrocytoma (A) preoperatively. (B) Six weeks following the completion of radiation therapy with the appearance of a new contrast enhancing CT abnormality outside the area of original tumor. PET scan images at this time showed no congruent area of hypermetabolism. (C) Six months following radiation, the contrast enhancing abnormality had disappeared without further treatment.

well without treatment. The enhancing abnormalities persisted on CT scans until approximately six months post treatment and then gradually resolved in all cases.

Patient no. 7 developed progressive aphasia and right hemiparesis during the second week of BUdR radiosensitization and radiation therapy. He underwent surgical decompression and resection of tumor. Tissue specimens were obtained for BUdR DNA incorporation analysis. DNA assay of the tumor tissue revealed a BUdR for thymidine substitution ranging from 2.2% to 5.0% in different regions of the tumor. The systemic venous plasma BUdR level in this patient was 0.11 micrograms/mL with an infusion rate of 500 mg/m$^2$/day of BUdR.

There have been no vascular complications from the presence of the IA pump system. Expected side effects of myelosuppression, ipsilateral forehead dermatitis, anorexia, weight loss, and fatigue have been seen. Onychomadesis occurred in seven patients. No patient has required dose reduction due to myelotoxicity, although a white count nadir of 1,500, platelet count of 28,000, and hematocrit of 25 occurred in patient no. 9 necessitating transfusion of two units of packed red blood cells and two units of platelets. This patient was receiving 600 mg/m$^2$/day of BUdR. The most severe side effect noted has been a blepharitis, iritis, and conjunctivitis of the orbit ipsilateral to the BUdR infusion seen, to a varying degree, in all patients. Patient no. 7, receiving 500 mg/m$^2$/day of BUdR, had chronic eye irritation with a coagulase positive staphylococcal organism that responded to predforte ophthalmic drops. He then developed corneal ulceration and a posterior vitreous chamber leak with blindness, necessitating eye enucleation.

In the past, systemic venous BUdR blood levels after IA infusion have been measured in all patients and have varied from 0.07 to 0.20 micrograms/mL at an infused dose of 400 to 600 mg/m$^2$/day. Increasing the daily BUdR dose produced a variable response in the venous blood level. Assuming minimal regional brain extraction, the systemic venous blood levels obtained with IA infusion give a total body clearance that resulted in an estimated $R_d$ of BUdR of 5 to 16, similar to that calculated by Russo et al.[2]

## Discussion

In the past, IA BUdR infusion has been limited by the vascular toxicity of percutaneous infusion.[13-15] Our primate study of IA

BUdR with concurrent external beam radiation showed no asymmetric hemispheric pathology ipsilateral to IA BUdR infusion when compared to the noninfused hemisphere in the BUdR group or to the IA hemisphere receiving buffer solution in the control group (Greenberg et al., submitted for publication). Based on these results, our Phase I study was undertaken to assess the feasibility of delivering continuous infusion IA BUdR concurrent with radiation therapy for the treatment of malignant gliomas.

The DNA assay results in patient no. 7 of 2.2% to 5.0% BUdR-thymidine substitution in tumor tissue DNA is comparable to BUdR incorporation in DNA found to be necessary for radiosensitization by Thomas et al.[24]

There has been moderate enhancement of normal tissue effects on the skin outside the radiated portal. Blepharitis and conjunctivitis do not occur with focal brain external beam irradiation alone and are likely due to an altered blood supply to the orbit. The distal external carotid is ligated during pump catheter placement.[1] With the altered surgical anatomy, the internal carotid artery through orbital collaterals of the ophthalmic artery probably supplies the majority of blood to the forehead and eye. These structures receive considerable BUdR, and since they have a high mitotic rate, will incorporate BUdR. The scatter of radiation to the orbit and ambient UV light is probably enough radiation in the sensitized tissues to produce local toxicity. An effort will be made to reduce this toxicity by the development of topical thymidine eye drops and ointment. Topical thymidine will compete with the arterial BUdR exposure to skin and eye for incorporation into DNA of these normal tissues.

Studies of IV administered BUdR have found the escalation of dose beyond 700 mg/m$^2$/12 hours to be limited by systemic myelosuppression.[25,26] Systemic toxicity has not been a limiting factor in our study of IA BUdR, with only one patient experiencing moderately severe myelosuppression.

The occurrence of new contrast-enhanced abnormalities on early follow-up CT scans is of uncertain significance. The areas of CT contrast enhancement in two patients were correlated with PET scan images, which revealed no congruent regions of hypermetabolism. Subsequent follow-up CT scans revealed resolution of these abnormalities in all cases. This may represent a delayed subacute effect of the combined therapy of BUdR and external beam radiation. The evanescent CT abnormalities did not correlate with clinical neurological deterioration in these patients. To our knowledge, these findings have not been described following conventional external beam radiation therapy.

Response to treatment at this early point cannot be determined. Two patients are disease free at 13 and 14 months, and three patients have developed clear evidence of tumor progression based on CT scan and clinical criteria. The short duration of follow-up prevents further outcome analysis in the remaining patients.

In summary, our preliminary Phase I clinical study has shown the feasibility of administering continuous IA doses of BUdR with concomitant external beam radiation treatment over an eight-week period. It is hoped that with the accrual of additional patients and a Phase II study, the efficacy of this multimodality therapy can be ascertained.

## Summary

A permanently implantable Infusaid pump system has been developed for safe continuous intraarterial (IA) carotid BUdR infusion.[1] BUdR is delivered IA in the carotid system because of its regional advantage $(R_d)$.[2] In previous studies, BUdR has been shown to be an effective radiation sensitizer in rapidly dividing cells.

In July 1985, a clinical study was initiated for the treatment of malignant astrocytomas of the brain with IA BUdR infusion with concurrent partial brain radiation to 5940 cGy. Nine patients have been treated on this protocol with IA BUdR doses of 400 to 600 mg/m²/day. Three of the nine patients have had progression of their tumor. Median follow-up is 8.5 months with a maximum of 14 months. No vascular complications or severe systemic side effects have occurred, and all patients have completed the planned course of treatment. At this preliminary point, efficacy cannot be determined. Continuous IA infusion of BUdR is feasible, safe, and represents a potential means of enhancing the effectiveness of radiotherapy in the treatment of malignant astrocytomas.

Acknowledgment: This work is supported in part by the National Institutes of Health grants R01 CA33768 and P01 NS15655; the John Masterson Brain Tumor Research Fund; and the Intermedics/Infusaid Corporation.

# References


1. Phillips TW, Chandler WF, Kindt GW, Ensminger WD, Greenberg HS, et al. (1982). New implantable continuous administration of bolus dose intracarotid drug delivery system for the treatment of malignant gliomas. Neurosurgery 11:213−218.
2. Russo A, Gianni L, Kinsella TJ, et al. (1984). A pharmacologic evaluation of intravenous delivery of 5-bromodeoxyuridine to patients with brain tumors. Cancer Res 44:1702−1705.
3. Djordjevic B, Szybalski W. (1960). Genetics of human cell lines. III. Incorporation of 5-bromo and 5-iododeoxyuridine into the deoxyribonucleic acid of human cells and its effect on radiation sensitivity. J Exp Med 112:509−531.
4. Szybalski W. (1974). X-ray sensitization by halopyrimidines. Cancer Chemother Rep 58:539−557.
5. Walker MD, Green SB, Byar DP, et al. (1980). Randomized comparisons of radiotherapy and nitrosoureas for the treatment of malignant glioma after surgery. N Eng J Med 303:1323−1329.
6. Shapiro JR, Yang WA, Shapiro WR. (1982). Heterogeneous chemosensitivities of subpopulations of human malignant gliomas. Cancer Res 42:992−998.
7. Walker MD, Alexander E, Hunt WE, et al. (1978). Evaluation of BCNU and/or radiotherapy in the treatment of anaplastic gliomas: A cooperative clinical trial. J Neurosurg 49:333−343.
8. Sheline GE, Wara UM, Smith V. (1980). Therapeutic irradiation and brain injury. Int J Radiat Oncol Biol Phys 6:1215−1228.
9. BUdR. (1980). Clinical Brochure, IND 2197, NSC 38297, July.
10. Greer S. (1960). Studies on ultraviolet irradiation of Escherichia Coli containing 5-bromouracil in its DNA. J Gen Microbiol 22:618−634.
11. Erikson RL, Szybalski W. (1961). Molecular radiobiology of human cell lines: I. Comparative sensitivity to x-rays and ultraviolet light cells containing halogen-substituted DNA. Biochem Biophys Res Commun 4:258−261.
12. Mohler WC, Elkind MM. (1963). Radiation response to mammalian cells grown in culture III. Modification of x-ray survival of Chinese hamster cells by 5-bromodeoxyuridine. Exp Cell Res 30:481−491.
13. Brown JM, Goffinet DR, Cleaver JE. (1971). Preferential radiosensitization of mouse sarcoma relative to normal skin by chronic intra-arterial infusion of halogenated pyrimidine analogs. JNCI 47:75−89.
14. Hoshino T. (1974). Radiosensitization of brain tumors. In: Deely TJ ed, Modern Radiotherapy and Oncology−Central Nervous System Tumours, London, England, Butterworths, pp 170−183.
15. Sano K, Sato F, Hoshino T, Hagai M. (1965). Experimental and clinical studies of radiosensitizers in brain tumors, with special reference to BUdR—antimetabolite continuous regional infusion—radiation therapy (BAR therapy). Neur Med Chir 7:51−72.

16. Sano K, Nagai M, Arai T, Hoshino T. (1972). Follow-up results of BAR therapy of malignant brain tumors. Proceedings of the Fourth European Congress of Neurosurgery. I Fusek and Z Kunc, eds, Excepta Medica, Amsterdam, pp 71−75.

17. Bagshaw MA, Doggett RLS, Smith KC, Kaplan HS, Nelsen TS. (1967). Intra-arterial 5-bromodeoxyuridine and x-ray therapy. *Radiology* 99:886−894.

18. Doggett RLS, Bagshaw MA, Kaplan HS. (1967). Combined therapy using chemotherapeutic agents and radiotherapy. In: Wood CAP, Deely TJ, eds, *Modern Trends in Radiotherapy*, London, Butterworth, pp 107−131.

19. Kriss JP, Revesz L. (1962). Distribution and fate of bromodeoxyuridine and bromodeoxycytidine in the mouse and rat. *Cancer Res* 2:254−265.

20. Kriss JP, Maruyama Y, Tung LA, Bonds D, Revesz L. (1963). The fate of 5-bromodeoxyuridine, 5-bromodeoxycytidine, and 5-iododeoxycytidine in man. *Cancer Res* 23:260−268.

21. Eckman WW, Patlak CS, Fenstermacher JD. (1974). A critical evaluation of the principles governing the advantage of intra-arterial infusions. *J Pharmacokinet Biopharmacokinet* 2:257−285.

22. Stetson PL, Shukla UA, Amin PR, Ensminger WD. (1985). High performance liquid chromatographic method for the determination of bromodeoxyuridine and its major metabolite, bromouracil, in biological fluids. *J Chromtogr* 341:217−222.

23. Stetson PL, Maybaum J, Shukla UA, Ensminger WD. (1986). Simultaneous determination of thymine and 5-bromouracil in DNA hydrolysates using gas chromatography-mass spectrometry and selected-ion monitoring. *J Chromatogr* 375:1−9.

24. Thomas GH, Maloney MA, Cleaver JE. (1982). Sensitization of mouse L cells to ultraviolet light by low amounts of bromodeoxyuridine. *Radiation Res* 91:145-154.

25. Kinsella TJ, Russo A, Mitchell JB, et al. (1984). A phase I study of intermittent intravenous bromodeoxyuridine (BUdR) with conventional fractionated irradiation. *J Radiat Oncol Biol Phys* 10:69-76. 10:69−76.

26. Kinsella TJ, Mitchell JB, Russo A, Aiken M, et al. (1984). Continuous intravenous infusions of bromodeoxyuridine as a clinical radiosensitizer. *J Clin Oncol* 2:1144−1150.

# Chapter 22

# Central Venous Ports in Immunocompromised Children: Complications Should be Avoided by Proper Experience


Eeva-Liisa Maunuksela
Jukka Rajantie
Marti A. Siimes
Kirsi-Marja Lähteenoja


## Introduction

Advanced oncologic therapy has improved the prognosis of children with leukemia dramatically and that of patients with solid tumors to some extent. However, this development does not mean that there is less suffering related to malignancy. Modern aggressive chemotherapy demands frequent intravenous injections and infusions together with blood sampling. During the course of therapy the child will often become sensitized for all kinds of procedures.[1] The fear of injection pain is one of the biggest subjective problems,

From: Ensminger WD, Salem JL (eds): *Infusion Systems in Medicine.* Mount Kisco, Ny, Futura Publishing Co., Inc., © 1987.

according to the information based on questionnaires given to 42 children after cessation of a three-year chemotherapy regimen for leukemia. The fear interferes with small, simple procedures, making them difficult. This is time consuming for the personnel and evokes further anxiety in the child.

In 1982 we initiated a program aimed at avoiding unnecessary pain and offering good analgesia for children on the Hematology—Oncology ward. Local anesthetic creme is used prior to blood drawing and venous cannulations.[2] All bone marrow aspirations and needle biopsies are done under an adequate analgesia or anesthesia.[3] Further, analgesics are used liberally for pain periods. As a part of this program, we have, since August 1984, implanted central venous ports for children. The port provides an easy access to the central veins, allowing injection of irritant and concentrated substances. It also permits easy aspiration of blood for laboratory samples. Over a peripheral intravenous infusion, it allows the child to use both hands freely, which is an important point during the long hospital stay.

On the other hand, a central venous port-system is a foreign body that may result in infections and other complications. Implantation of a port in a child demands general anesthesia. Only limited information is available on the specific considerations of implantation, benefits, and disadvantages of this kind of central venous access in pediatric patients.[4,5]

## Patients

We have implanted 56 central venous ports in 52 children. Forty-eight of the children had a malignant disease: 13 leukemia and 35 solid tumors. The age and weight of the patients together with the details of the diagnoses are shown in Table 1.

## Methods

The first 30 implantations were performed by use of PORT-A-CATH (PAC) (Pharmacia Laboratories, NJ). The catheter diameter was 2.79/1.02 mm in 29/30 cases. The subsequent implantations included 18 Vascular Access Ports (VAP) (Norfolk Medical Products, Illinois), two Implantofix (Braun Melsungen AG, FRG), two PAC,

**Table 1**
**The Mean Age and Weight (range) and Diagnoses of the Patients**

| | | | | |
|---|---|---|---|---|
| Age, years | 7.4 | (0.3−16.0) | | |
| Weight, kg | 28.9 | (6.7−60.0) | | |
| | | | | |
| Diagnosis: | | | | |
| *Malignancies* | | | *Other Diseases* | |
| Leukemia | 13 | | Aplastic anemia | 2 |
| Lymphoma | 4 | | Cystic fibrosis | 1 |
| Hodgkin's disease | 3 | | Tyrosinemia | 1 |
| Osteosarcoma | 6 | | | |
| Rhabdomyosarcoma | 4 | | | |
| Synovial sarcoma | 2 | | | |
| Wilm's tumor | 2 | | | |
| Brain tumor | 7 | | | |
| Yolk sac tumor | 2 | | | |
| Other tumors | 5 | | | |
| Total number of patients | 48 | | | 4 |

and four PAC Pediatric in 22 children. One PAC was exchanged to a broviac-type catheter and later back to VAP. One child had three port implantations, and another child had two implantations due to the malfunction and/or infection.VAP and Implantofix were chosen because their size was smaller or configuration more favorable in small children. After PAC Pediatric became available, we used it as a first choice for small children. Its advantages include a relatively large membrane, low-rounded configuration, and simple implantation because of the easy-to-connect separate silicone catheter.

Prior to the implantation, a coagulation profile was obtained in all patients. Attempts were made to correct major derangements, especially low platelet count. No prophylactic antibiotic was used. The operation was always performed under general anesthesia occasionally in connection with other diagnostic or operative procedures. The central venous access was obtained by percutaneous puncture of the internal jugular vein (42 cases) using Desilet 7.0−8.0Fg introducters (Vygon, France) for PAC and COOK peel-off 5.5−7.0 Fg introducers for VAP and Implantofix. Cut down of the internal jugular (6 cases) or external jugular vein (8 cases) was performed primarily in cases with increased bleeding tendency or after an unsuccessful percutaneous puncture. The pocket for the port was prepared subclavicularly on either side.

## Results

The cumulative duration of the central venous access was 14,322 days by October 31, 1986, with a range from 4 to 785 days and with a mean of 276 days/patient (Fig. 1). Fourteen ports have been used longer than one year. Cytostatic drugs and intravenous fluid therapy have been administrated in 48 ports. The port has been used primarily for repeated administration of red blood cells in two cases and for intravenous antibiotics in one case. All ports were used for blood sampling.

All patients and parents except one (patient 28) considered the port system to be a practical and comfortable device. Currently, there are 27 functioning ports in use. The port has been electively extracted after discontinuation of chemotherapy in nine cases. The port was transformed to a broviac type catheter using a steel connecting pin in two other cases (patients 14 and 21). Both of these children were prepared for autologous bone marrow transplantation, which demanded continuous intravenous infusions and parenteral nutrition. In the first of the two cases, the catheter was switched back to a central venous port after the successful operation. Nine patients died of their primary disease with a port. No complications associated with the implantation or use of the central venous port were observed in 39 of the 52 children.

### Complications

The summary of the complications is shown in Table 2. There were three *technical failures*, two of them early in the series (patients 4 and 5). In the first case, the catheter was too long, and the tip gradually migrated into the pulmonary artery. It was operatively shortened to an appropriate length. In the second case, there was a tear in the silicone catheter, probably done with the tunnelling needle, at the jugular puncture site. Two months after the implantation, the catheter was obstructed. The lesion was diagnosed using contrast media and x-ray. The catheter part was exchanged. The third technical complication was a catheter embolization into the

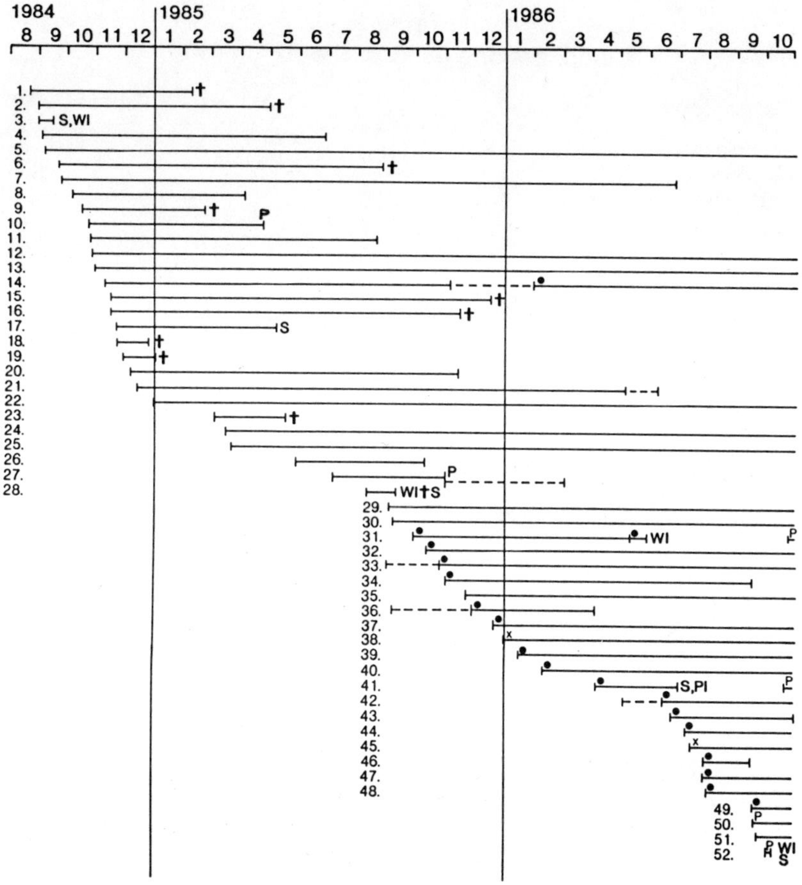

**Figure 1:** Follow-up of the 56 central venous ports implanted in 52 children in the Children's Hospital, University of Helsinki. 1, Port-A-Cath; p, Port-A-Cath Pediatric; o, Vascular-Access-Port; x, Implantofix; S, Sepsis; WI, wound infection; P, perforation of the skin; PI, pocket infection; T, death.

right heart during a splicing procedure (patient 27). The event was suspected after seeing some extrasystoles in the ECG and documented by an x-ray picture. The embolized catheter was then extracted in the catheterization laboratory under the same anesthesia. A broviac type catheter was inserted through the femoral vein. Prophylactic antibiotics were given. The patient healed well with no further complications.

**Table 2**
**Complications in 13 of the 52 Children**

| Complication | | *Number of cases* |
|---|---|---|
| Technical | | x) 3 |
| Hematomas | | 3 |
| Perforation of the skin | | x) 2 |
| Extravasation | | o) 1 |
| Infection | | 6 |
|   Surgical infection | o) 2 | |
|   Implantation during sepsis | 1 | |
|   Wound infection | 1 | |
|   Pocket infection, sepsis | 1 | |
|   Sepsis | 1 | |
| Total | | 15 |

Two children had two different complications.
x, skin perforation and catheter embolization
o, extravasation and surgical infection

## Hematomas

Patients 16, 34, and 51 had postoperative hematomas, one on the puncture site, one in the pocket, and the last one in the sternocleidomastoid muscle. Neither of them caused further complications or demanded extraction of the port.

## Skin Perforations

Two ports perforated the skin. The tenth implantation was in a 12.5 kg thin child. There was some tension over the port's edges after implantation. The port perforated the skin after six months and was extracted. The wound healed well. The other perforation occurred 103 days after implantation following a hematoma formation, possibly due to a local trauma, in the port-bearing pocket (patient 27). It was decided to extract the port and to use the central part of the catheter after connecting it with a broviac type catheter. The catheter embolization described above occurred on this event. Both of the perforated ports were PACs.

## Extravasation

After successful use of a port of 7.5 months, a needle misplacement resulted in extravasation of antibiotics and obstruction of the central venous port system in a 1.5 year-old boy (patient 31) with cystic fibrosis. The system was excised and a new port implanted during the same anesthesia. This port was probably contaminated during the surgery and is further described under infectious complications.

## Infectious Complications

A total of six infectious complications were recorded. This represents 11.5% of the patient population or 1 per 2,389 central venous access days. Two of the infections were associated with surgery, the second port of patient 31 and patient 52. In the latter case, the source of contamination was probably an inadequately covered x-ray tube used intraoperatively. The port no. 3 was implanted because of very poor venous access during the second relapse of acute lymphatic leukemia in a five-year-old girl. The patient had been diagnosed with *Staph. epid.* septicemia seven days earlier, even if she had been considered to be cured by antibiotics before the procedure. However on the first day after the implantation, the same type of *Staph. epid.* was cultured from her blood samples. The wound opened on the third day, and the *Staph. epid.* was cultured from the wound. The port was extracted on the eighth day. The *Staph.* was again cultured from the port. The patient died in sepsis six days later.

Patient 28 was a 1.8 year-old boy who fell down and hurt his chin shortly after implantation of the central venous port. The wound was sutured but infected. It was noted that while taking a shower, the infected material ran from the chin over the fresh implantation wound, which was then infected. The central venous port system was not used, but because it did not perforate through the wound, it was not extracted. Thirty days after implantation, the child died suddenly with a clinical picture of sepsis. In autopsy, the port-bearing pocket was not infected, and there was no bacterial growth in the samples from the port. However, *Staph. aureus.* was cultured from blood.

Disobeying our general recommendations, a 9-month-old baby (patient 41) had a cytostatic infusion for six days without changing the angled huber-point needle. After the needle was removed, the skin was noticed to be red and swollen. Two days later, the baby was brought into the hospital with septic fever (Fig. 2). Blood culture was taken and antibiotics were started. The C-reactive protein concentration (CRP) rose up to 100, fever remained high, and redness around the port was widened. After *Staph aureus.* grew in the blood culture, the port was extracted. The same type of staphylococcus was cultured from the pus in the port-bearing pocket. After extraction, the fever and CRP soon normalized, and the baby healed well. A new port has now been implanted.

Patient 17 had an infected wound with a metal fixation plate on his thigh with *Staph. epidermidis septicaemia* (Fig. 3). The sepsis was thought to be sustained by the port, which had been implanted 5.5 months earlier. After extraction of the port, the fever and CRP normalized rapidly. The pocket wound and later, the thigh healed without complications. Patient 46, a 3.5 year-old boy with tyrosinemia had a *Staph. aureus* sepsis documented in an-

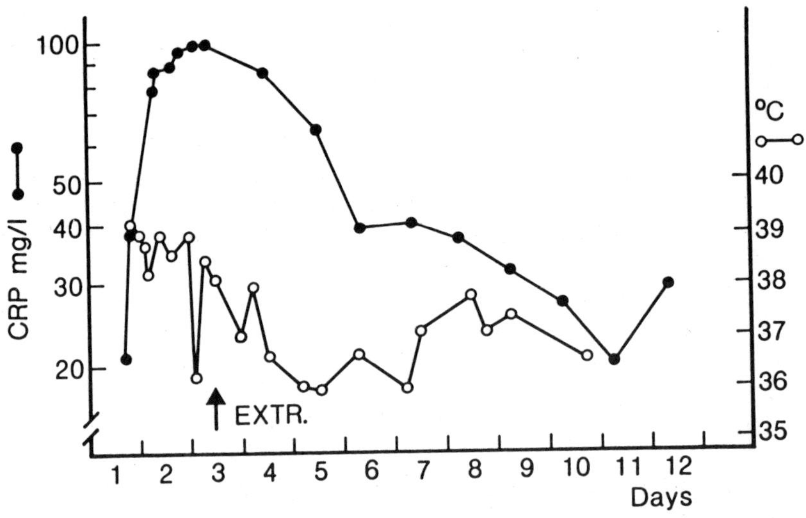


**Figure 2:** Body temperature and the concentration of C-reactive protein (CRP) in patient 41 with *Staph. aureus* infection of the port-bearing pocket and septicemia. Blood culture was taken (positive) on the first day antibiotics were started. The port was extracted on the third day. CRP is used as one indicator of bacterial infection in our hospital.[11]

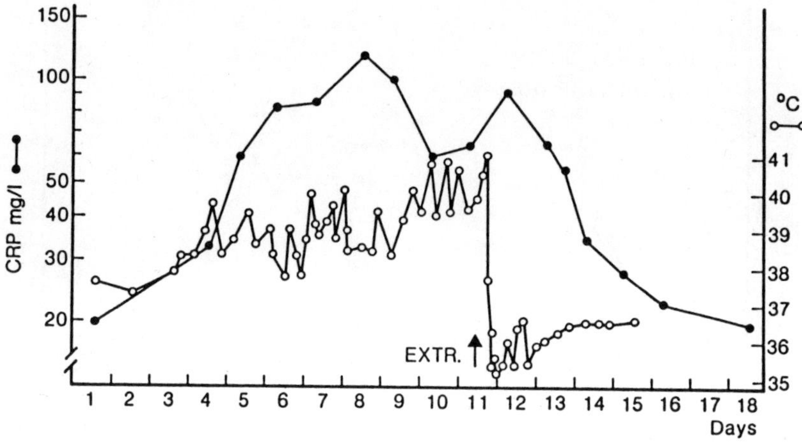



**Figure 3:** Body temperature and CRP (see legend to Fig. 2) in patient 17 with *Staph. epidermidis* septicemia. Blood cultures were positive on the fourth and sixth days. Antibiotics were started on the sixth day. The port was extracted on the eleventh day.

other hospital (Fig. 4). Despite antibiotic therapy, the general condition of the child worsened. The port was suspected to sustain the infection and it was removed. The child needed ventilatory support and was taken to the intensive care unit (ICU). As seen in Figure 4, the port was obviously not the cause of the infection. The child developed a therapy-resistant pneumonia and died 17 days later in the ICU.

## Discussion

The relatively low incidence of infectious complications and patient comfort have been the major arguments for use of a totally implantable central venous port in adults.[6,7] In our experience, the patient compliance was good. The attitudes tended to be more positive in patients who had experienced a long chemotherapy using peripheral veins. After minor problems in the beginning of the series, the ports functioned well. For primary acceptance of the children, it was important to have an angled Huber-point needle with an infusion connection in the port during the implantation. Thus, touching the still-hurting implantation wound could be avoided

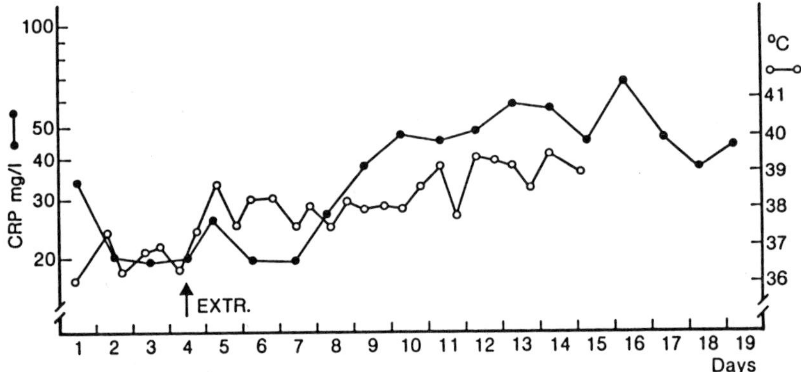


**Figure 4:** Body temperature and CRP (see legend to Fig. 2) in patient 46. *Staph. aureus* was cultured from the blood in another hospital on day 4, when antibiotics had been started. On the day of port extraction, all cultures were negative.

during the first days. We also ordered an antipyretic analgesic with fixed time intervals for the three first days. The maximum interval between flushings of the port has routinely been one month. There have been no port obstructions. Technical failures occurred in the beginning of the series. Experience helps to reduce them; therefore, these operations have been concentrated in a few hands in our hospital.

The incidence of six infectious complications per 14,332 observation days compared favorably with the experience of other centers.[8,9] The implantation during sepsis could have been avoided with our present experience. Long-lasting intravenous nutrition may increase the risk of obstruction and sepsis in the central venous port system. The lipid and protein components may form clots, with electrolytes and drugs tending to obstruct the angled Huber-point needle. The flow in the port chamber is sluggish and turbulent collecting clotted particles on the edges if not regularly flushed. These particles on the chamber wall, together with glucose, are an excellent media for growth of accidental bacteria in an environment where systemic antibiotics and leucocytes have no access. If the Huber-point needle remains on the same site for several days, it often errodes the skin, creating a route for infection to enter the port-bearing pocket. To insert a correctly proportioned needle through healthy skin and change it frequently together with appropriate needle fixation are important details to protect the port and pocket from contamination and extravasation. It is our impression that the needle change should be performed at less than 48-hour intervals to prevent this pattern of complications.

In our opi.ion, there is necessarily no reason to believe that totally implantable central venous ports would be less prone to infection than Dacron-cuffed silicone catheters under continuous intravenous nutrition. After our first-year experience, we do not implant central venous ports in children who need intravenous infusion for several weeks. For these cases, we use a broviac-type central venous catheter, which may be subsequently switched to a port through a minor subcutaneous procedure in cases when only intermittent venous access is needed. The central venous port has successfully been switched to a broviac type catheter or vice versa on six occasions in five patients during the last year.

The decision to extract or retain a port when the patient has a documented septicemia is difficult. We have presented some cases where it was not possible to cure the patient with antibiotics but extraction of the port was immediately effective. There are three other patients who were clinically cured from documented septicemia and whose blood cultures became negative while the port system was still in place. Two of these ports were extracted; one is retained and without bacterial growth. We do not know any reliable parameter to predict the outcome of septicemia with an implanted central venous port.

Until now there have been no thrombotic complications in our patients. This finding is in contrast to the adult data.[8,10] It might be due to the young age and generally lower incidence of thrombotic episodes in any children. The use of the internal jugular vein instead of the subclavian vein might also be of importance. In two cases there has been an autopsy finding of a circular fibrous mass around the silicone catheter.

The indications for use of a central venous port have changed during the time period we have been using the system. At the start of the series, the port was implanted in children who had poor venous access due to long-lasting chemotherapy. Often, the malignant disease had relapsed, and the prognosis for the child was no longer good. In nine patients who died of their primary disease with a port, the implantation had been done during the first year of the series. In addition, the early patients were often sensitized to all painful procedures. These patients appreciated the port because it made blood sampling and intravenous injections easier. However, there were often some derangements in the coagulation profile, which caused technical difficulties during the implantation. Further, the healing of wounds might have been disturbed during aggressive chemotherapy.

At the start of the series, it was agreed with the child and the family to extract the port at cessation of the chemotherapy. Thus, the extraction became a symbol of being cured and it could hardly be postponed. Today, we represent the port system as a more or less permanent device for venous access. Only two of the ports implanted after the first year have been electively extracted.

With our present experience, we consider implanting a central venous port prophylactically when a long-lasting and frequently administered chemotherapy is foreseen, for a small child needing prolonged intravenous therapy or if venous access is poor or the child is exceptionally anxious of venous cannulation. This has resulted in implantations earlier during the course of a malignant disease. For patients with solid tumors, the port is often implanted in association with diagnostic surgical procedures. This allows the wounds some time to heal prior to the start of chemotherapy. The port has also been successfully implanted in young children needing repeated intravenous therapy, including blood transfusions in two patients with aplastic anemia and antibiotics in a patient with cystic fibrosis. In the series there are 11 children weighing less than 15 kg. The youngest two babies were only four months of age. This also indicated the usefulness of the port in some infants. In fact, we do not see any age limitations for central venous port implantation for a full-term baby.

The central venous port is an important advancement in the treatment of children needing frequent venous access. Many of the complications that have taken place in our patients during the first year should be avoided by our current experience. Prior indications, skillful implantation, and meticulous aseptic technique when injecting into the port should also help to keep the incidence of complications at an acceptable level.

---

## References


1. Jay SM, Ozolins M, Elliot CH. (1983). Assessment of children's distress during painful medical procedures. *Health Psychol* 2:133.

2. Manuksela E-L, Korpela R. (1986). Double blind evaluation of the lignocaine-prilocain cream (EMLA) in children. Effect on pain associated with venous cannulation. *Br J Anaesth* 58:1242.
3. Maunuksela E-L, Rajantie J, Siimes MA. (1986). Flunitrazepam-fentanylinduced sedation and analgesia for bone marrow aspiration and needle biopsy in children. *Acta Anaesthesiol Scand* 30:409.
4. McGovern B, Solenberger R, Reed K. (1986). A totally implantable venous access system for long-term chemotherapy in children. *J Pediatr Surg* 20:725.
5. Van der Staak F, Bokkerink J, Lippens R, et al. (1986). Totally implantable systems for intravenous drug delivery. Experiences in children with cancer. *Z Kinderchir* 41:39.
6. Gyves JW, Ensminger WD, Niederhuber JE, et al. (1984). A totally implanted injection port system for blood sampling and chemotherapy administration. *JAMA* 251:2538.
7. Dauplat J, Condat P, Giraud B. (1985). Totally implantable venous access system in long-term chemotherapy. *Int Surg* 70:251.
8. Bothe A Jr, Piccione W, Ambrosino JJ, et al. (1984). Implantable central venous access system. *Am J Surg* 147:565.
9. Brinker H, Saeter G. (1986). Fifty-five patients years' experience with a totally implanted system for intravenous chemotherapy. *Cancer* 57:1124.
10. Starkhammar H, Bengtsson M. (1985). Totally implanted device for venous access. *Acta Radiol Oncol* 24:173.
11. Peltola HO. (1982). C-reactive protein for rapid monitoring of infections of the central nervous system. *Lancet* 1:980.

# Other Applications

# Chapter 23

# Optimal Control of Antiarrhythmic Drug Infusion


Thomas E. Bump
Jeffrey Brown
Charles Yurkonis
Alain Guezennec
Robert C. Arzbaecher


## Introduction

Rapid infusions of antiarrhythmic drugs are useful in many clinical settings. Bolus-plus-drip infusions of lidocaine and bretylium are often used for acute control of ventricular arrhythmias, and bolus infusions of verapamil are often used to terminate paroxysmal supraventricular tachycardia. Unfortunately, it has not been possible to safely administer procainamide, quinidine, or disopyramide in this manner. These latter drugs must be given more slowly, and therapeutic levels are typically not produced until half an hour or more has elapsed from the onset of administration.[1-3] As a consequence, we do not yet have satisfactory pharmacologic techniques for rapidly treating arrhythmias that do not respond to lidocaine, bretylium, or verapamil. For example, we do


*From:* Ensminger WD, Selam JL (eds): *Infusion Systems in Medicine.* Mount Kisco, NY, Futura Publishing Co., Inc.,©1987.

not yet have a good method for rapid pharmacologic conversion of atrial fibrillation to sinus rhythm.

The purpose of the present study was to develop pharmacologic techniques for rapidly terminating atrial fibrillation. Specifically, we tested the hypothesis that we could rapidly produce and maintain therapeutic plasma concentrations of procainamide and disopyramide by delivering the drugs through exponentially tapered infusion. Kruger-Thiemer and subsequent investigators have shown that this type of infusion is the best way to produce therapeutic concentrations immediately and maintain them.[4-7] We evaluated the ability of this approach to terminate atrial fibrillation in an animal model.

## Methods

### Procainamide

This part of the study used a conscious canine preparation and involved two stages: pharmacokinetic characterization and evaluation of pharmacokinetically-based, exponentially-tapering infusion. On the first experimental day, each of three dogs was restrained in a sling. Two intravenous lines were established, one for infusion of procainamide and one for obtaining blood samples. After control blood samples were obtained, a procainamide infusion was begun. This infusion was designed to produce a plasma concentration of 8 mg/L and consisted of a bolus of 2.5 mg/kg over one minute followed by a steady infusion of 0.065 mg/kg/min for 3 to 4 hours. Blood samples were obtained at the following intervals during the infusion: 1, 2, 3, 4, 5, 6, 7, 8, 9, 10, 12, 14, 16, 20, 30, 40, 50, 60, 75, 90, 105, 120, 150, 180, 210, and 240 minutes. After this procedure, · all lines were removed, and the animal was allowed to recover.

Plasma concentrations of procainamide were determined for each blood sample, using the SYVA EMIT enzyme immunoassay technique. The plasma concentrations were then used for calculations of pharmacokinetic parameters using our modified version of the nonlinear regression program BMDO7R, which uses Gauss-Newton procedures for least square estimation and is modified to use stepwise linear regression in order to avoid singularity problems. The program requires user-supplied evaluations of the fitted function and partial derivatives with respect to the parameters. The program adjusts the pharmacokinetic parameters in order to minimize the mean squared error. Our pharmacokinetic modeling assumed two compartments, and the calculated parameters included the sizes of both compartments and the rates of elimination and transfer between the central and tissue compartments.

On a second experimental day, at least one week after the first, we evaluated the technique of exponentially tapering infusion. Dogs were again restrained, and two intravenous lines were established. After control blood samples were obtained, an exponentially tapering infusion of procainamide was begun. The infusion was designed to give a plasma concentration of 8 mg/L of procainamide and was based on the previously calculated pharmacokinetic properties of the animal. Again, frequent blood samples were obtained, with the same schedule as above.

## Disopyramide

This part of the study used an anesthetized, closed-loop canine preparation, and involved two stages: pharmacokinetic characterization, and automatic termination of atrial fibrillation by exponentially-tapered, pharmacokinetic-based infusion of disopyramide. On the first experimental day, mongrel dogs of either sex were anesthetized with ACE-promazine and sodium pentobarbital (20 to 30 mg/kg, supplemented as needed). Each dog was intubated and ventilated by a positive pressure Harvard pump. A femoral arterial line was established for obtaining blood samples. Two intravenous lines were established for infusing acetylcholine and disopyramide, respectively. First, acetylcholine (0.3 mg/kg/min.) was infused. After five minutes, an infusion of disopyramide phosphate was delivered through the other line. This infusion was designed to produce a plasma concentration of disopyramide of 4 mg/L and consisted of 1.2 mg/kg over one minute followed by a steady infusion of 0.066 mg/kg/min. for three hours. Arterial blood samples were obtained prior to disopyramide and at the following intervals during infusion: 15, 30, and 45 seconds and 1, 2, 3, 4, 5, 7, 10, 15, 20, 25, 30, 45, 60, 75, 90, 105, 120, 150, and 180 minutes into the infusion. After this procedure, all lines were removed, and the dog was allowed to recover.

Plasma concentrations of disopyramide were determined for each blood sample, using the same technique as described above for procainamide. Pharmacokinetic properties were also calculated using the same techniques described above.

On a second experimental day, at least one week after the first, we evaluated our ability to automatically terminate atrial fibrillation. Dogs were again anesthetized with ACE-promazine and sodium pentobarbital, intubated, and ventilated by a Harvard respirator. An arterial and two venous lines were established. A Cordis 5 French bipolar J-shaped electrode catheter was inserted into a jugular vein, and the catheter tip was positioned in the right atrial appendage under fluoroscopic control. A 6 French USCI quadripolar electrode catheter was inserted, and its tip was positioned in the right ventricular apex under fluoroscopic control. Both catheters were connected to amplifiers of a multichannel recorder and oscilloscope (Electronics for Medicine VR-12). Signals were filtered at 30 and 500 Hz. A surface electrocardiographic lead was also monitored and recorded.

Outputs of the atrial and ventricular recording amplifiers were connected to an Intel iPDS microcomputer on which we have implemented our previously described algorithms for arrhythmia detection and analysis.[8,9] These algorithms diagnose atrial fibrillation when the atria depolarize at a rate of more than 330 beats per minute.

An infusion of 0.3 mg/kg/min. acetylcholine was started. The atrial leads were disconnected from the recording equipment and connected to a programmable stimulator. A train of 20 stimuli with a cycle length of 50 ms, each with a width of 2 ms and an amplitude of 5 volts, was delivered to the right atrium. This technique, a modification of protocols reported by other investigators,[10,11] caused sustained atrial fibrillation in all cases. The atrial catheter was then reconnected to the recording amplifier. After 15 minutes, the infusion of acetylcholine was turned off and sinus rhythm was restored. In no case did atrial fibrillation terminate spontaneously before the infusion of acetylcholine was stopped.

We now enabled the arrhythmia detector to trigger an infusion of disopyramide whenever it had detected one minute of atrial fibrillation. After at least five minutes of sinus rhythm, an infusion of 0.3 mg/kg/min. acetylcholine was restarted, and atrial fibrillation was reinduced by the same pacing protocol as above. After one minute of atrial fibrillation, the detection algorithm triggered a pharmacokinetically-based infusion of disopyramide. This infusion was designed to produce a plasma concentration of disopyramide of 5 mg/L, and was based on the previously determined pharmacokinetic properties of the dog. The target level of 5 mg/L was chosen because it falls in the high therapeutic range for humans and dogs.[12–14] The infusion was performed using an infusion pump, which was turned on and off by a program running on the same Intel iPDS computer on which the arrhythmia detection algorithms were implemented.

The infusions of disopyramide and acetylcholine were both continued for an hour. The time from onset of infusion to termination of atrial fibrillation was recorded. Arterial blood samples were obtained before infusion of disopyramide and at the following time-points during infusion: 15, 30, and 45 seconds and 1, 2, 3, 4, 5, 7, 10, 15, 20, 25, 30, 45, and 60 minutes.

## Results

### Procainamide

As expected, bolus-plus-drip infusions of procainamide produced a rapid rise in plasma concentration followed by a significant undershoot (Fig. 1). The pharmacokinetic characteristics of procainamide in each dog, calculated from the plasma concentra-

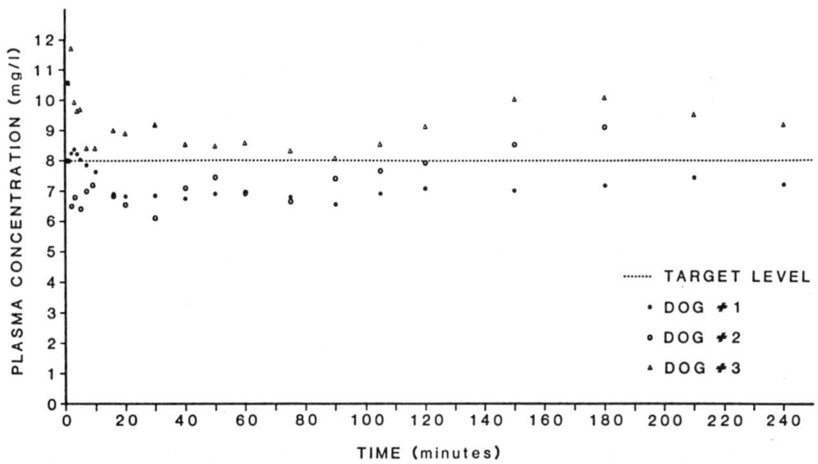


**Figure 1:** Plasma concentrations of procainamide produced in one dog by a bolus-plus-drip infusion.

tions produced by the bolus-plus-drip experiments, are presented in Table 1. The mean elimination rate constant ($\lambda_{01}$) was 0.0347 $\pm$ 0.0151 min.$^{-1}$. The mean rate constant for transfer from the central to the peripheral compartment ($\lambda_{12}$) was 0.948 $\pm$ 0.276 min.$^{-1}$. The mean rate constant for transfer from the peripheral to the central compartment ($\lambda_{21}$) was 0.1443 $\pm$ 0.0659 min.$^{-1}$. The mean volumes of the central and peripheral compartments ($V_1$ and $V_2$) were 0.1748 $\pm$ 0.0420 L/kg and 1.199 $\pm$ 0.061 L/kg, respectively.

The plasma concentrations of procainamide, which were produced by exponentially tapering infusion, are presented in Figure 2. The mean plasma concentrations of procainamide at 5, 30, 60, 120, and 180 minutes were 8.0 $\pm$ 1.7, 7.4 $\pm$ 1.6, 7.5 $\pm$ 1.0, 8.0 $\pm$ 1.0, and 8.8 $\pm$ 1.5 mg/L, respectively. Indicators of the accuracy of the pharmacokinetically-based infusions are presented in Table 2.

## Disopyramide

Bolus-plus-drip infusions of disopyramide produced rapid rises in plasma concentration followed by significant undershoots (Fig. 3). The pharmacokinetic characteristics for disopyramide in each dog, calculated from plasma concentrations produced by bolus-plus-drip infusions, are presented in Table 3. The mean elimi-

**Table 1**
**Pharmacokinetics of Procainamide in Dogs**

| Dog no. | $V_1$ (L/kg) | $V_2$ (L/kg) | $\lambda_{01}$ (min.$^{-1}$) | $\lambda_{12}$ (min.$^{-1}$) | $\lambda_{21}$ (min.$^{-1}$) |
|---|---|---|---|---|---|
| 1 | 0.1847 | 1.188 | 0.0342 | 1.228 | 0.1910 |
| 2 | 0.1286 | 1.264 | 0.0512 | 0.677 | 0.0689 |
| 3 | 0.2109 | 1.144 | 0.0210 | 0.939 | 0.1731 |
| Mean | 0.1748 | 1.199 | 0.0347 | 0.948 | 0.1443 |
| $\pm$ S.D. | $\pm$0.0420 | $\pm$0.061 | $\pm$0.0151 | $\pm$0.276 | $\pm$0.0659 |

Abbreviations: $V_1$ = volume of central compartment; $V_2$ = volume of peripheral compartment; $\lambda_{01}$ = rate constant for elimination; $\lambda_{12}$ = rate constant for transfer from the central to the peripheral compartment; $\lambda_{21}$ = rate constant for transfer from the peripheral to the central compartment.

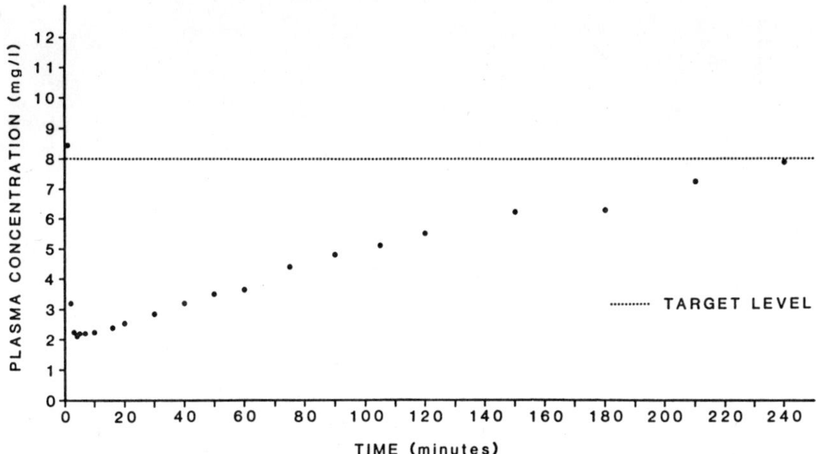


**Figure 2:** Plasma concentrations of procainamide produced in three dogs by pharmacokinetically-based, exponentially tapering infusion.

### Table 2
### Exponentially Declining Infusion of Procainamide

| Dog No. | Early Max (mg/L) | Late Max (mg/L) | Undershoot (mg/L) | Time to 90% (min) |
|---|---|---|---|---|
| 1 | 10.6 | 8.1 | 6.6 | < 1.0 |
| 2 | 8.0 | 9.2 | 6.1 | < 1.0 |
| 3 | 11.7 | 10.1 | 8.1 | < 1.0 |
| Mean ± SD | 10.1 ± 1.9 | 9.1 ± 1.0 | 6.9 ± 1.0 | < 1.0 |

Abbreviations: Early Max = maximum plasma concentration in first 5 minutes of infusion; Late Max = maximum plasma concentration following the first 5 minutes of infusion; Undershoot = minimum plasma concentration following the initial peak in plasma concentration; Time to 90% = duration of infusion required to produce a concentration of 7.2 mg/L.

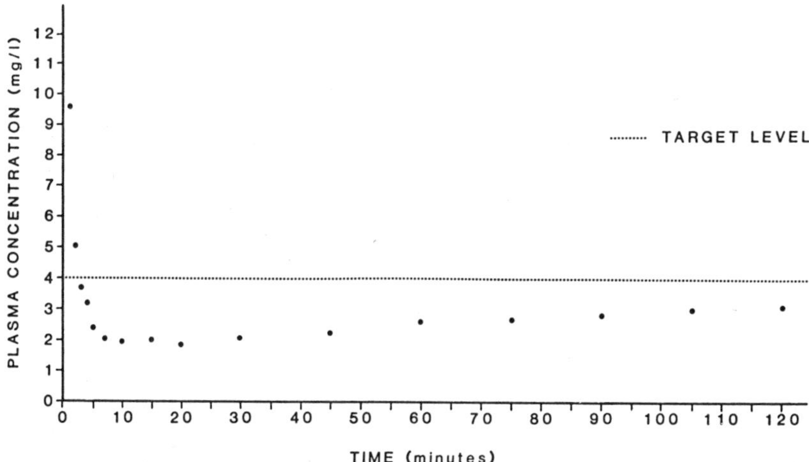


**Figure 3:** Plasma concentrations of disopyramide produced in one dog by a bolus-plus-drip infusion.

## Table 3
## Pharmacokinetics of Disopyramide in Dogs

| Dog no. | $V_1$ (L/kg) | $V_2$ (L/kg) | $\lambda_{01}$ (min.$^{-1}$) | $\lambda_{12}$ (min.$^{-1}$) | $\lambda_{21}$ (min.$^{-1}$) |
|---|---|---|---|---|---|
| 4 | 0.0882 | 1.136 | 0.1195 | 0.5983 | 0.04647 |
| 5 | 0.1127 | 2.488 | 0.1280 | 0.2876 | 0.01303 |
| 6 | 0.0787 | 1.416 | 0.1989 | 0.5467 | 0.03038 |
| 7 | 0.0541 | 0.730 | 0.1488 | 0.5879 | 0.04169 |
| 8 | 0.0793 | 2.579 | 0.0524 | 0.3252 | 0.01000 |
| Mean | 0.0826 | 1.670 | 0.1295 | 0.4691 | 0.0283 |
| ± S.D. | ± 0.0211 | ± 0.826 | ± 0.0530 | ± 0.1504 | ± 0.0165 |

Abbreviations: $V_1$ = volume of central compartment; $V_2$ = volume of peripheral compartment; $\lambda_{01}$ = rate constant for elimination; $\lambda_{12}$ = rate constant for transfer from the central to the peripheral compartment; $\lambda_{21}$ = rate constant for transfer from the peripheral to the central compartment.

nation rate constant ($\lambda_{01}$) was $0.0826 \pm 0.0211$ min.$^{-1}$. The mean rate constant for transfer from the central to the peripheral compartment ($\lambda_{12}$) was $0.4691 \pm 0.1504$ min.$^{-1}$. The mean rate constant for transfer from the peripheral to the central compartment ($\lambda_{21}$) was $0.0283 \pm 0.0165$ min.$^{-1}$. The mean volumes of the central and peripheral compartments ($V_1$ and $V_2$) were $0.0826 \pm 0.0211$ L/kg and $1.670 \pm 0.826$ L/kg respectively.

In all five dogs, the combination of 0.3 mg/kg/min. intravenous acetylcholine and a single train of atrial pacing at a cycle length of 50 ms was sufficient to induce sustained atrial fibrillation, which did not terminate until the infusion of acetylcholine was stopped or until disopyramide was administered. In all five dogs, the arrhythmia detection algorithms correctly diagnosed both sinus rhythm and atrial fibrillation.

The plasma concentrations produced by exponentially-tapering infusion are presented in Figure 4. These infusions caused termination of atrial fibrillation in all five dogs after $2.8 \pm 1.6$ minutes (Figure 5). The plasma concentrations of disopyramide at 5, 10, 30,

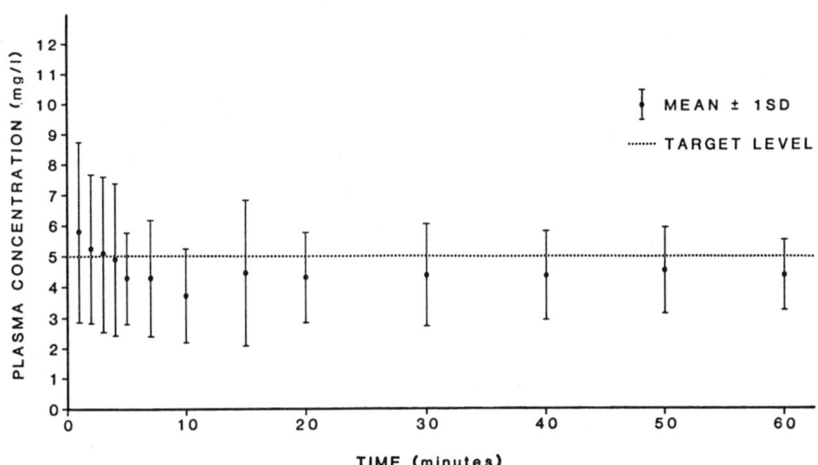



**Figure 4:** Plasma concentrations of disopyramide produced in five dogs by pharmacokinetically-based, exponentially-tapering infusion.

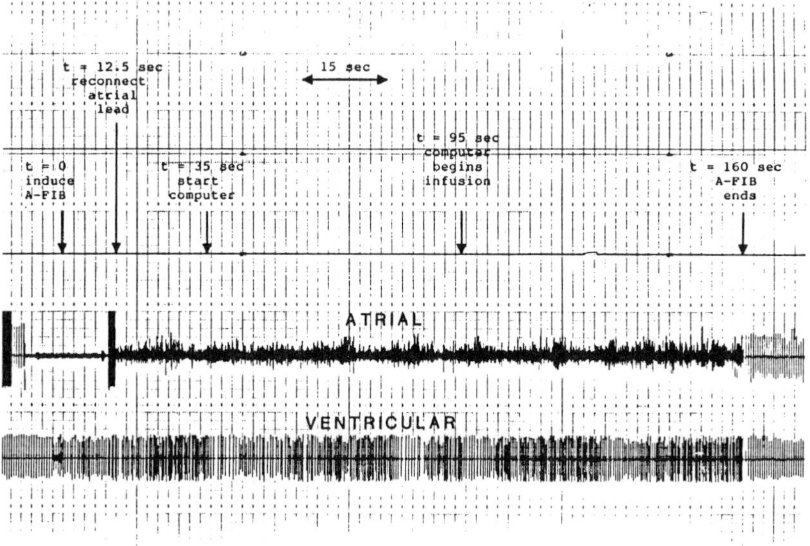


**Figure 5:** Simultaneous recordings of atrial and ventricular electrograms during termination of induced atrial fibrillation by an automatic infusion of disopyramide.

60, and 180 minutes were 4.3 ± 1.5, 3.7 ± 1.5, 4.4 ± 1.7, and 4.4 ± 1.1 mg/L, respectively. Indicators of the accuracy of the pharmacokinetically-based infusions are presented in Table 4.

## Discussion

All presently available antiarrhythmic therapies have their limitations. We believe that a significant potential role exists for an implantable device that would be capable of detecting arrhythmias and of responding by delivering a pharmacokinetically-based, exponentially-tapering infusion of antiarrhythmic drug. We have had success with detection of arrhythmias by a microprocessor-based algorithm that uses information from leads in the atrium and ventricle.[8,9] In the present study, we found that the algorithm for arrhythmia detection had no trouble in diagnosing sinus rhythm and atrial fibrillation as long as the atrial electrodes were in good position.

**Table 4**
**Exponentially Declining Infusion of Disopyramide**

| Dog No. | Early Max (mg/L) | Late Max (mg/L) | Undershoot (mg/L) | Time to 90% (min) | Conversion (Min) |
|---|---|---|---|---|---|
| 4 | 13.7 | 6.2 | 3.6 | $< 0.5$ | 5.0 |
| 5 | 6.4 | 5.2 | 3.5 | $< 1.25$ | 1.1 |
| 6 | 7.8 | 8.3 | 6.2 | $< 0.75$ | 3.1 |
| 7 | 4.4 | 3.2 | 2.4 | — | 3.5 |
| 8 | 3.6 | 4.1 | 2.2 | — | 1.3 |
| Mean $\pm$ SD | 7.2 $\pm$ 4.0 | 5.4 $\pm$ 2.0 | 3.6 $\pm$ 1.6 | — | 2.8 $\pm$ 1.6 |

Abbreviations: Same as in Table 2 except Time to 90% = duration of infusion required to produce a plasma concentration of 4.5 mg/L; Conversion = duration of infusion required to convert to sinus rhythm.

We also found that therapeutic levels of procainamide and disopyramide can be rapidly produced and can then be maintained through use of exponentially-tapering infusion. In our small series of dogs, we achieved better control over levels of procainamide than over levels of disopyramide. A possible reason for this difference could be that the dogs receiving procainamide were conscious, were not receiving anesthetics or acetylcholine, and did not have arrhythmias induced. The dogs that were given disopyramide received the same dose of acetylcholine during pharmacokinetic characterization as they received during exponential infusion, but the poorer control of disopyramide compared to procainamide might have been the result of confounding effects of anesthesia, acetylcholine, or arrhythmia. Another possibility is that the pharmacokinetic behavior of disopyramide is less well represented by a two-compartment model than is the case with procainamide.

An automatic implantable antiarrhythmic drug infusor would be particularly well suited for the management of patients with paroxysmal atrial fibrillation. Aggressive therapy against paroxysmal atrial fibrillation is justified, because persistent atrial fibrillation is associated with embolic phenomena, including stroke,[15] and is associated with an unacceptably high risk of overall mortality and cardiovascular mortality.[16,17] None of the presently available drugs, devices, or surgical techniques for paroxysmal atrial fibrillation is ideal. Chronic antiarrhythmic drug therapy is often employed for prophylaxis, but is difficult to comply with, and exposes patients to significant risks and inconvenience. Intermittent drug therapy, taken as needed for attacks of atrial fibrillation, has been suggested[18] but requires that patients be able to diagnose accurately their own cardiac rhythm. Intermittent oral drug therapy, furthermore, is limited by the lagtime between drug ingestion and drug effect; and intermittent intravenous drug therapy requires unpleasant and expensive visits to emergency rooms or doctors' offices. Implantable antitachycardia pacemakers cannot terminate atrial fibrillation, and while implantable defibrillators may be able to terminate atrial fibrillation,[19] they only do so by delivering shocks that are unpleasant for conscious patients. There is no direct surgical approach against atrial fibrillation. Many of these problems and limitations could be overcome by a device that could deliver a pharmacokinetically based, self-limited infusion of an antiarrhythmic drug in response to the presence of paroxysmal atrial fibrillation.

The present report is the first to describe the management of atrial fibrillation with automatic detection of arrhythmia followed by automatic exponential infusion of an antiarrhythmic drug. The present results are promising enough to warrant a larger scale investigation of this technique. Furthermore, since little memory is required by our programs for arrhythmia detection and exponential infusion of drug, the technique appears suitable for a programmable implantable arrhythmia detector and infusor.

This work was supported in part by a grant from the National Institutes of Health, Bethesda, Maryland: HL-32131.

---

# References


1. Mason JW, Winkle RA. (1978). Electrode-catheter arrhythmia induction in the selection and assessment of antiarrhythmic drug therapy for recurrent ventricular tachycardia. *Circulation* 58:971−985.
2. Horowitz LN, Josephson ME, Farshidi A, Spielman SR, Michelson EL, Greenspan AM. (1978). Recurrent sustained ventricular tachycardia. 3. Role of the electrophysiologic study in selection of antiarrhythmic regimens. *Circulation* 58:986−997.
3. Kerr CR, Prystowsky EN, Smith WM, Cook L, Gallagher JJ. (1982). Electrophysiologic effects of disopyramide phosphate in patients with Wolff-Parkinson-White syndrome. *Circulation* 65:869−878.

4. Kruger-Theimer E. (1968). Continuous intravenous infusion and multicompartment accumulation. *Eur Pharmaco* 4:317–324.
5. Collins SM, Arzbaecher RC. (1979). Feedback control in the management of cardiac arrhythmias. *ISA Transactions* 18:95–100.
6. Jelliffe RW. (1983). Computer-controlled administration of cardiovascular drugs. *Prog Cardiovasc Dis* 26:1–14.
7. Riddell JG, McAllister CG, Wilkinson GR, Wood AJ, Roden DM. (1984). A new method for constant plasma drug concentration: Application to lidocaine. *Ann Intern Med* 100:25–28.
8. Arzbaecher R, Bump T, Jenkins J, Glick K, Munkenbeck F, Brown J, Nandhakumar N. (1984). Automatic tachycardia recognition. *PACE* 7:541–547.
9. Munkenbeck FC, Bump TE, Arzbaecher RC. (1986). Differentiation of sinus tachycardia from paroxysmal 1:1 tachycardias using single late diastolic atrial extrastimuli. *PACE* 9:53–64.
10. Folle L, Bianchi–DeGuiria A, Baglietto J, Espinosa L, Venturini N. (1974). Standardized model for the production of experimental atrial fibrillation. *Experientia* 30:669–670.
11. Whittington J, Cross M, Raftery E. (1979). An effective conscious animal model of atrial fibrillation. *Cardiovasc Res* 13:105–112.
12. Gallagher JJ, Pritchett ELC, Benditt DG, Wallace AG. (1977). High dose disopyramide phosphate: An effective treatment for refractory ventricular tachycardia. *Circulation* 55,56:III–25.
13. Niarchos AP. (1976). Disopyramide: Serum level and arrhythmia conversion. *Am Heart J* 92:57–64.
14. Patterson E, Gibson JK, Lucchese BR. (1980). Electrophysiologic effects of disopyramide phosphate on reentrant ventricular arrhythmia in conscious dogs after myocardial infraction. *Am J Cardiol* 46:792–799.
15. Wolf PA, Dawber TR, Thomas HE, Kannel WB. (1978). Epidemiological assessment of chronic atrial fibrillation and risk of stroke: The Framingham study. *Neurology* 28:973–977.
16. Gajewski J, Singer R. (1981). Mortality in an insured population with atrial fibrillation. *JAMA* 245:1540–1544.
17. Kannel W, Abbott R, Savage D, McNamara P. (1982). Epidemiologic features of chronic atrial fibrillation. *N Engl J Med* 306:1018–1022.
18. Margolis B, DeSilva RA, Lown B. (1980). Episodic drug treatment in the management of paroxysmal arrhythmias. *Am J Cardiol* 45:621–626.
19. Reid P, Mower M, Mirowski M, Watkins L, Juanteguy J, Platia E, Griffin L. (1983). Correction of atrial tachyarrhythmias with the automatic implantable cardioverter defibrillator. *Circulation* 68:III–4.

# Chapter 24

# Chronobiologic Engineering

Franz Halberg

## Introduction

This paper introduces the fledgling science of chronobiology very briefly, but with extensive references. It then illustrates the importance of this science for engineering aimed at health care.

Chronobiology deals with the cyclic patterns that occur in all living organisms and explores the relationships of these rhythms to prediction, prevention, diagnosis, and treatment of diseases or abnormalities more broadly. Virtually all organisms exhibit about-daily (circadian) cycles of body core and surface temperature and of chemical variables in blood, urine, and tissues. Several decades of research worldwide have established that medical diagnoses can be subject to a much higher proportion of false positives and false negatives when only single samples are taken at arbitrary times of the day instead of taking rhythms into account. Moreover, treatments (radiation, chemotherapy, and other medications) have been shown to have markedly different efficacy and safety depending upon the pattern of administration within the day.

Many persons believe that medicine stands on the threshold of a revolution in diagnosis and treatment, based on the combination of several emerging technologies, including chronobiologic under-

From: Ensminger WD, Selam JL (eds): *Infusion Systems in Medicine*. Mount Kisco, NY, Futura Publishing Co., Inc.,©1987.

standing of the health effect of rhythms; availability of portable, personal, long-term ambulatory monitors of biologic variables such as blood pressure, the ECG, or EEG undergoing changes that recur spontaneously and as responses; availability of database systems to acquire and analyze volumes of data obtained from personal monitors; availability of statistical procedures to analyze and model the biologic rhythms and from them to devise optimal dosage time patterns for specific individuals; availability of portable, programmed devices to administer therapy, e.g., by physiologic rate-adjusted cardiac pacemakers or drug pumps.

These developments represent an exciting potential for engineering and health-care personnel both in research and in practical applications. The employment of chronobiologic methods in routine medical screening, diagnosis, prognosis, treatment, and, most important, disease prevention, remains a challenge to be met.

*Chronobiology is not only:*

1. A naked eye study in time plots of *physiologic variation,* encountered at all organization levels, from molecular over organismic to ecologic, in microorganisms, unicells, and pluricellulars, including human beings[1-67];

2. The critical *control* in all of biology, namely the requirement that one takes ubiquitous rhythms into account once one realizes their critical pertinence to any cost-effective biologic test[3,4];

3. An added indispensable, objective, computer-aided inferential statistical estimation of the characteristics of *biologic trends* with development and aging,[7] including changes recurring with a broad mathematical spectrum of frequencies, the (algorithmically) validated *rhythms*[4,8];

4. A generally applicable biologic methodology including, with the *design* of conditions for data sampling and analyses in ordinary as well as special lighting and other *environments,*[17,43-46] the computer-aided *hardware* and *software* for *data collection*[36,47] as well as for chronobiometry;

5. A set of procedures for biologic, including medical research and practice yielding improved old and new dynamic endpoints, e.g., for human blood pressure or ciruclating hormones. A single measure and a mean of casual measures with its standard error are the currently used endpoints. A midline-estimating statistic of rhythm, the MESOR, M, a rhythm-adjusted mean, is usually more reliable than the conventional mean based on casual samples. As

compared to the mean, the M is usually associated with a smaller standard error since part of the overall variability is assigned in *chronobiometry* to added endpoints. These are the period(s) ($\tau$) of rhythms and, at each $\tau$, measures of extent and timing of change, the amplitude, A, and acrophase, 0, of the fundamental $\tau$, as well as the (A,Ø)s of the harmonics of each $\tau$ that together with the characteristics of the fundamental $\tau$, quantify the waveform[4,41−43];

6. A basis for medical or other action based on *statistical inference* yielding probabilities (P-values) describing the reliability of findings for the given *individual*. With each endpoint of rhythm, a standard error is computed and (in view of the availability of the chronobiologic time series [rather than single measurements]), one can then test for the statistical significance of any changes—in any one or several of the rhythm characteristics—for the given individual[63,64];

7. An approach resolving some of the individual's *interactions with the socioecologic environment*, such as physiologic synchronization or desynchronization, frequency division and/or multiplication, variance transposition or rhythm scrambling (dissimilation) in the face of complex (circadian-circaseptan-circannual) schedules in shiftwork[25] or transmeridian travel[26];

8. The resolution of *rhythms* with periods that are only an approximate (*circa* = about) match of environmental cycles, and that under conditions of isolation differ (usually with statistical significance) from their environmental counterparts, e.g., the solar day, lunar day, lunar month, and solar year. Such free-running periods, whether they are discovered after a manipulation of the environment[17,18] or of the organism,[19−21] represent a first indirect line of evidence for the heritability of *circa*-rhythms. Their periods are of about one day, the *circadians*[3,4]; of about a week, the *circaseptans*[21−23]; of about one month, the *circatrigintans*[24]; and of about a year, the *circannuals*[18]);

9. A way to *quantify health positively*, inside the range of usual variation, by measuring, e.g., blood pressure rhythm characteristics and other changes such as trends (rather than indicating only the absence of unusual values [outside the "normal range"] and/or the absence of signs and symptoms of overt disease)[60,62−64];

10. A way to assess the *risks* of developing diseases such as breast cancer, alcoholism, other chemical dependencies, anxiety, and cardio-, cerebro-, certain reno-, and retinovascular diseases. Constellations of rhythm stage-dependent endocrine and systemic classifiers may serve for this purpose[63−66];

11. A paradigm of *preventive medicine*, e.g., with assessment, already in the newborn, of the risk of developing high blood pressure later in life, by the half-hourly monitoring for 48 hours of blood pressure and heart rate, followed by chronobiometry, which allows the separation by the circadian amplitude of groups of newborns with a positive versus negative family history of high blood pressure[37,39,63];

12. A way toward *self-help* in preventive as well as in medically guided curative health care, by individuals whatever their ethnic or socioeconomic background, whether they dispose only of traditional or also of modern tools. Once data collection and interpretation with modern tools is accomplished in research, the use of traditional tools can proceed in the light of experience gained with new technology[36];

13. A study of time-patterned *variation in pathology*. Pertinent examples abound in human medicine, such as nocturnal versus diurnal blood pressure elevation,[10,63] epilepsy,[11,12] asthma,[13] or filariasis[14];

14. A basis for *screening*, e.g., of deviant blood pressure, such as a deviant timing or extent of change in odd-hour hypertension or circadian amplitude-hypertension[10,63];

15. A basis for *diagnosis*, e.g., of Addison's disease or Cushing's syndrome by sampling blood for circulating cortisol in the morning or evening, respectively[60];

16. A basis for *prognosis*, e.g., of hypercortisolism,[61] accelerated blood pressure elevation, or sudden, presumably cardiac death,[62] by reliance on rhythm characteristics, rather than only a mean of casual time-unspecified measurements of blood pressure;

17. A way to optimize the *utilization of calories*, exploiting different effects upon body weight gain, e.g., as a function of consuming all daily calories within one hour of awakening or not before 12 hours after awakening[4,51];

18. A dimension for classical chemical and physical *treatment modes*, e.g., of cancer by timed radiotherapy,[57] of high blood pressure with beta-blocking agents or diuretics,[10,63] of asthma with corticosteroids,[58] and a host of other conditions, with timing complementary to dosing[57,59];

19. A *focus* on the eminently multifrequency rhythmic immune system[58] and its earliest changes as it erodes toward diseases such as cancer or the acquired immune deficiency syndrome (AIDS). Since many individuals who carry an infectious agent, e.g., a virus,

do not exhibit overt pathology, one might speculate that one of the larger challenges of our day for *chronoimmunopharmacology* lies in the particular field of (about-daily, -weekly, -monthly, and -yearly) rhythmically recurring deficits in immunity and their chronobiologic mechanism;

20. A way to reduce if not avoid the *toxicity*[52-58] of physical stimuli, such as radiation or a host of drugs. Cases in point are the cardiac drug ouabain, corticosteroids, psychiatric normalizers, anesthetic agents, and cancer chemotherapy with agents such as doxorubicin, cisplatin, arabinosyl cytosin, vincristine, cyclophosphamide, and melphalan. The body's resistance to many other kinds of agents is documented to undergo rhythmic change;

21. A set of mechanisms for multiple rhythmic interactions, the so-called *feedsidewards in biologic networks*,[4,44,45] that substitute for oversimplified feedbacks in axes. Feedsidewards represent interactions among three or more physiologic entities and result in several orders of (a) spontaneous, (b) reactive, (c) modulatory, and (d) harmonically frequency-dividing and/or -multiplying rhythms. When these rhythms are isolated outside the body, they are referred to as $\alpha$-, $\beta$-, $\gamma$- and $\delta$-rhythms; the latter two categories of rhythms can account for directionally different yet predictably recurring effects, e.g., amplification, no-effect and attenuation, for instance, of hormone production or action[48-50];

22. A study of feedsideward-derived *chronomodulation*, consisting of effects as different as stimulation versus inhibition of DNA synthesis in healthy bone by the same hormone analogue[49] or the acceleration versus retardation of tumor growth by an immunotherapeutic agent,[43,50] in both cases as a function of the timing of agent administration;

23. A focus by *genetic engineering*, e.g., on mutants of fruit flies that lack a circadian rhythm and exhibit it again after gene transfer[5,6] by examining the extent of reconstitution of circadians in a broader ultradian-to-infradian rhythm spectrum[28,29];

24. A focus on *heritability*, e.g., of circadians, by studies on monozygotic twins reared apart, demonstrating that within-twin-pair differences in rhythm characteristics are smaller than among-twin-pair differences, notwithstanding the different geographic environments in which the twins were brought up and continue to live until the time of study[27];

25. A view of the *Darwinian evolution* of species that acquired a time structure of rhythms, in health as well as disease, including

some rhythmic changes that represent an apparent match of geophysical environmental periodicities, such as the day, month, and year[15,16];

26. A way to look at an *internal evolution* of life on earth as a feature not only of environmental adaptation but also of integration within a microorganism, unicell, or pluricellular organism. For instance, circaseptan time structures that have no known geophysical environmental counterpart, are encountered in the time to death from natural or experimental infections,[30] in the time to the rejection of mammalian transplants[32–34] (in multiples of about seven days), the blood pressure of the human newborn,[37,39] and the response patterns to shifts of environmental cycles[2,31,32];

27. A fledgling *science* in its own right with a substantial body of stimulating if as yet incomplete facts, integrated by unifying mechanisms such as cephaloendocrine and cellular feedsidewards and chronomodulation, leading to new principles such as internal evolution, and offering procedures for various applications throughout human and veterinary medicine, animal husbandry, agriculture, and other fields of biology.

Chronobiology is all of these.

## Illustrative Chronobiologic Challenge to Engineering Chronotherapy

The right devices for chronotherapy must be portable and miniaturized so that they do not interfere with daily life.[69–78] Moreover, the devices should be programmable, so that in a day and age of real problems in compliance, one relies on modern technology rather than on the patient's discipline and memory. Totally implantable devices for drug infusion are becoming available, are replacing the bulky infusion machine and may be better-tolerated than external pumps.[78]

The question then arises from the viewpoint of chronobiology whether drug administration should be continuous or patterned. Continuous administration does not result in constant blood concentrations, since drug metabolism, interactions, and excretion are all periodic.[34,36,59] Rather than aiming at drug concentrations that relate only to the aforementioned factors, a rational approach can be used, derived from studies on experimental animals.

One method for testing anticancer treatments in the laboratory is to administer a drug every three hours over a 24-hour span in order to bathe the body frequently if not continually with the anti-cancer substance, and thus to catch any cancer cells that might enter a certain drug-sensitive stage of their cell division cycles. The drug then has the best chance to inhibit or kill the cancer cell. Unfortunately, healthy tissue is also destroyed by the drug. This results in undesired, life-threatening damage, e.g., to the bone marrow, along with the desired reduction in number of cancer cells. The abstract Figures 1 and 2 portray the available evidence and

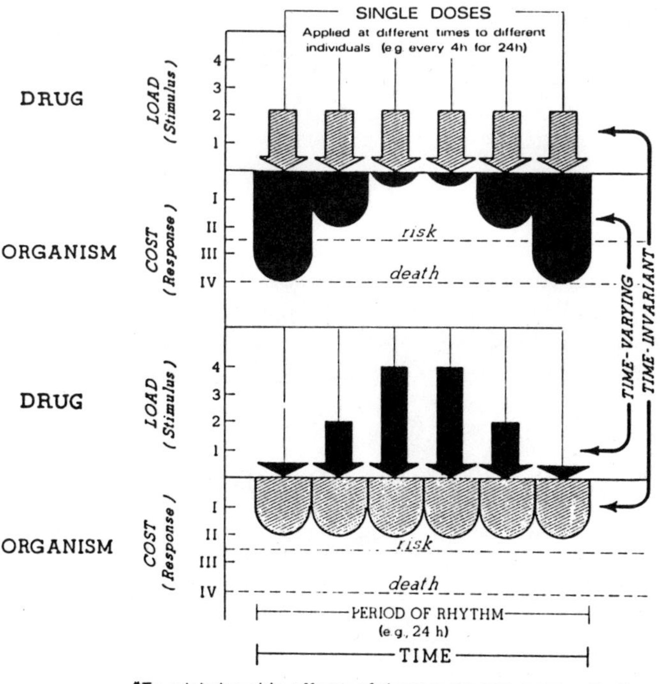



**Figure 1:** Abstract schemes representing a wealth of information on the importance of rhythm stage in the outcome of a desired or undesired response, including death. © 1973 by Halberg.[8,55]

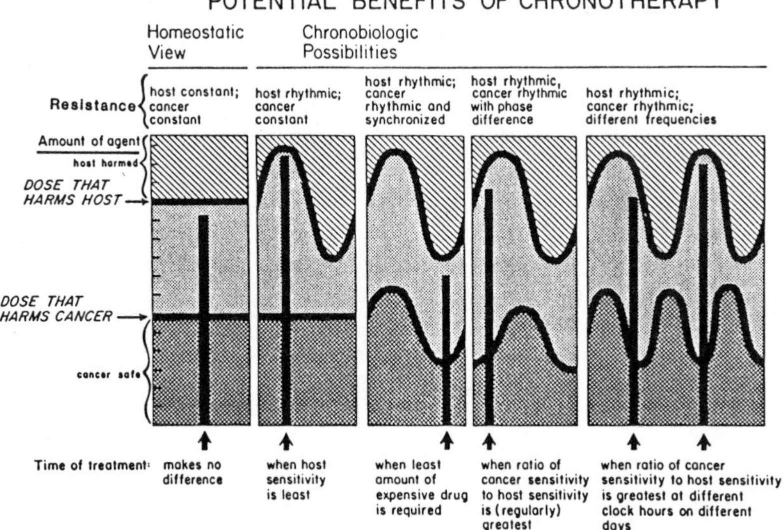


**Figure 2:** Further abstract summaries of decades of work from many laboratories documenting the rational basis of cancer chronotherapy. © 1973 by Halberg.[8,55]

rationale underlying chronotherapy in general. It is well known for many agents, including drugs, that a given dose of a potentially harmful agent can be tolerated better at one time than at another time. It seems reasonable, therefore, to vary dosing with timing (Fig. 3).

## Chronotherapy via the Drug Pump

An implantable and externally programmable pump such as that in Figures 4 through 8 was used on 21 outbred beagle dogs to administer cyclosporine with one of several circadian sinusoidal schedules or at a constant rate. The dogs were kept in 12 h of light alternating with 12 h of darkness. This experiment is described in part in Figure 9.[34-36] Untreated dogs only live for 5 to 7 days (not shown). This average of about six days can be improved by treatment with cyclosporine, as shown in Figure 9. Four animals suffice to document the point of a statistically significant improvement

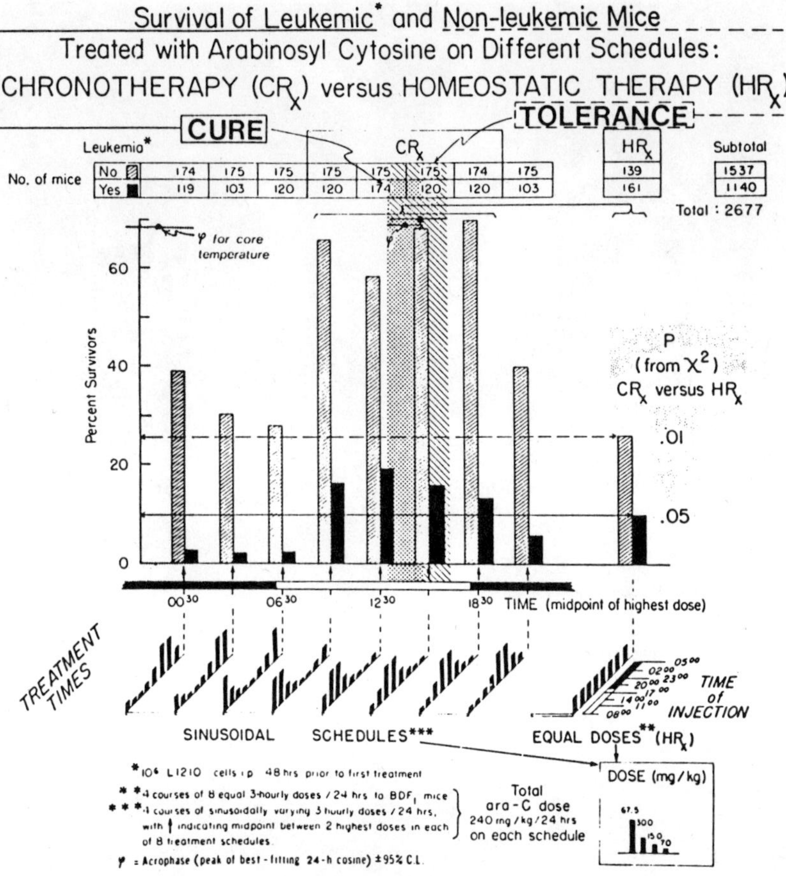



**Figure 3:** Homeostatic (equal-dose) versus chronobiologic (sinusoidal) treatment of leukemia. The stage of circadian rhythms at the time of exposure to a fixed dose of a potentially noxious stimulus (including antimitotic agents) dramatically tips the scale between death and survival. Such observations were made under standardized conditions, including continuous darkness, to document that rhythms were not simply a function of the lighting regimen or of the time of day. On the basis of such results, a chronotherapy of cancer was considered promising. Several chronobiologists met with a group from the National Cancer Institute (USA) early in the 1970s to draw up acceptable rules for testing the effectiveness of chronotherapy on laboratory animals. It was decided to compare survival times following the administration of an anticancer drug, ara-C, given in four courses of homeostatic (fixed-dose) versus chronobiologic (sinusoidally-varying dose) schedules. This study demonstrated that chronotherapy with ara-C as compared to conventional therapy was less toxic when tested on intact mice and was superior in prolonging the survival time of leukemic mice.[55] This figure summarizes an early study on both tolerance and cure rate. © 1973 by Halberg.[55]

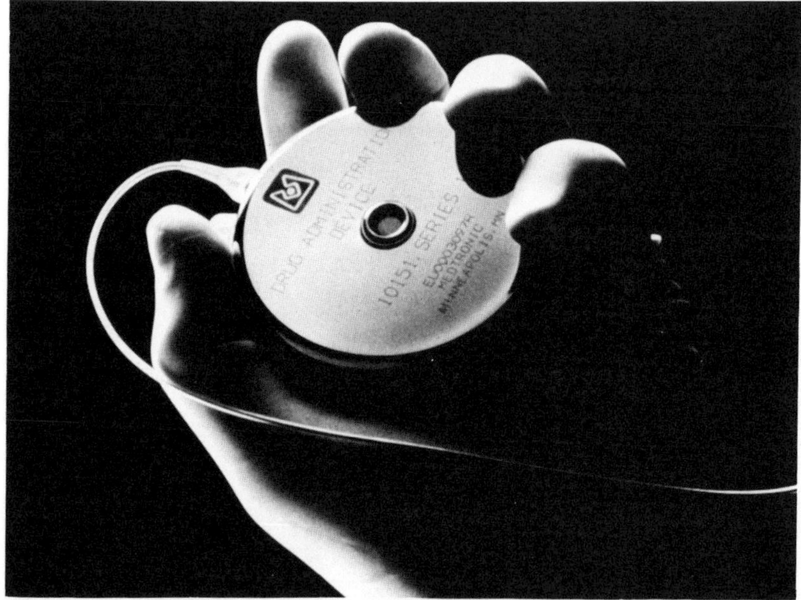


**Figure 4:** Hand-held implantable externally programmable Medtronic pump. Courtesy of Medtronic Inc., Minneapolis, MN.

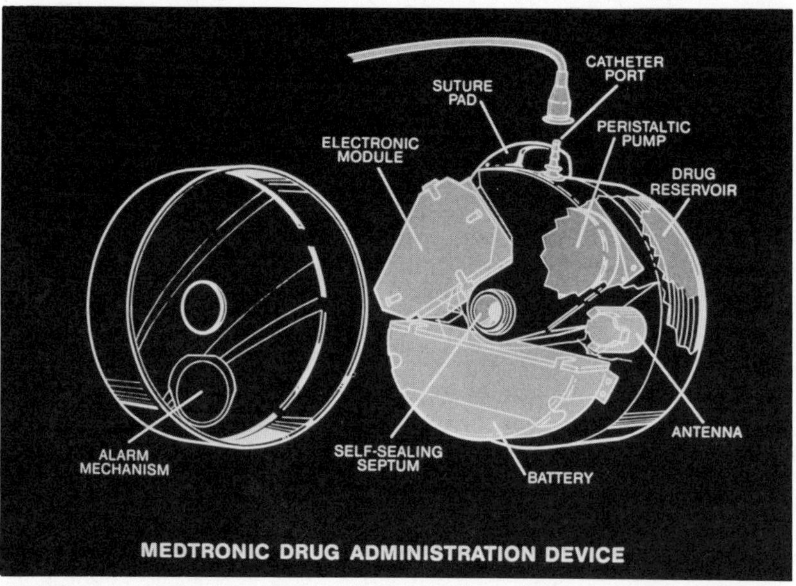


**Figure 5:** Exploded internal view of an implantable drug administration pump.

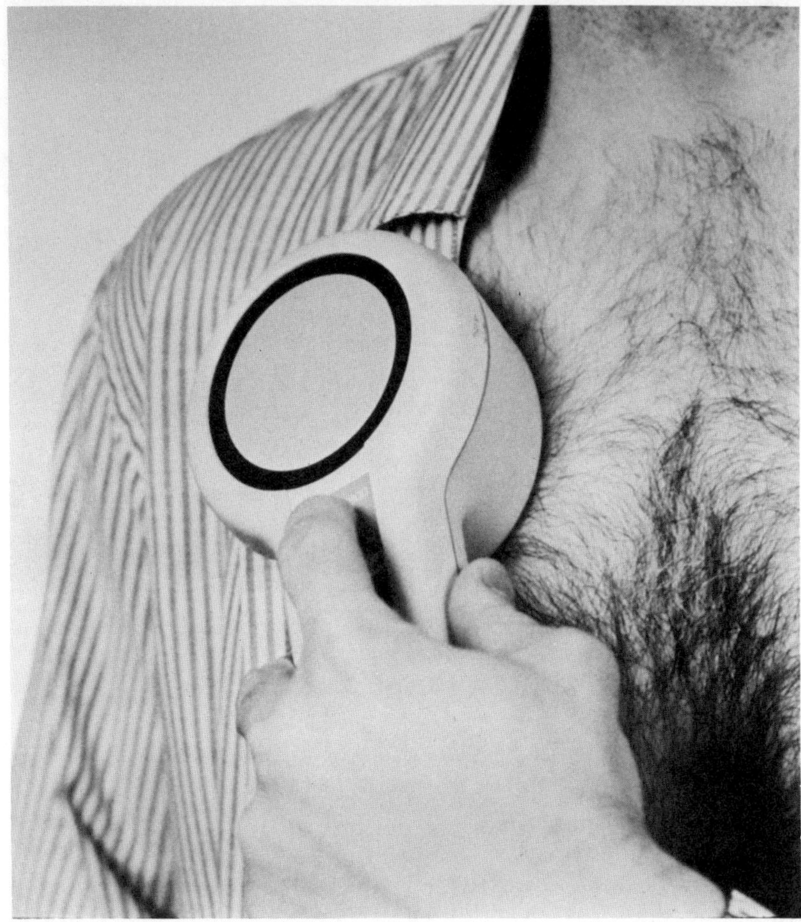

**Figure 6:** Illustrative programmer WAND location for telemetry link to an implanted pump.

from cyclosporine given by continuous infusion, as compared to the nine untreated dogs ($P < 0.01$).[36] This improvement is kept to a modest prolongation so as not to unduly prolong the suffering of the animals and the cost. Against these two reference standards (one from untreated dogs, the other from dogs treated with cyclosporine infused at a constant rate), the results obtained with the sinusoidal schedules given via the drug pump can be compared. With the pump and programmer described in Figures 4 through 7,

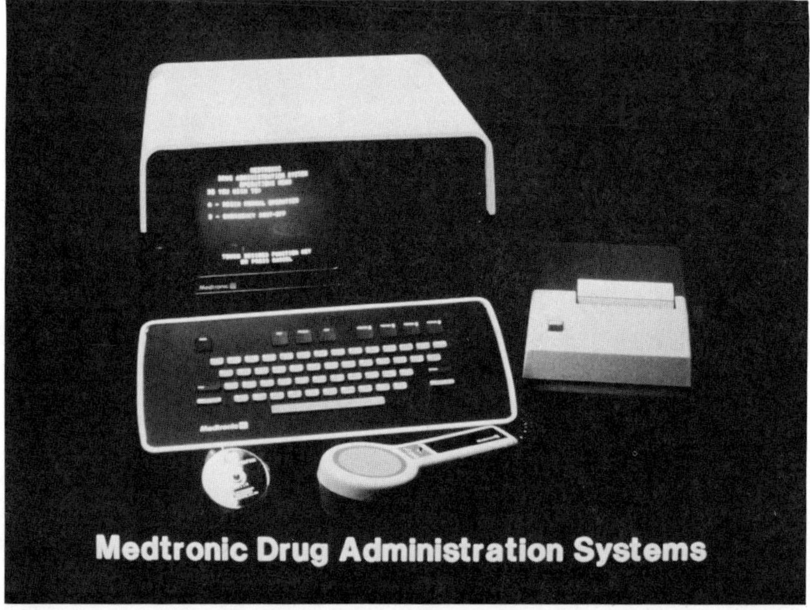



**Figure 7:** External programmer of implantable pump, used to vary rate of cyclosporine (or any other) infusion according, e.g., to circadian quasi-sinusoidal schedules (see Figure 14).

one can indeed implement the several sinusoidal schedules shown in the bottom half of Figure 9 (cf. also complex schedule in Fig. 8). The sinusoidal timing of cyclosporine consisted of gradually increasing and then decreasing doses. Different dogs received the peak daily dose at a preselected circadian stage. Daily treatment with a sinusoid peaking at the right time, shortly after the middle of the daily dark span, greatly increased the effect obtained as compared to the effect of the same daily dose injected at a constant rate or injected with the sinusoidal schedule peaking at the wrong time (during the light span in the laboratory).

Figure 10 introduces the results from the application cosinor of the method of data analysis[8,41,42] by showing the 24-h cosine curve best fitting the data obtained with different sinusoidal schedules (shown in Fig. 9). With the fit shown in Figure 10, one can test whether the amplitude of the fitted cosine curve is likely to be zero. In rejecting the zero-amplitude assumption (result not shown), the rhythm can indeed be validated, as is the case for the results on

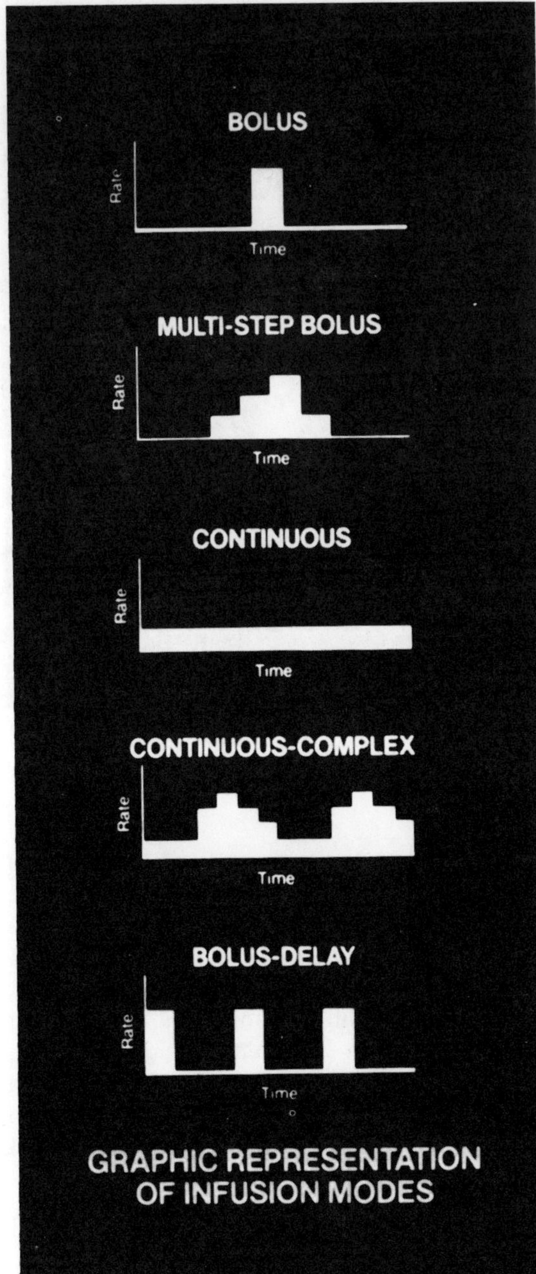


**Figure 8:** Comparison of various modes of operation of an implantable pump. The continuous complex mode is not complex enough if it is to accommodate at least circadian and circaseptan intermodulations (see text).

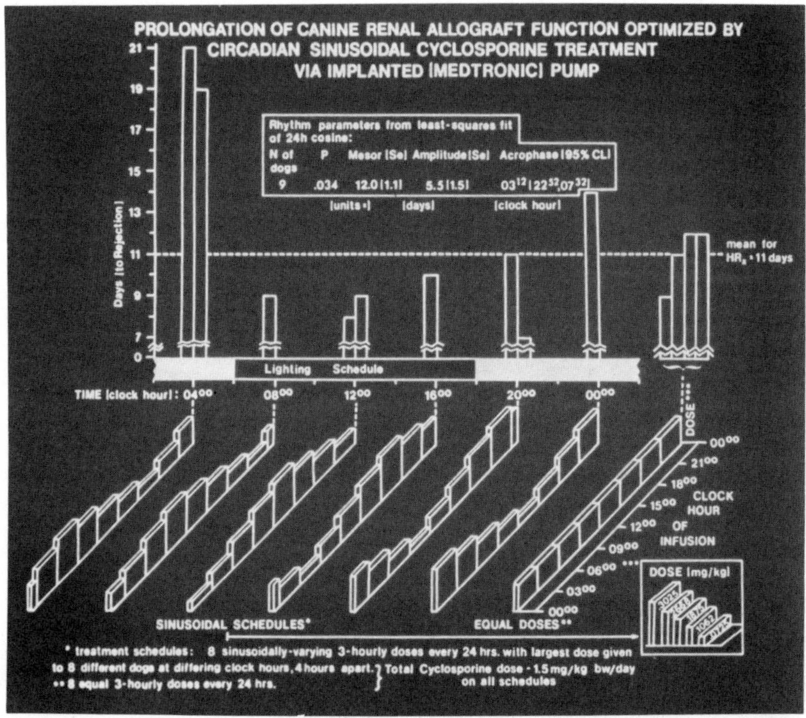


**Figure 9:** Treatment with sinusoidally varying doses, with different time location of high and low doses, has different effects. Studies by Cavallini et al.[34–36]

cyclosporine in this figure. One can then proceed to an estimation of rhythm characteristics, also shown in Figure 10; it can be seen that the amplitude is of 5.23 days. This amplitude is one-half of the total predictable change due to the organism's rhythmic response, i.e., the extent of change that can be exploited by drug timing. The double amplitude or the total predictable change (not the range of overall variability) is 10 days. The best treatment time derived from these results is also given by the acrophase, an indication of the lag from some arbitrary zero-time (in this case midnight) of the peak in the curve best-approximating all data. It does appear that this best time is 2h, 24 min. after the time reference (i.e., after midnight).

Figure 11 shows the results already shown in Figures 9 and 10 in a different way, namely along polar coordinates, as a step toward the estimation of the uncertainty of the joint rhythm characteristics.

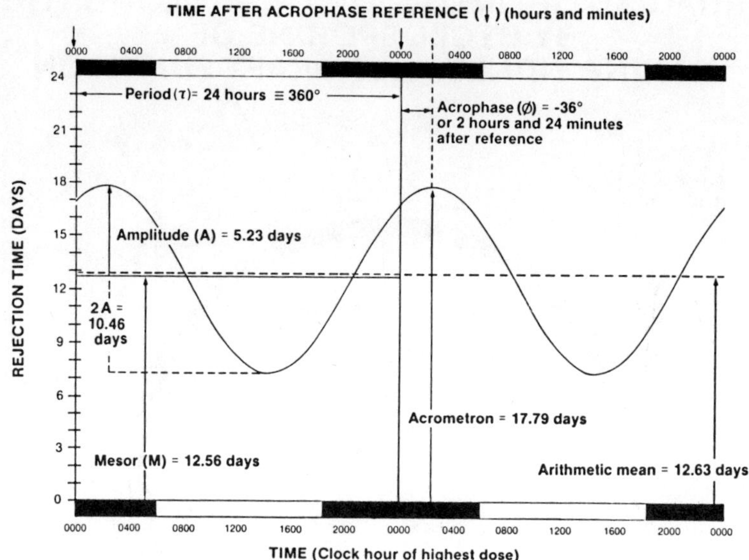


**Figure 10:** A presentation of rhythm parameters, estimated by the 24-h cosine curve fit, approximates the extent of gain or loss with timing. Studies by Cavallini et al.[34-36]

These characteristics are displayed on a clockface. Midnight is shown on top, noon at the bottom, and 6 a.m. and 6 p.m. are shown on the sides. Negative degrees are shown in a clockwise fashion so that midnight corresponds to 0°, 0600 to −90°, noon to −180°; other times are readily computed if it is realized that 360° are equated to 24 hours, 15° to 1 hour and hence 1° to 4 minutes. A confidence region for the uncertainty of the best time for highest concentrations of the sinusoidal cyclosporine schedule is also represented, in Figure 12, as the elliptical region around the tip of the vector representing the amplitude-acrophase pair.

Once the cyclosporine sinusoid peaking at night was known to be associated with best results, whereas a sinusoid peaking around noon yielded the worst results, two different treatment times were used for follow-up work with oral doses aimed to check on the degree of generality of the result. These were so chosen that one led to blood concentrations that peaked at the anticipated best circadian stage (around 0230); the second peaked about 12 hours later, at the anticipated worst circadian stage. By the choice of these oral

# CIRCADIAN OPTIMIZATION OF PROLONGATION BY CYCLOSPORINE OF CANINE KIDNEY ALLOGRAFT FUNCTION

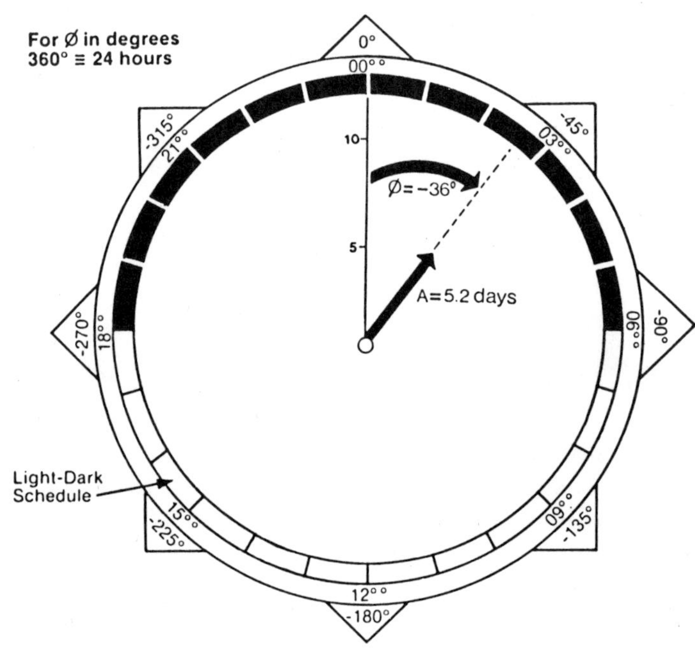


**Figure 11:** Rhythm parameters are given in polar plot as length and angle of a vector. Studies by Cavallini et al.[34-36]

treatment times, allowance was made for differences in route of administration, for reproducing the time courses of the desired and the undesired cyclosporine concentrations in blood. Pharmacokinetic studies indicated that the intended timing of changing blood concentrations was indeed achieved.[34,36]

This follow-up study on kidney-allografted dogs validated, with the oral administration of cyclosporine, the results obtained earlier by the use of the pump. As a start, 10 dogs were paired; each had one kidney removed and discarded, while the other kidney was removed and transplanted into its partner in the pair. Within each pair, one dog was assigned to one treatment time while the other

## CIRCADIAN OPTIMIZATION OF PROLONGATION
## BY CYCLOSPORINE OF
## CANINE KIDNEY ALLOGRAFT FUNCTION

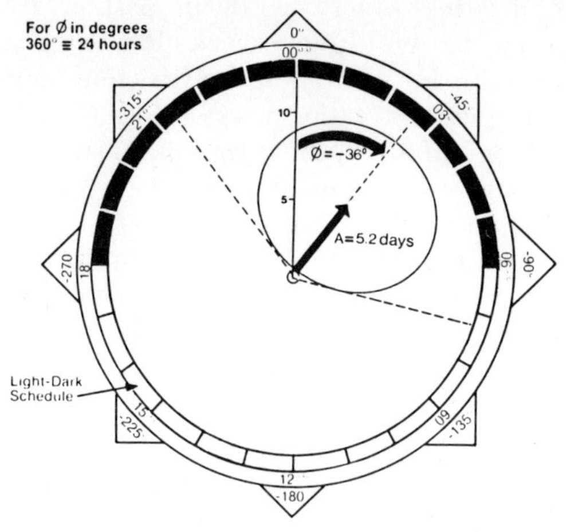


| P | No. Obs. | PR | Mesor SE (Days to Rejection) | Amplitude(A) (95% CL) | Acrophase(Ø) |
|---|---|---|---|---|---|
| 0.041 | 8 | 72 | 12.6   1.1 | 5.2   (.3,10.2) | -36° (-321,-108) |

P = Probability of hypothesis:   Amplitude = 0;   No. obs. = Number of observations
PR = Percent Rhythm (percentage of variability accounted for by cosine curve)
95% CL = Conservative 95% confidence limits derived from cosinor ellipse

**Figure 12:** Uncertainty of parameters is shown by 95% confidence region. Studies by Cavallini et al.[34–36]

was assigned to the other treatment time. In an attempt to delay, if not prevent, the transplanted kidney from being rejected, cyclosporine was given orally once each day for as long as the kidney functioned. One dog in each pair received the drug at 0830 every day, while the second dog received the drug at 2030.

Treatment notwithstanding, all dogs receiving cyclosporine in the morning had rejected their grafted kidney by 10 days after surgery. Rejections in this group started as early as 6 days after surgery and were roughly comparable to those of the earlier series. Of the five dogs treated in the evening, the predicted right time, only one dog had rejected the transplanted kidney at 15 days after surgery. Even in this case, there is a 50% increase over the longest graft survival time for dogs receiving the drug in the same dose in the morning (at the wrong treatment time). The grafts in the other four dogs treated in the evening (at the right time) were still functioning at the time of the first summary. One of these dogs had lived for more than a month after surgery, while its partner, treated at the wrong time, had rejected within one week after surgery. These statistically highly significant results on the first five pairs were confirmed by follow-up work on other pairs of dogs (Fig. 13[35,36]).

A high-technology product, the drug pump, served in this case as a tool for therapy research leading the way toward a conventional (oral) therapy mode optimized according to circadian rhythms. It has been shown in the interim, however, that much added gain can be derived from a therapy with cyclosporine also optimized according to built-in about-7-day circaseptan rhythms. When multiple circadian and circaseptan patterns, Figure 14, are to be adminis-

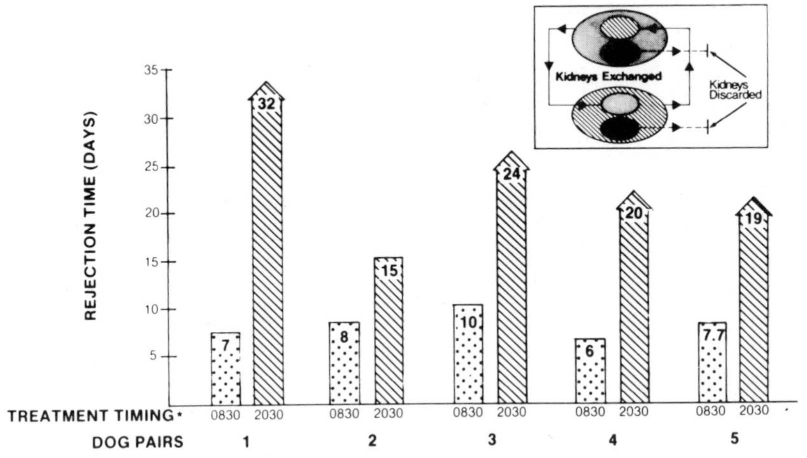


**Figure 13:** In dogs kept in light from 0600 to 1800, treated either at 0830 or at 2030 with a single daily oral dose of 12.5 mg/kg cyclosporine, the evening dose is over twice as effective as the morning dose in prolonging kidney allograft function. A pharmacokinetic difference is not detected at these particular treatment times. Studies by Cavallini et al.[34-36]

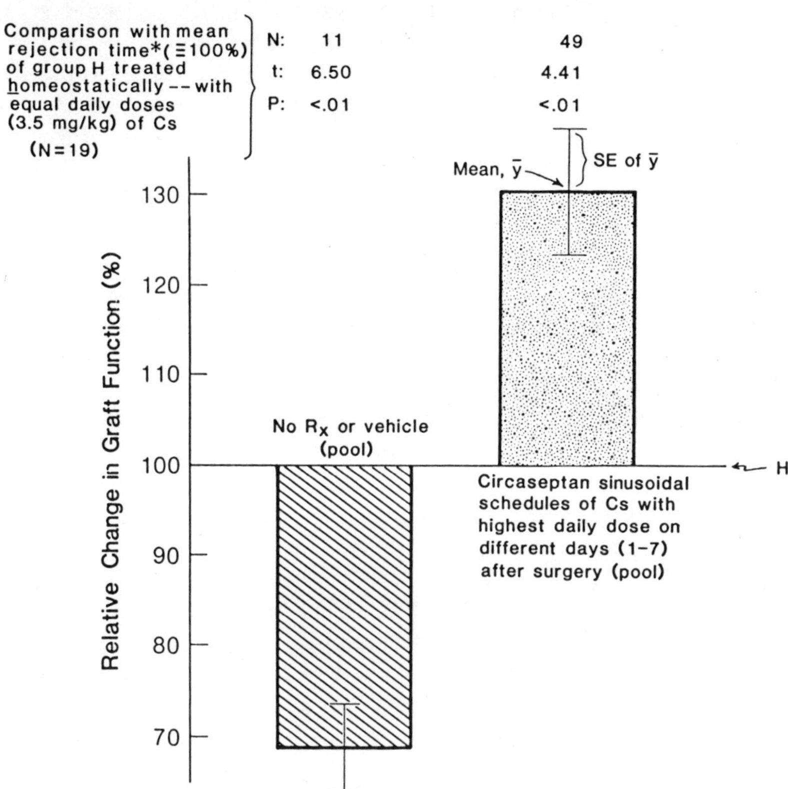



**Figure 14:** As compared to treatment with equal daily doses, circaseptan dosing schedules (that vary quasi-sinusoidally with a 7-day cycle, irrespective of the timing of the highest dose) prolong graft function.

tered, drug pumps become an indispensable tool. In combination with the use of marker rhythms, they can provide the properly timed "peaks and valleys" in drug concentration, as these are needed for an optimal therapeutic effect (Figs. 13 and 14).

For some of the work with ara-C in Figure 3, a former laboratory staff member, an Olympic runner (he had to be one!), administered the sinusoidal drug patterns. His effort was considerable: he injected 270 mice within 180 minutes; that is, he injected each mouse within less than 60 seconds. At this feverish pace, he continued reinjecting these groups of 270 mice every three hours, for 48 hours. He repeated this 48-hour marathon after a rest day for three more cycles. Even his stamina would not have sufficed for the addition of a second, about-7-day, (circaseptan) pattern to the circadian one. The same demanding patterns, however, are now easily and automatically implemented in the patient by an implantable externally programmable pump. Indeed, more complex schedules than a single set of increasing and decreasing doses during 24 hours can and should be given with the pump in view of the exhaustive evidence documenting the clinical importance of circadian-circaseptan intermodulation.[35,36]

The next task is to administer drugs according to marker rhythms monitored automatically. Monitored information should be analyzed as one goes, and results of analyses should govern the pattern of drug administration. This "closing of the loop" between the dispenser (the pump) and the sensor (of the organism) constitutes a desirable development. As yet only a limited number of marker rhythms, such as those of the ECG, EEG, blood pressure, respiration, motor activity, and body temperature can be monitored automatically around the clock. The need to collect data manually is now eliminated in these instances, but the need to analyze them automatically remains. Even with this qualification, marker rhythmometry is particularly useful when the period of a patient's pertinent rhythm(s) is different from precisely 24 hours, as can be the case for electrocardiographic abnormality.[36] The data from ambulatory monitoring devices have to be properly analyzed to test the possible merits of various applications in fields including, among others, cardiology and immunology as well as cancer. Eventually, there may be pacemaker−pump systems for properly scheduled, i.e., timed electrical and pharmacologic combination treatment. It seems reasonable to suggest, on the basis of available evidence, that all treatment should be timed, in any event.

# Another Challenge to Chronobioengineering:  A Blood Pressure and Related Cardiovascular Summary, the Sphygmochron*

The range of blood pressure variability in health is as large as (or even larger than) the difference between systolic and diastolic pressure. When analyzed chronobiologically, part of this variability is predictable in that it can be objectively characterized by sensitive parameters of extent (the amplitude) and timing (the acrophase and, in the case of long series, the period) of rhythmic change. Although part of this predictable or rhythmic variability occurs with changes in activity or posture, the circadian blood pressure rhythm persists in recumbency.[63]

The great variation in blood pressure was recognized before the turn of the century; chronobiologists have long advocated that part of this variability can be rendered predictable by assessing rhythm characteristics. This task can be aided by modern instrumentation for monitoring and analysis. The issue of whether one should rely on manual or automatic blood pressure measurement is being discussed, however, apart from assessing any predictable variability, as a matter of cost-effectiveness. The availability of new instrumentation prompts the question of whether it is worth monitoring around the clock to obtain a more reliable mean rather than a casual pressure. From a chronobiologic viewpoint, a much broader issue is not only how, but also how often and when to measure and whether to interpret data *homeostatically* or *chronobiologically*.[79]

*Homeostasis* focuses upon *the* blood pressure, relying on casual measurements such as those recommended in the World Health Organization (WHO) Guidelines. For a test of a mild blood pressure elevation, defined as 90−104 mmHg diastolic, without organ damage and "to provide a safe classification of patients," the International Society of Hypertension joins WHO in recommending the criterion of the mean of two (casual) diastolic measurements. If the mean of these is 90 mmHg or above, further measurement pairs on at least two further days over four weeks are recommended. If the mean values of these are above 100 mmHg, drug treatment is to start. If in turn these means are below 100 mmHg, further measure-

---

*Sphygmo−:* of or relating to the circulating pulse, notably blood pressure; *chronos:* time.

ments over three months and behavioral intervention, but not drug treatment, are recommended. If the overall mean is now above 95 mmHg, drug treatment is recommended; if the mean is below 95 mmHg, behavioral intervention is prescribed with further observations over three months. It is left to the individual to pick the time of measurements.

*Chronobiology* focuses upon both the predictable and the global dynamics of *the variation in blood pressure* and detects pressure elevations that are likely to be missed if one measures at only one or another convenient time of day. Some treated or untreated cases show elevations during odd hours when measurements, as a rule, are not taken. To detect such cases, systematic manual or preferably automatic around-the-clock measurement is required. With such series available, one takes into account a usually large circadian variation that, under ambulatory conditions in clinically healthy North American men, averages well over 60 mmHg systolic and over 50 mmHg diastolic. Part of this variation is resolved as predictably rhythmic by the fit of cosine functions with periods of 24 hours and submultiples thereof. The characteristics (MESOR, amplitudes and acrophases of the 24-hour and additional harmonics—10 of them if the data are densely obtained from automatic measurements) constitute a section of blood pressure-related cardiovascular summaries, the so-called sphygmochrons, shown as a short form (S), Figures 15 and 16, or long form (L), Figure 17, respectively. On the face of the form, peer group reference limits for rhythm characteristics are given for the fit of a 24-hour (form-S) or for that of both a 24- and 12-hour (form-L) cosine curve. The key is on the back of the short form, Figure 17, and in the upper right-hand corner of the long form. On the back of the form, one can add results related to further harmonics and to comparisons of single or multiple rhythm parameters with so-called paradesms, one kind of chronodesm, and displays for the interpretation of time-specified single values in the light of time-specified 90% prediction limits—other chronodesms. Chronodesms are best based on data for a peer-group with the same ethnicity, age, and gender. Chronodesms vary with the conditions of measurement, e.g., as a function of whether the subject is ambulatory, room-restricted, sitting, or recumbent. For each case, the chronobiologic approach has to provide a separate set of reference intervals (and eventually should provide conversion factors) for single blood pressures that are time-specified; for the characteristics of the fundamental and additional harmonics (whereby the

# SPHYGMOCHRON™

**BLOOD PRESSURE (BP) AND RELATED CARDIOVASCULAR SUMMARY.**

(Circadian Sphygmochron; from *sphygmo-*, of or relating to the circulating pulse, notably blood pressure, and *chronos*, time)

**COMPUTER COMPARISON MONITORING PROFILE OVERTIME PROJECTED AGAINST PEER GROUP LIMITS**

Name ___________________  Patient # ___________  No. of Profiles: ___________

Age _______  Sex ☐ M ☐ F  Monitoring From ___________  To ___________ , 19 _______

**TIMES OF**

Awakening: Day of Profile ___________  Activity[1] ___________  Breakfast ___________

Habitually

Diet[2,3]

Going to Sleep: Day of Profile ___________  Shift Schedule. Yes ☐  Lunch ___________

Habitually

Dinner ___________

Drugs[3] ___________  If Yes, Explain: ___________

Snack ___________

**CHRONOBIOLOGIC CHARACTERISTICS**

| | SYSTOLIC BP (mmHg) | | DIASTOLIC BP (mmHg) | | HEART RATE (bpm) | |
|---|---|---|---|---|---|---|
| | PATIENT VALUE | PEER GROUP REFERENCE LIMITS | PATIENT VALUE | PEER GROUP REFERENCE LIMITS | PATIENT VALUE | PEER GROUP REFERENCE LIMITS |
| ADJUSTED 24-h MEAN (MESOR) | | RANGE | | RANGE | | RANGE |
| PREDICTABLE CHANGE (DOUBLE AMPLITUDE) | | RANGE | | RANGE | | RANGE |
| TIMING OF OVERALL HIGH VALUES (ACROPHASE) | | RANGE | | RANGE | | RANGE |

| | SYSTOLIC | DIASTOLIC | HEART RATE |
|---|---|---|---|
| PERCENT TIME OF ELEVATION | | | |
| EXTENT OF EXCESS | (mmHg x hour) | (mmHg x hour) | (bpm x hour) |
| 10 YEAR CUMULATIVE EXCESS | (mmHg x hour) (in 100,000's units) | (mmHg x hour) (in 100,000's units) | (bpm x hour) |
| TIMING OF EXCESS | | | |

**INTERVENTION NEEDED**

☐ No

☐ Yes  ☐ Drug  ☐ Non-Drug

**MORE MONITORING NEEDED**

☐ Annually

☐ As soon as possible

☐ Other specify ___________

PREPARED BY ___________  DATE ____ / ____ / ____



**Figure 15:** Front of sphygmochron-S, the short form of a blood pressure and related cardiovascular summary.

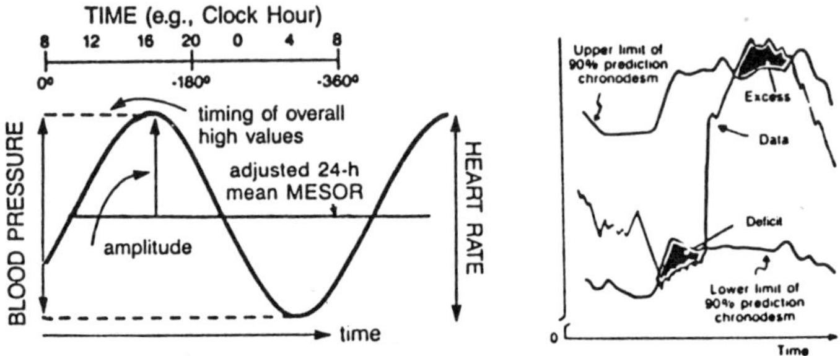


**MESOR, (M)** rhythm-adjusted mean (midline-estimating statistic of rhythm), defined as average value of rhythmic function (e.g., cosine curve) fitted to data; expressed in same units as original data. Note that MESOR will differ from arithmetic mean if data are unequidistant (e.g., concentrated near crest of rhythm) and/or cover non-integral number of cycles.

**AMPLITUDE, (A)** half of total predictable change in rhythm, defined by rhythmic function fitted to data; expressed in original or "relative" units, e.g., as percentage of series mean or MESOR.

**ACROPHASE, (Ø)** lag from reference time of rhythm's crest-time, defined by rhythmic function fitted to data; usually expressed in (negative) degrees, with 360° = period, 0° = reference time; customary time units (e.g., clock-hours and minutes, days, weeks, months or years); physiologic units (e.g., number of heart beats, respiratory or menstrual cycles) also appropriate for rhythm synchronized with corresponding period.

**Figure 16:** Back of sphygmochron-S, the short form of a blood pressure and related cardiovascular summary.

waveform is also accounted for); and in addition, for excess or deficit assessed on the basis of a data set as a whole, compared to the appropriate (earlier-determined) individualized and/or peer-group chronodesms. Automated measurements are superior to self-measurements at the outset, until a personal set of reference values is established, with both automatic and manual self-measurement under real-life conditions. As a complement, monitoring under standardized conditions is also desirable, to assess both the spontaneous and reactive blood pressure dynamics.

The use of the sphygmochron starts with newborn monitoring. The conventional approach does not work, in that a mean or a standard deviation of extensive series (such as half-hourly measurements for 48 hours) does not separate groups of newborns with a positive versus negative family history of high blood pressure, Figure 18. As Figures 19 and 20 show, however, the chronobiologic approach does so by the criterion of a circadian amplitude.[37] The difference in linear trend during the first two days of life is not shown in the normalized data of Figure 19 and their analysis in Figure 20. The trend is unmasked in part as the onset of the about-

**BLOOD PRESSURE AND RELATED CARDIO-VASCULAR MONITORING SUMMARY OVER TIME*** (Circadian Sphygmochron; from *sphygmo-*, of or relating to the circulating pulse, notably blood pressure, and *chronos*, time)

Name ___________

Age ___  [M] [F]  Sex   From __________ To __________, 19____

TIMES OF

Awakening _______   Activity[1] _______   Diet[2,3] _______

Drugs[3] _______

Going to Sleep _______

MESOR, (M) rhythm-adjusted mean (midline-estimating statistic of rhythm), defined as average value of rhythmic function (e.g., cosine curve) fitted to data, expressed in same units as original data. Note that MESOR will differ from arithmetic mean if data are unequidistant (e.g., concentrated near crest of rhythm) and/or cover non-integral number of cycles.

AMPLITUDE, (A) half of total predictable change in rhythm, defined by rhythmic function fitted to data, expressed in original or "relative" units, e.g., as percentage of series mean or MESOR.

ACROPHASE, (∅) lag from reference time of rhythm's crest-time, defined by rhythmic function fitted to data, usually expressed in (negative) degrees, with 360° = period, 0° = reference time, customary time units (e.g., clock-hours and minutes, days, weeks, months or years), physiologic units (e.g., number of heart beats, respiratory or menstrual cycles) also appropriate for rhythm synchronized with corresponding period.

**CHARACTERISTICS[4]**

| | MESOR | 24-hr AMPLITUDE | 24-hr ACROPHASE | 12-hr AMPLITUDE | 12-hr ACROPHASE |
|---|---|---|---|---|---|
| SBP mmHg | | | | | |
| DBP mmHg | | | | | |
| PP mmHg | | | | | |
| MAP mmHg | | | | | |
| HR bpm | | | | | |
| SBPxHR mmHg x bpm | | | | | |

SBP = Systolic Blood Pressure, DBP = Diastolic Blood Pressure, PP = Pulse Pressure (SBP-DBP), MAP = Mean Arterial Pressure, HR = Heart Rate, bpm = beat per minute.

**INDICES OF DEVIATION**

TIME (CLOCK HOURS)

**INDEX OF EXCESS [4,5]**   PTE   **TIMING OF EXCESS**

h = hour   PTE = Percent Time Elevation

| | Index of Excess | PTE | Timing of Excess |
|---|---|---|---|
| SBP mmHg xh | | | |
| DBP mmHg xh | | | |
| PP mmHg xh | | | |
| MAP mmHg xh | | | |
| HR bpm xh | | | |
| SBPx HR mmHg x bpm x h | | | |

**INTERVENTION NEEDED** [ ] [ ]
YES   NO

1) Unusually long standing or lying-down during waking; unusual activity, such as exercise, etc.; 2) Salt, calories, other, etc.; 3) Kind and amount, if any; 4) Rectangles on baselines indicate acceptable range; other rectangles serve for values off-scale; 5) Values calculated with respect to ☐ chronodesmic limits (time-specified 90% prediction limits) or with respect to ☐ fixed limits, determined on the basis of the median acrometron (MESOR + amplitude, i.e., highest predictable value) of a peer group: check this box ☐ if index of deficit rather than excess.

* Crosses on form indicate results from your individualized cardiovascular monitoring profile; if numbers (instead of crosses) are used, they refer to several stages of your monitoring, along with results of tests for any change in circadian parameters. (See comments on reverse side, that may also refer to rhythms other than circadian and/or trends.)

PREPARED BY _______   DATE (YR, MO, DAY) _______



**Figure 17:** Sphygmochron-L, long form of a blood pressure and related cardiovascular summary.

Double circadian amplitude (2A, left) but not the
MESOR (M, right) separates groups of newborns with
a positive versus a negative family history of high
blood pressure (BP), while numerically the difference
(△) in 2A (left) is smaller than that in M (right).*

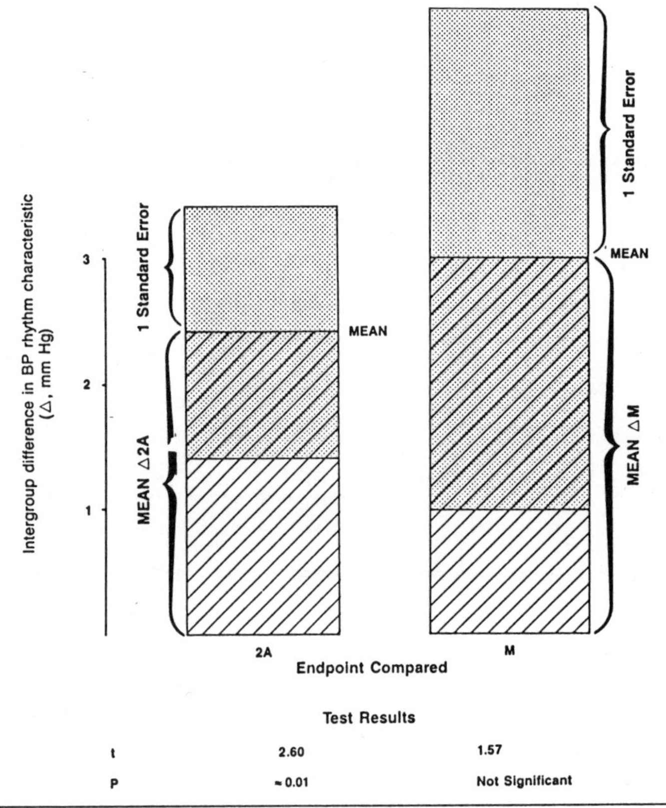


* The smaller standard error of the △2A, as compared to that of △M, accounts for the better resolution of △2A.

**Figure 18.**

7-day rhythm shown in Figure 21; again, one finds that the chronobiologic approach, i.e., the circaseptan amplitude, just as does the
circadian one, distinguishes the groups with a positive versus negative family history of high blood pressure, when the mean value
does not work (Fig. 18).

Data collection and summary by sphygmochron should start at

A great challenge lies in recognizing cardiovascular risk at birth on the basis of the precocious development of the circadian and circaseptan blood pressure (BP) amplitudes. In ongoing research, the newborn's BP and heart rate are being monitored automatically for 48 hours. The data are analyzed chronobiologically. Whether the index can be changed by preventive measures instituted on the pregnant woman acting *in utero* alone is a topic for research. The results thus far show a circadian variation apparent to the naked eye in neonates with a family history of high blood pressure (right) but not in those without such a family history (left). In the preparation of this display, the original data of each series are first expressed as percent of their series mean. Thereafter, they are stacked for consecutive hours of an idealized day and averaged.

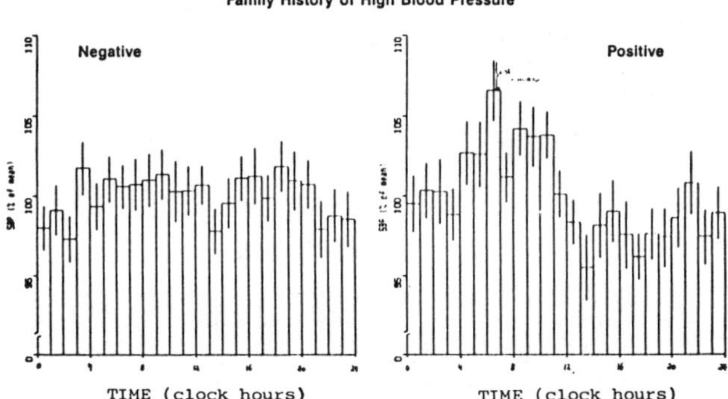



**Figure 19.**

birth and continue in family and school. Primary and again secondary schooling can serve for the teaching of instrumentation use, data self-analysis, and self-interpretation. For this purpose, the engineering community again faces the task of developing an autochronor in which self-measurements or simple automatic measurements are introduced and analyzed by chronobiometry.[65] Once chronobiologic literacy wedded to computer literacy becomes obligatory, the criteria of the sphygmochron lead not only to an early detection of overt disease, but also to a recognition of risk elevation. Thus, non-drug treatment can be recommended, before blood pressures exceed

A linear increase and a circaseptan feature characterize systolic blood pressure (SBP) of newborns observed during the first week of life.*

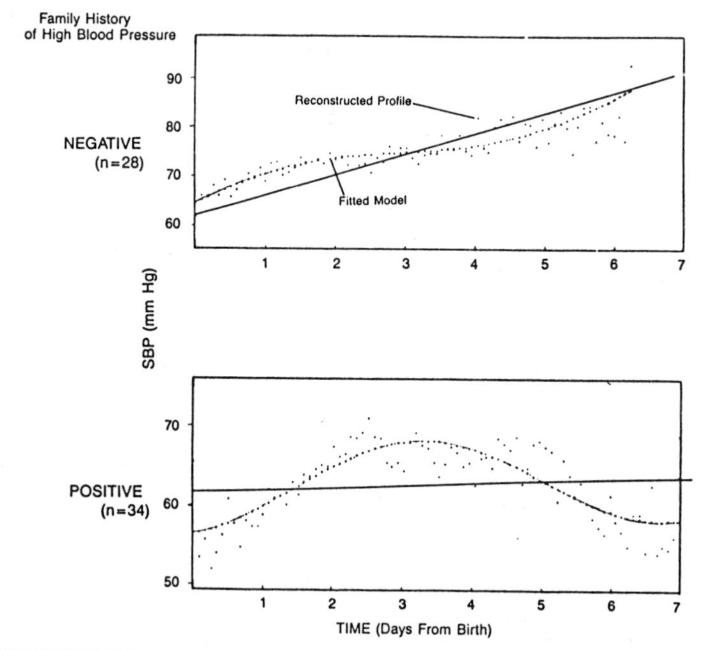


*Weekly profile reconstructed from a data pool contributed by newborns starting 48-h monitoring (at 30-min intervals) at different times after birth. Model fitted to reconstructed profile:

$$Y(t) = a_0 + a_1 t + A \cos\left(\frac{2\pi t}{168} + \phi\right) + e(t)$$

Circadian aspect handled separately in Section XI, is ignored for these reconstructions of circaseptan structure.

**Figure 20.**

currently recommended limits. This is warranted in view of insurance company statistics. These already reveal, with pressures for men and women starting at 118 and 114 mmHg systolic and 72 and 71 mmHg diastolic, respectively, an increase in blood pressure-related morbidity and early mortality as the value of blood pressure increases.[80]

At even lower pressures, it is possible to distinguish, with chronobiologic methods, those found (by epidemiologic questionnaire) to be at a high versus low risk of developing a high blood

The many displays of the chronobiologist need not remain a matter of research. As illustrated earlier, these so-called cosinor methods describe the rhythm by a vector. The length of this directed line corresponds to the extent of change, the amplitude. The orientation of the vector shows the timing of high values. The uncertainty of the summary is also given, as a confidence region around the vector's tip. On the left is the cosinor summary for blood pressures (BP) from a group of neonates with a negative family history of high BP; the confidence region of the vector covers the center of the display. By contrast, for the group of neonates with a positive family history of high BP on the right, the cosinor plot shows that a rhythm is found, as seen from the fact that the confidence region of the vector does not cover the center of the plot and thus the zero-amplitude (i.e., the no circadian rhythm) hypothesis, is rejected.

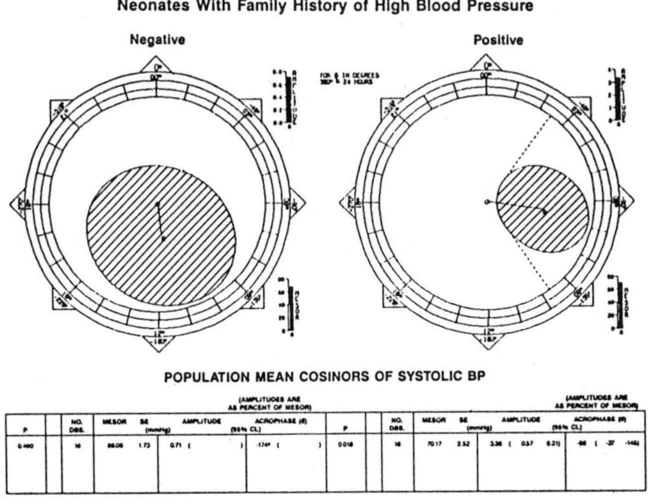


| | | | (AMPLITUDES ARE AS PERCENT OF MESOR) | | | | | | (AMPLITUDES ARE AS PERCENT OF MESOR) | |
|---|---|---|---|---|---|---|---|---|---|---|
| P | NO. OBS. | MESOR  SE (mmHg) | AMPLITUDE | ACROPHASE (φ) (95% CL) | P | NO. OBS. | MESOR  SE (mmHg) | AMPLITUDE | ACROPHASE (φ) (95% CL) |
| 0.490 | 16 | 96.06  1.73 | 0.71 ( ) | -174° ( ) | 0.018 | 16 | 70.17  2.52 | 3.36 ( 0.57  6.21) | -86 ( -37  -148) |

**Figure 21.**

pressure later in life. Thus, measurements at 10-minute intervals for 24 hours in recumbency on women in high versus low-risk groups reveal a circannual mean, in mmHg, of 108 versus 100 systolic and 69 versus 64 diastolic, respectively.[10] Chronobiologically, novel characteristics of genetic and reactive components of time structure, are quantified in human blood pressure for preventive as well as curative intervention. At the bottom of each sphygmochron, any such need is also indicated on the basis of statistical inference applied to the individual.

## Epilogue

The detailed references indicating the scope of chronobiology should stimulate those in the fields of health and engineering to join forces so that progress is made far beyond the illustrative examples chosen herein. If rhythms are the dynamics of all life, the scope of bioengineering may well be to assess rhythm alterations that are harbingers of earliest risk elevation. The harbingers, in turn, should prompt preventive intervention before elevated risk turns into overt disease. Rather than being concerned primarily or even exclusively with the treatment of catastrophic disease, as we are now, we may invest a major effort into chronobioengineering for health maintenance.

## References


1. Halberg, F, Conner RL. (1961). Circadian organization and microbiology: Variance spectra and a periodogram on behavior of *Escherichia coli* growing in fluid culture. *Proc Minn Acad Sci* 29:227.
2. Schweiger H-G, Berger S, Kretschmer H, et al. (1986). Evidence for a circaseptan and a circasemiseptan growth response to light/dark cycle shifts in nucleated and enucleated *Acetabularia* cells, respectively. *Proc Natl Acad Sci USA* 83:8619.
3. Scheving LE. (1976). The dimension of time in biology and medicine—chronobiology. *Endeavour* 35:66.
4. Halberg F. (1983). Quo vadis basic and clinical chronobiology: Promise for health maintenance. *Am J Anat* 168:543.
5. Hamblen M, Zehring WA, Kyriacou CP, et al. Germ-line transformation involving DNA from the period locus in *Drosophila melanogaster*:overlapping fragments that restore circadian and ultradian rhythmicity to per° and per⁻ mutants. *J Neurogenetics*, in press.
6. Young MW, Jackson FR, Shin H-S, et al. (1985). A biological clock in *Drosophila*. *Cold Spr Harb Symp Quant Biol* 50:865.
7. Halberg F. (1981). Biologic rhythms, hormones and aging. In: Vernadakis A, Timiras PS, eds, *Hormones in Development and Aging*, Spectrum Publications, New York, p 451.
8. Halberg F. (1969). Chronobiology. *Ann Rev Physiol* 31:675.

9. Kanabrocki EL, Scheving LE, Halberg F, et al. (1973). Circadian variations in presumably healthy men under conditions of peace time army reserve unit training. *Space Life Sci* 4:258.
10. Halberg F, Halberg E, Carandente F, et al. (1986). Dynamic indices from blood pressure monitoring for prevention, diagnosis and therapy. In: ISAM 1985, Proc Int Symp Ambulatory Monitoring, Padua, March 29–30, 1985, CLEUP Editore, 1986, p 205.
11. Halberg F. (1978). The chronobiology of convulsive disorders. *Totus Homo* 10:20.
12. Cornélissen G, Halberg F, Engel R, et al. (1986). Chronobiology of paroxysmal central nervous system disorders. In: Halberg F, Reale L, Tarquini B, eds, Proc 2nd Int Conf Medico-Social Aspects of Chronobiology, Florence, Oct 2, 1984, Rome, Istituto Italiano di Medicina Sociale, p 185.
13. Halberg F. Chronobiology and the lung: Implications and applications. Introductory remarks, SEPCR Symposium, Nov 16–18, 1986, Wiesbaden, FRG, in press.
14. Engel R, Halberg F, Dassanayake WLP, et al. (1958). 24-hour rhythms in blood eosinophils and in *Wuchereria bancrofti* microfilariae before and after $\Delta^1$ 9α-fluorocortisol. *Nature* (Lond) 181:1135.
15. DeMairan J. (1729). Observation botanique. *Histoire de L'Academie Royale des Sciences*, p 35.
16. Darwin C. (1859). On the origin of species by means of natural selection or the preservation of favored races in the struggle for life. London, Murray.
17. Halberg F, Nelson W, Runge WJ, et al. (1971). Plans for orbital study of rat biorhythms. Results of interest beyond the Biosatellite program. *Space Life Sci* 2:437.
18. Sundararaj BI, Vasal S, Halberg F. (1982). Circannual rhythmic ovarian recrudescence in the catfish *Heteropneustes fossilis* (Bloch). In: Takahashi R, Halberg F, Walker C, eds, *Toward Chronopharmacology*, Proc 8th IUPHAR Cong and Sat Symposia, Nagasaki, July 27–28, 1981, Oxford/New York, Pergamon Press, p 319.
19. Halberg F (1954). Beobachtungen über 24 Studen-Periodik in standardisierter Versuchsanordnung vor und nach Epinephrektomie und bilateraler optischer Enukleation. 20th meeting of the German Physiologic Society, Homburg/Saar, September, 1953. *Ber ges Physiol* 162:354.
20. Halberg F. (1959). Physiologic 24-hour periodicity: General and procedural considerations with reference to the adrenal cycle. *Z Vitamin-, Hormon- u Fermentforsch* 10:225.
21. Halberg F, Engeli M, Hamburger C, et al. (1965). Spectral resolution of low-frequency, small-amplitude rhythms in excreted 17-ketosteroid; probable androgen-induced circaseptan desynchronization. *Acta Endocrinol* (Kbh) (Suppl) 103:5.
22. Halberg F, Halberg E, Halberg Francine, et al. (1985). Circaseptan (about 7-day) and circasemiseptan (about 3.5-day) rhythms and contributions by Ladislav Dérer. 1. General methodological approach and biological aspects. *Biológia* (Bratislava) 40:1119.
23. Halberg F, Halberg E, Halberg Francine, et al. (1986). Circaseptan (about

7-day) and circasemiseptan (about 3.5-day) rhythms and contributions by Ladislav Dérer. 2. Examples from botany, zoology and medicine. *Biológia* (Bratislava) 41:233.

24. Ferin M, Halberg F, Richart RM, et al, eds. (1974). *Biorhythms and Human Reproduction*, John Wiley & Sons, New York, p 665.

25. NIOSH Research Symposium, Shift-Work and Health, Cincinnati, 1976.

26. Scheving LE, Halberg F, eds. (1980). *Chronobiology: Principles and Applications to Shifts in Schedules*. Alphen aan den Rijn, The Netherlands, Sijthoff and Noordhoff.

27. Hanson BR, Halberg F, Tuna N, et al. (1984). Rhythmometry reveals heritability of circadian characteristics of heart rate of human twins reared apart. *Cardiologia* 29:267.

28. Dowse HB, Hall JC, Ringo JM. Circadian and ultradian rhythm in period mutants of Drosophila melanogaster. *Behav Genetics* (in press).

29. Halberg F, Marques N, Cornélissen G, et al. Circaseptan biologic time structure reviewed in the light of contributions by Laurence K. Cutkomp and Ladislav Dérer. In press.

30. Sánchez de la Peña S, Halberg F, Schweiger H-G, et al. (1984). Circadian temperature rhythm and circadian-circaseptan (about 7-day) aspects of murine death from malaria. *Proc Soc Exp Biol Med* 175:196.

31. Marques MD, Cutkomp LK, Cornélissen G, et al. (1986). Life prolongation by circaseptan optimization of (simulated) shift(-work) schedules in the springtail, *Folsomia candida*. *J Minn Acad Sci* 51:15 (Abstr).

32. Hayes DK, Shade L, Cornélissen G, et al. (1985). Chronomodulatory infradian synchronization by *placebo* or ACTH 1-17 of *Musca autumnalis* mortality on shifted lighting regimens. In: Neuroimmunomodulation, Proc. 1st Int. Workshop on NIM, Bethesda, MD, Nov. 27–30, 1984, Bethesda, IWGN, 1985, p 150 and Chronobiologia 12:361.

33. Halberg F, Halberg E, Herold M, et al. (1982). Toward a clinospectrometry of conventional and novel effects of ACTH 1-17—Synchrodyn®—in rodents and human beings. In: Takahashi R, Halberg F, Walker C, eds, *Toward Chronopharmacology*, Proc 8th IUPHAR Cong and Sat Symposia, Nagasaki, July 27–28, 1981, Oxford/New York, Pergamon Press, p 119.

34. Cavallini M, Halberg F, Cornélissen G, et al. (1986). Organ transplantation and broader chronotherapy with implantable pump and computer programs for marker rhythm assessment. *J Contr Rel* 3:3.

35. Liu T, Cavallini M, Halberg F, et al. (1986). More on the need for circadian, circaseptan and circannual optimization of cyclosporine therapy. *Experientia* 42:20.

36. Halberg F. (1987). Perspectives of chronobiologic engineering. In: Scheving LE, Halberg F, Ehret CF, eds, *Chronobiotechnology and Chronobiological Engineering*. Dordrecht, The Netherlands, Martinus Nijhoff, p 1.

37. Halberg F, Cornélissen G, Bingham C, et al. (1986). Neonatal monitoring to assess risk for hypertension. *Postgrad Med* 79:44.

38. Halberg F, Halberg E, Halberg J, et al. (1986). Chronobiology, the indispensable control in bioscience: Chronobioengineering for social medicine. Proc III Int Symp Social Diseases and Chronobiology, Florence, Nov 29, 1986, in press.

39. Cornélissen G, Halberg F, Tarquini B, et al. (1986). Blood pressure rhythmometry during the first week of human life. Proc. III Int. Symp. Social Diseases and Chronobiology, Florence, Nov. 29, 1986, in press.
40. Halberg F. (1985). Book review: *The Seven Day Circle* by Eviatar Zerubavel. Chronobiologia 12:369.
41. Halberg F, Tong YL, Johnson EA. (1967). Circadian system phase—An aspect of temporal morphology; procedures and illustrative examples. Proc. Int. Congress of Anatomists. In: *The Cellular Aspects of Biorhythms*, Symposium on Biorhythms, Springer-Verlag, p 20.
42. Halberg F, Bingham C. (1986). The scope and promise of chronobiology and biostatistics: Interpenetrating, inseparable disciplines. Proc. Biopharmaceutical Section, Am. Statistical Assn., 1986, in press.
43. Halberg E, Halberg F. (1980). Chronobiologic study design in everyday life, clinic and laboratory. *Chronobiologia* 7:95.
44. Sánchez de la Peña S, Halberg F, Halberg E, et al. (1983). Pineal modulation of ACTH 1-17 effect upon murine corticosterone production. *Brain Res Bull* 11:117.
45. Sánchez de la Peña S, Halberg F, Ungar F, et al. (1983). Circadian pineal modulation of pituitary effect on murine corticosterone *in vitro*. *Brain Res Bull* 10:559.
46. Halberg F. (1985). Chronobiological aspects of the 24th International Industrial Pharmacy Conference, Boerne, Texas. *Chronobiologia* 12:175.
47. Halberg F. (1987). Chronobiology: Professional wallflower or paradigm of biomedical thought and practice? In: Pauly JE, Scheving LE, eds, *Advances in Chronobiology, Part A*, Proc. XVII Int Conf Int Soc Chronobiol, Little Rock, Ark., USA, Nov. 3−7, 1985, Alan R. Liss, New York, p 1.
48. Halberg F, Sánchez de la Peña S, Cornélissen G. (1985). Circadian rhythms and the central nervous system. In: Redfern PH, Campbell I, Xavier JA, Martin KF, eds, *Circadian Rhythms in the Central Nervous System*, Proc IX Conf IUPHAR, Sat Symp, Bath, England, August 4−5, 1984, Macmillan, p 57.
49. Walker WY, Russell JE, Simmons DJ, et al. (1985). Effect of an adrenocorticotropin analogue, ACTH 1−17, on DNA synthesis in murine metaphyseal bone. *Biochem Pharmacol* 34:1191.
50. Levi F, Halberg F, Chihara G, et al. (1982). Chronoimmunomodulation: Circadian, circaseptan and circannual aspects of immunopotentiation or suppression with lentinan. In: Takahashi R, Halberg F, Walker C, eds, *Toward Chronopharmacology*, Proc 8th IUPHAR Cong and Sat Symposia, Nagasaki, July 27−28, 1981, Oxford/New York, Pergamon Press, pp 289−311.
51. Halberg F, Halberg E, Carandente F. (1976). Chronobiology and metabolism in the broader context of timely intervention and timed treatment. Diabetes Research Today, Meeting of the Minkowski Prize Winners, Symposia Medica Hoechst 12 (Capri), FK Schattauer Verlag, Stuttgart/New York, p 45.
52. Halberg F. (1960). Temporal coordination of physiologic function. *Cold Spr Harb Symp Quant Biol* 25:289.
53. Halberg F, Spink WW, Albrecht PG, et al. (1955). Resistance of mice to

*brucella* somatic antigen, 24-hour periodicity and the adrenals. *J Clin Endocrinol* 15:887 (Abstr.).

54. Halberg F, Johnson EA, Brown BW, et al. (1960). Susceptibility rhythm to *E. coli* endotoxin and bioassay. *Proc Soc exp Biol* (NY) 103:142.

55. Halberg F, Haus E, Cardoso SS, et al. (1973). Toward a chronotherapy of neoplasia: Tolerance of treatment depends upon host rhythms. *Experientia* (Basel) 29:909.

56. Scheving LE, Haus E, Kühl JFW, et al. (1976). Close reproduction by different laboratories of characteristics of circadian rhythm in 1-β-D-arabinofuranosylcytosine tolerance by mice. *Cancer Res* 36:1133.

57. Halberg F, Gupta BD, Haus E, et al. (1977). Steps toward a cancer chronopolytherapy. In: Proc. XIV Int. Cong. Therapeutics, Montpellier, France, L'Expansion Scientifique Française, p 151.

58. Halberg F. (1974). Protection by timing treatment according to bodily rhythms—An analogy to protection by scrubbing before surgery. *Chronobiologia* 1 (Suppl 1):27.

59. Halberg F. (1982). Chronopharmacology and chronotherapy. In: Carpenter DO, ed, *Cellular Pacemakers*, John Wiley & Sons Inc., New York, p 261.

60. Halberg F, Halberg E, Nelson W, et al. (1982). Chronobiology and laboratory medicine in developing areas. In: Khayat NH, Montalbetti N, Ceriotti G, Bonini PA, eds, Proc. 1st African and Mediterranean Congress of Clinical Chemistry, Dolphin, Milan, p 113.

61. Lipsett MB, Halberg F. (1987). Endocrine disorders: Need for new instrumentation. In: Scheving LE, Halberg F, Ehret CF, eds, *Chronobiotechnology and Chronobiological Engineering*. Dordrecht, The Netherlands, Martinus Nijhoff, p 86.

62. Orth-Gomér K, Cornélissen G, Halberg F, et al. (1986). Relative merits of chronobiologic vs. conventional monitoring of ventricular ectopic beats (VEB). In: Halberg F, Reale L, Tarquini B, eds, Proc 2nd Int Conf Medico-Social Aspects of Chronobiology, Florence, Oct 2, 1984, Rome, Istituto Italiano di Medicina Sociale, p 767.

63. Halberg F, Cornélissen G, Halberg E, et al. (1987). Chronobiology of human blood pressure. Medtronic Continuing Medical Education Seminars.

64. Hermida RC, Halberg F, Halberg E. (1986). Closer to a psychoneuroendocrine hemopsy? *Biochim Clin* 10:1053.

65. Bingham C, Arbogast B, Cornélissen Guillaume G, et al. (1982). Inferential statistical methods for estimating and comparing cosinor parameters. *Chronobiologia* 9:397.

66. Scarpelli PT, März W, Cornélissen G, et al. (1986). Blood pressure self-measurement in schools for rhythmometric assessment of hyperbaric impact to gauge pressure 'excess,' In: ISAM 1985, Proc Int Symp Ambulatory Monitoring, Padua, March 29–30, 1985, CLEUP Editore, p 229.

67. Halberg F, Sánchez de la Peña S, Fernandes G. (1983). Immunochronopharmacology. In: Hadden J, Chedid L, Dukor P, Spreafico F, Willoughby D, eds, *Advances in Immunopharmacology*, Oxford, Pergamon Press, p 463.

68. Buchwald H, Rohde T, Schneider R, et al. (1980). Long-term, continu-

ous intravenous heparin administration by an implantable infusion pump in ambulatory patients with recurrent venous thrombosis. *Surgery* 88:507.

69. Buchwald H, Varco RL, Rupp WM, et al. (1981). Treatment of a type II diabetic by a totally implantable insulin infusion device. *Lancet* p 1233.
70. Dakhil S, Ensminger W, Kindt J, et al. (1981). Implanted system for intraventricular drug infusium in central nervous system tumors. *Cancer Treat Rep* 65:401.
71. Ensminger W, Niederhuber J, Dakhil S, et al. Total implanted drug delivery system for hepatic arterial chemotherapy. *Cancer Treat Rep* 65:393.
72. Ensminger W, Niederhuber J, Gyves J, et al. (1982). Effective control of liver metastases from colon cancer with an implanted system for hepatic arterial chemotherapy. *Proc. ASCO* 1:94 (Abstr.).
73. Greatbatch W. (1983). Engineering and instrumentation in the manufacture and patient delivery of drugs. *Med Instrumentation* 17:9.
74. Pipp TL, Warrick J. (1983). Infusion devices (infusion pumps). *Crit Care Intl*, April, p 4.
75. Prestele K, Funke H, Möschl R, et al. (1983). Development of remotely controlled implantable devices for programmed insulin infusion. *Life Support Sys* 1:23.
76. Schade DS, Eaton RP, Edwards WS, et al. (1982). A remotely programmable insulin delivery system. Successful short-term implementation in man. *JAMA* 247:1848.
77. Spencer WJ. (1981). A review of programmed insulin delivery systems. *IEEE Trans Biomed Eng* BME-28:237.
78. Halberg F, Delmore P, Halberg Francine, et al. (1986). A blood pressure and related cardiovascular summary: The sphygmochron. In Tarquini B, Vergassola R, eds, III Int. Symposium, Social Diseases and Chronobiology, Florence, Nov. 29, p 3.
79. 1986 Guidelines for study of mild hypertension (1986). *Bull WHO* 64:31.
80. Lew EA. (1974). High blood pressure, other risk factors and longevity: The insurance viewpoint. In: Laragh JH, ed, *Hypertension Manual*, New York, Dun-Donnelley, p 43.

# Chapter 25

# Local Delivery of Antibiotics Via an Implantable Pump in the Treatment of Osteomyelitis

Clayton R. Perry
Kenneth Davenport
Mark K. Vossen

## Introduction

An implantable drug pump has become available for use in humans. We are evaluating this pump as a means of delivering antibiotics locally in the treatment of osteomyelitis.

We have previously shown that various antibiotics maintain their stability in an implantable pump.[9] We have also shown in animals that we can achieve extremely high local and low systemic levels of antibiotic in normal and infected bone with an implantable pump, and that this method can eradicate experimentally-induced osteomyelitis.[8] This report details our experience using local delivery of amikacin or netilmicin via an implantable drug pump in conjunction with surgical debridement in the treatment of osteomyelitis. We emphasize that this is a method of antibiotic

From: Ensminger WD, Selam JL (eds): *Infusion Systems in Medicine.* Mount Kisco, NY, Futura Publishing Co., Inc.,©1987.

administration, and only increases the antibiotic concentration in the wound. The infection will not be eradicated unless the other aspects of therapy are addressed, in particular: excision of necrotic bone and soft tissue; coverage of soft tissue and skin defects; and stabilization of nonunions.[2,4,13]

## Materials and Methods

### Patient Selection

Sixty patients with osteomyelitis, as manifested by draining sinuses and positive deep wound cultures, were treated with surgical debridement and local delivery of antibiotics via an implantable pump. The first 21 patients are 12–27 months post pump removal. Baseline laboratory tests included: erythrocyte sedimentation rate; peripheral blood count; creatinine clearance; audiogram; and culture and sensitivity of organisms from the wound or sinus. The first seven patients had cultures obtained in the clinic. The subsequent 14 patients had surgical biopsies performed in the operating room.

### The Pump

The pump consists of two chambers. One is filled with drug, the other with freon. The chambers are separated by a collapsible metal bellows. As the freon changes from a liquid to a gas, it expands and compresses the chamber containing the drug. The drug is driven out of the outflow tube of the pump and into the outflow catheters.

### Implantation of Pump and Debridement

In order to decrease the risk of infecting the pump implant site, surgery was performed at one sitting, but in two stages: (1) implantation of the pump, and (2) debridement of necrotic bone and soft tissue. The patient was taken to the operating room with an impermeable drape over the draining sinus. The ipsilateral thigh, lower quadrant of the abdomen, or anterior aspect of the chest was prepped and draped. An implantable drug pump (Infusaid Model 400) was placed subcutaneously. The pump was filled with amikacin (19 patients) or netilmicin (two patients). Hemostasis was carefully maintained, as a postoperative hematoma might become infected. The outflow catheter was passed subcutaneously to the edge of the sterile area that was closest to the draining sinus. Here is was brought through the skin, coiled, and held in place with an adhesive drape. The pump pocket was irrigated with saline and bacitracin and closed. A sterile dressing was applied. The drapes were removed from the area to be debrided, and this area was prepped. Care was taken not to contaminate the sterile adhesive drape over the outflow catheter. Draping was accomplished so that the outflow catheter under the adhesive drape was included in the sterile field. All necrotic soft tissue and bone were debrided. As dead bone was excised, the underlying bone was irrigated, and the viable bone was identified by the presence of pinpoint bleeding. Small gouges or osteotomes were used, as opposed to high-speed burrs, in an attempt to avoid heat necrosis of viable bone. Devitalization of bone was avoided by minimizing periosteal stripping. Nonunions of the femur or tibia were stabilized with an external fixator if the pins could be placed outside of the infected area (three cases) or with a reamed intramedullary nail (three cases). The nonunion of the radius was stabilized with a splint. Sinus tracts were not excised. Following debridement, the adhesive drape was removed from over the outflow catheter, and the catheter was brought to the osteomyeltic defect subcutaneously. Flow through the catheter was checked by injecting antibiotic through the sideport of the pump. This was performed by an assistant who had regowned and regloved to avoid contaminating the pump site with organisms from the infected area. In these first 21 cases, primary wound closure was performed without additional soft-tissue procedures such as local flaps or free flaps. A drain was used if necessary.

## Postoperative Protocol

Postoperatively, the following parameters were monitored: amikacin levels in serum and wound drainage (wound drainage levels could be measured only if a drain was left in the wound); serum creatinine; peripheral blood count; and erythrocyte sedimentation rate. The pump was refilled percutaneously at intervals based on its flow rate. Amikacin (50 mg/mL) or netilmicin (14 mg/mL) was used to fill the pump. The first seven patients had their pumps removed at six weeks. The subsequent 14 patients had removal of their pump based upon clinical signs and their erythrocyte sedimentation rate. The clinical sign that we found most reliable was a well-healed, completely benign appearing surgical scar at the site of debridement. The erythrocyte sedimentation rate dropped during therapy and, empirically, we liked to see it below 20 mm/hr before pump removal. Two months after pump removal, an audiogram, creatinine clearance, and erythrocyte sedimentation rate were obtained. All patients continue to be seen at regular intervals.

## Results

### Patient History and Details of Therapy (Tables 1, 2, and 3)

Twenty-one adult patients were treated using the described regimen. The duration of symptoms ranged from one month to 22 years. The area involved was the tibia in nine cases, the femur in six cases, the hip in two cases, shoulder, knee, radius and elbow, in one case each. Seven patients had an infected nonunion (four tibia, two femur, and one radius). Seventeen cases were post-traumatic or postsurgical in origin; three cases involving the femur were hematogenous in origin; one case was a secondary infection of a draining sinus caused by tuberculosis of the hip. Nineteen patients had at least one previous unsuccessful "conventional treatment" combining surgical debridement and extended (at least four weeks) intravenous antibiotic therapy. Case 2 had undergone surgical biopsy and extended intravenous antibiotic therapy without a formal debridement, and case 6 had undergone surgery with only perioperative antibiotics. Six patients had previous local flap procedures. Intraoperative cultures indicated the infecting organism was *Staphylococcus aureus* alone in seven cases and in combination with gram negatives in nine cases. Five cases grew only gram negatives. Perioperative systemic antibiotics were used in all cases. They were discontinued when we felt the surgical wounds had stabilized. Five patients (cases 1, 4, 13, 14, and 15) received between 14 and 28 days of systemic antibiotics because of persistent infection. The remaining 16 patients received between 2 and 13 days of systemic antibiotics (mean = 6).

**Table 1**
**Patient History**

| Case No. | Patient Age (years) | Duration of Symptoms (years) | Etiology |
|---|---|---|---|
| 1 | 29 | 4 | post traumatic |
| 2 | 24 | 5 | hematogenous |
| 3 | 59 | 22 | hematogenous |
| 4 | 23 | 0.6 | post traumatic |
| 5 | 40 | 0.75 | post traumatic |
| 6 | 40 | 0.08 | hematogenous |
| 7 | 35 | 0.75 | post traumatic |
| 8 | 37 | 1.5 | post surgical |
| 9 | 59 | 3.5 | post traumatic |
| 10 | 23 | 0.9 | post traumatic |
| 11 | 31 | 4 | post traumatic |
| 12 | 59 | 11 | post traumatic |
| 13 | 25 | 0.75 | post traumatic |
| 14 | 44 | 1.2 | post traumatic |
| 15 | 50 | 2 | post traumatic |
| 16 | 41 | 15 | post traumatic |
| 17 | 59 | 20 | post tuberculosis |
| 18 | 21 | 2 | post traumatic |
| 19 | 20 | 2.5 | post traumatic |
| 20 | 46 | 4 | post traumatic |
| 21 | 41 | 1.66 | post traumatic |

## Amikacin Levels in Serum, and Wound Drainage (Table 4)

Nineteen patients had amikacin-filled pumps. The recommended systemic dose of amikacin for a patient with normal renal function is 15 mg/kg/day. We administered 5 ± 1.5 mg/kg/day. The serum amikacin levels ranged from less than 2.5 μg/mL to 8.2 μg/mL (8 μg/ml = recommended trough level). Two patients had single episodes of serum amikacin being 7.4 μg/mL, and 8.2 μg/mL; the other seventeen patients with amikacin-filled pumps always had levels below 5.5 μg/mL. Two patients had netilmicin-filled pumps. The recommended systemic dose of netilmicin is 4.0−6.5 mg/kg/day. We administered 1.5 mg/kg/day. The serum netilmicin levels ranged from 0.5 μg/mL to 3.5 μg/ml (5 μg/ml = recommended trough level). Eleven patients drained post-

**Table 2**
**Patient History**

| Case No. | Bone Involved | Previous Therapy |
|---|---|---|
| 1 | tibia | debridement × 5<br>extended IV therapy × 5 |
| 2 | femur | biopsy<br>extended IV therapy × 1 |
| 3 | femur | debridement × 5<br>extended IV therapy × 5 |
| 4 | tibia* | debridement × 2<br>muscle flap (soleus)<br>extended IV therapy × 1 |
| 5 | tibia | debridement × 1<br>muscle flap (gastrocnemius)<br>extended IV therapy × 1 |
| 6 | femur | debridement × 1 |
| 7 | distal humerus<br>proximal radius<br>proximal ulna | abdominal flap<br>debridement × 2<br>extended IV therapy × 1<br>extended po therapy × 1 |
| 8 | femur and<br>acetabulum | debridement × 3<br>extended IV therapy × 3 |
| 9 | femur* | debridement × 3<br>extended IV therapy × 3 |
| 10 | radius midshaft* | debridement × 1<br>extended IV therapy × 1 |
| 11 | shoulder | debridement × 4<br>muscle flap (pectoralis)<br>extended IV therapy × 4<br>extended po therapy × 2 |
| 12 | tibia | debridement × 2<br>extended IV therapy × 2<br>extended po therapy × 1 |
| 13 | tibia | debridement × 1<br>extended IV therapy × 1 |
| 14 | tibia* | debridement × 1<br>extended IV therapy × 1<br>extended po therapy × 1 |
| 15 | tibia* | debridement × 4<br>extended IV therapy × 1 |
| 16 | femur* | debridement × 2<br>extended IV therapy × 1 |
| 17 | hip | debridement × 4<br>extended IV therapy × 2<br>gentamicin beads × 2<br>extended po therapy × 3 |

**Table 2** *(Continued)*

| Case No. | Bone Involved | Previous Therapy |
|---|---|---|
| 18 | tibia | debridement × 4<br>muscle flap (gastrocnemius)<br>extended IV therapy × 4<br>extended po therapy × 3 |
| 19 | knee | debridement × 1<br>muscle flap (gastrocnemius)<br>extended IV therapy × 1<br>extended po therapy × 2 |
| 20 | tibia* | debridement × 5<br>extended IV therapy × 1<br>extended po therapy × 2 |
| 21 | femur | debridement × 1<br>extended IV therapy × 1<br>extended po therapy × 1 |

*These patients had an associated delayed or nonunion.

operatively for several days, and in all cases the amikacin levels of drainage fluid were always greater than the upper limit of the assay (55 µg/mL−5,000 µg/mL).

## Incidence of Side Effects (Table 5)

Ototoxicity was defined as a decrease in auditory acuity of 15 dB at two or more frequencies in both ears. There was no ototoxicity as demonstrated by pre- and postoperative audiograms. Nephrotoxicity was defined as a decrease in creatinine clearance from preoperative values that were within the normal range to values less than normal (70 mL/min.). The creatinine clearance dropped to 66 mL/min. and 55 mL/min. respectively post therapy in case 9 and case 20. At no time, during or after therapy, did either of these patients' serum creatinine exceed the upper limits of normal (1.5 mg/mL). All other post therapy creatine clearances were within normal limits. In case 17, the pump pocket became infected six weeks after implantation, necessitating removal. After removal and irrigation, the infection at the pump site cleared.

**Table 3**
**Cultures Pre- and Posttherapy**

| Case No. | Pretherapy Cultures | Therapy MIC of Organism of Amikacin ($\mu$g/mL) | Posttherapy Cultures of Drainage |
|---|---|---|---|
| 1 | Staph. aureus | $\leq 2$ | Staph. aureus |
|  | Enterococcus | >64 |  |
| 2 | Staph. aureus | $\leq 2$ | No drainage |
| 3 | Proteus mirabilis | $\leq 2$ | Bacteroides |
|  | Bacteroides | >64 |  |
|  | Enterococcus | >64 |  |
| 4 | Staph. aureus | < 4 | Pseudomonas |
|  | Pseudomonas aeruginosa | 4 |  |
| 5 | Staph. aureus | $\leq 2$ | Staph. aureus |
| 6 | Staph. aureus | $\leq 2$ | No drainage |
| 7 | Staph. aureus | $\leq 2$ | No drainage |
| 8 | Escherichia coli |  | No drainage |
| 9 | Staph. aureus | 8 | No drainage |
| 10 | Staph. aureus |  | No drainage |
| 11 | Pseudomonas aeruginosa | 4 | No drainage |
|  | Staph. aureus | 8 |  |
| 12 | Pseudomonas aeruginosa | 4 | No drainage |
|  | Staph. aureus | $\leq 2$ |  |
|  | Enterobacter | $\leq 2$ |  |
| 13 | Staph. aureus | 8 | No drainage |
|  | Enterococci | >64 |  |
| 14 | Staph. aureus | 4 | No drainage |
| 15 | Staph. aureus | 8 | No drainage |
|  | Proteus mirabilis | 2 |  |
|  | Pseudomonas aeruginosa | 4 |  |
| 16 | Proteus mirabilis | 4 | No drainage |
|  | Staph. aureus | 4 |  |
| 17 | Staph. aureus | < 4 | Staph. aureus |
|  | Pseudomonas aeruginosa | < 4 | Escherichia coli |
| 18 | Klebsiela pneumonia | < 1 | No drainage |
|  | Enterococcus | > 6 |  |
|  | Proteus mirabilis | 4 |  |
| 19 | Proteus mirabilis | < 4 | No drainage |
|  | Escherichia coli | < 2 |  |
|  | Serratia marseaus | < 2 |  |
| 20 | Staph. aureus |  | No drainage |
|  | Enterobacter cloacae | < 1 |  |
|  | Pseudomonas aeruginosa | < 1 |  |
| 21 | Pseudomonas aeruginosa | 4 | No drainage |

Pretherapy cultures were the results of tissue biopsies at the time of pump implantation.

**Table 4**
**Amikacin Levels in Serum and Wound Drainage**

| Case No. | Serum Amikacin Level Range | Amikacin Level in Drainage ($\mu$g/mL) and Postop Day | |
|---|---|---|---|
| 1 | < 2.5−4.8 | > 2,000 | 2 |
| 2 | < 2.5−5.2 | > 1,000 | 3 |
| 3 | < 2.5−7.4 | > 5,000 | 8 |
| 4 | < 2.5−3.3 | No postop drainage | |
| 5 | < 2.5−3.2 | > 55 | 2 |
| 6 | < 2.5−3.3 | > 1,010 | 3 |
| 7 | < 2.5−3.2 | No postop drainage | |
| 8 | < 2.5−8.2 | > 80 | 2 |
| 9 | < 2.5−5.5 | > 1,000 | 4 |
| 10 | < 2.5− | No postop drainage | |
| 11 | < 2.5− | > 1,000 | 2 |
| 12 | < 2.5−4.2 | No postop drainage | |
| 13 | < 2.5−3.1 | > 1,000 | 2 |
| 14 | < 2.5−2.8 | > 55 | 2 |
| 15 | < 1.0−2.0 | No postop drainage | |
| 16 | 0.4−2.3 | > 50 | 3 |
| 17 | < 2.0−4.9 | No postop drainage | |
| 18 | 2.2−3.8 | No postop drainage | |
| 19 | 0.7−2.1 | No postop drainage | |
| 20 | 0.5−3.5 | No postop drainage | |
| 21 | 3.5−7.06 | No postop drainage | |

Serum amikacin levels were obtained every other day until the levels had stabilized; they were then obtained weekly. Wound drainage levels were obtainable only if the wound was draining, and were always higher than the upper limit that the radio-immuno assay. The levels over which toxic side effects may occur is 8 $\mu$g/mL for amikacin and 40 $\mu$g/mL for netilmicin.

## Eradication of Infection (Table 6)

The twenty-one patients are 12 to 27 months post explantation of the pump. A draining wound is our primary indication of infection. We consider a wound to be draining if there is any defect in the skin, at any time after termination of therapy. Whether or not pus or serous fluid is expressed at the time of examination, such a defect in the skin indicates that there is an infection present. All 21 patients stopped draining during therapy. Five patients resumed draining after pump removal, case 3 and 17 immediately, case 1

**Table 5**
**Incidence of Side Effects**

| Case No. | Change in Audiogram | Pretherapy Creatinine Clearance (mL/min.) | Posttherapy Creatinine Clearance (mL/min.) |
|---|---|---|---|
| 1 | no | 141 | 105 |
| 2 | no | 75 | 136 |
| 3 | no | 102 | 93 |
| 4 | no | 130 | 104 |
| 5 | no | 90 | 71 |
| 6 | no | 84 | 126 |
| 7 | no | 134 | 105 |
| 8 | no | 70 | 77 |
| 9 | no | 92 | 66 |
| 10 | no | 92 | |
| 11 | no | 135 | 92 |
| 12 | no | 68 | 70 |
| 13 | no | 89 | 66 |
| 14 | no | 58 | 91 |
| 15 | no | 121 | 81 |
| 16 | no | 90 | 123 |
| 17 | no | 108 | 100 |
| 18 | no | 120 | 117 |
| 19 | no | 62 | 93 |
| 20 | no | 105 | 55 |
| 21 | no | 110 | 115 |

Significant change in the audiogram is defined as a decrease in auditory acuity of 15 decibels at 2 or more frequencies in both ears. Renal toxicity is defined as a drop in creatinine clearance from normal preoperative levels (>70 mL/min.) to less than normal postoperative levels.

after two months, case 5 after 11 months, and case 4 after 18 months.

Pretherapy erythrocyte sedimentation rates were above 20 mm/h in sixteen of the nineteen patients in whom it was measured preoperatively. The erythrocyte sedimentation rate two months after pump removal was less than 20 mm/h in 13 of the 21 patients. Of the eight patients with erythrocyte sedimentation rates of 20 mm/h or greater, four have drained (cases 1, 3, 5, and 17), one patient (case 8) has a pain-free allograft hip, which may account for her elevated erythrocyte sedimentation rate. Three patients (15, 16, and 21) have erythrocyte sedimention rates of 30, 24, and 33 mm/h. These patients have no clinical signs of infection.

**Table 6**
**Eradication of Infection**

| Case No. | Drainage Preop | Drainage Post-therapy | Erythrocyte Sedimentation Rate; Pre-therapy (mm/hr) | Erythrocyte Sedimentation Rate; 2−3 mos. Posttherapy (mm/hr) | Length of Follow-up (mos.) |
|---|---|---|---|---|---|
| 1 | yes | yes | 25 | 20 | 18 |
| 2 | yes | no | 27 | 9 | 18 |
| 3 | yes | yes | — | 30 | 18 |
| 4 | yes | yes | 40 | 13 | 18 |
| 5 | yes | yes | 10 | 31 | 18 |
| 6 | yes | no | 120 | 10 | 18 |
| 7 | yes | no | — | 17 | 17 |
| 8 | yes | no | 23 | 63 | 14 |
| 9 | yes | no | 97 | 6 | 13 |
| 10 | yes | no | 1 | 1 | 12 |
| 11 | yes | no | 13 | 4 | 12 |
| 12 | yes | no | 22 | 11 | 11 |
| 13 | yes | no | 30 | 6 | 10 |
| 14 | yes | no | 24 | 12 | 7 |
| 15 | yes | no | 56 | 30 | 15 |
| 16 | yes | no | 110 | 24 | 15 |
| 17 | yes | yes | 32 | 33 | 15 |
| 18 | yes | no | 42 | 15 | 14 |
| 19 | yes | no | 53 | 5 | 14 |
| 20 | yes | no | 53 | 7 | 14 |
| 21 | yes | no | 32 | 33 | 12 |

All patients stopped draining during therapy. Cases 3 and 17 started to drain immediately after the pump was removed. Case 1 started to drain 2 months after the pump was removed. Case 5 drained 11 months after the pump was removed, and case 4 drained 18 months after the pump was removed. Pretherapy erythrocyte sedimentation rates were not obtained for cases 3 and 7. Follow-up is calculated from the date of pump removal.

We were able to obtain union in six of seven patients with nonunions. Case 9 had a nonunion of a supracondylar femur fracture and a fused knee. His femur was stabilized with an external fixator post debridement; although he has no clinical signs of infection, the nonunion has persisted. Six of the seven patients with nonunions have not drained following therapy. Case 4 had a reamed nail inserted in his tibia, and he has subsequently drained 18 months after pump removal.

## Duration of Hospitalization and Therapy (Table 7)

Total hospitalization was calculated by adding the days spent in the hospital for the initial debridement and pump implantation, and the days spent in the hospital for pump removal. Hospitalization ranged from 5 to 52 days with a mean of 23 days. Duration of therapy ranged from 32 to 140 days with a mean of 63 days. Three patients were treated as inpatients for various reasons, noncompliance (case 5), persistent infection (cases 3 and 4).

**Table 7**
**Hospitalization**

| Case No. | Total Days in Hospital | Total Days of Therapy |
|---|---|---|
| 1 | 33 | 42 |
| 2 | 12 | 42 |
| 3 | 43 | 43 |
| 4 | 34 | 32 |
| 5 | 52 | 42 |
| 6 | 29 | 42 |
| 7 | 19 | 42 |
| 8 | 20 | 76 |
| 9 | 9 | 119 |
| 10 | 5 | 55 |
| 11 | 8 | 91 |
| 12 | 10 | 48 |
| 13 | 11 | 111 |
| 14 | 46 | 140 |
| 15 | 40 | 125 |
| 16 | 26 | 112 |
| 17 | 35 | 48 |
| 18 | 8 | 48 |
| 19 | 8 | 110 |
| 20 | 7 | 90 |
| 21 | 7 | 48 |
| Mean | 23 | 63 |

Case 3 had been admitted for other medical problems; therefore, his hospitalization is calculated from the day of surgery to pump removal.

## Discussion

Surgical debridement of necrotic tissue is necessary if osteomyelitis is to be treated successfully. Once the necrotic bone and soft tissue are excised, antibiotics are usually used to sterilize the wound. The intravenous route is the most commonly used method of antibiotic administration.[4] However, intravenous administration has several disadvantages: venous access is not always easy to obtain, and the site can become irritated or infected; patients must be carefully monitored; therefore, hospitalization is often necessary; side effects to the antibiotics can occur; and most importantly, the maximum local wound level of antibiotic is limited by the systemic level of antibiotic that can be tolerated by the patient. Local antibiotic administration has been attempted in a response to the disadvantages of intravenous administration.[5-7] The most commonly used method of local antibiotic administration is to mix the antibiotics with polymethylmethacrylate (PMMA).[2,3,11] The fact that the dead space, which frequently results from a thorough surgical debridement, can be filled with the PMMA antibiotic composit is a significant advantage. Drawbacks to this method are: only a limited amount of antibiotic can be administered; therefore, local levels are high initially, but rapidly fall[12]; PMMA inhibits the activity of white cells[10]; and there is no way (short of removing the PMMA) of changing the antibiotic or of stopping therapy.

This study was undertaken to evaluate the treatment of osteomyelitis with surgical debridement and local antibiotic therapy via an implantable pump. The parameters studied were the incidence of toxic side effects to the antibiotics used in the pump, the duration of hospitalization and of therapy, and eradicaton of infection. The 21 patients selected all had osteomyelitis with draining sinuses, radiographic changes, and positive cultures.

The occurrence of toxic side effects to antibiotics administered over a protracted period of time is a definite possibility. This is particularly true of the aminoglycosides. There was no significant change between pre- and post-therapy audiograms. Two patients' creatinine clearances dropped to 66 mL/min., and 55 mL/min., 4 and 15 mL/min. below normal range. Serum creatinines were monitored weekly in all patients and were always within the limits of normal. The low incidence of side effects is due to the low systemic levels of antibiotics.

Hospitalization in 13 of the patients was significantly shortened. The other eight were hospitalized for nearly the usual amount of time because of persistent drainage or noncompliance. We were very concerned with these initial patients that an unexpected side effect might occur; therefore, we were conservative in terms of discharging patients. However, as experience is gained, more of the treatment will be as an outpatient.

All 21 patients stopped draining for a time. This indicates that we were able to at least suppress the infection with this therapy. Five of our patients resumed draining, and we consider our therapy to have failed in these patients. The remaining 16 patients have not drained since the pump was removed, and 12 of these patients have erythrocyte sedimentation rates below 20 mm/h. Case 8 has not drained since surgery, and we feel that her persistently elevated erythrocyte sedimentation rate is due to the presence of an allograft hip. Cases 15, 16, and 21 have persistently elevated erythrocyte sedimentation rates, and although they have no clinical signs of infection, we suspect that they may drain in the future. It is impossible to predict whether any of these patients are cured; however, we feel this high rate of suppression of infection achieved with the described therapeutic regimen is our most significant finding. The success of this method is due to the high local levels of antibiotic, not the sustained low serum levels. This is illustrated by cases 9, 11, 13, 15, and 16, all of whom grew *Staphylococcus* with an MIC to amikacin higher than the patient's peak serum concentration of amikacin (Tables 3 and 4). The possibility exists that our patients were responding not to the antibiotic delivered by the pump, but to the perioperative systemic antibiotics and the surgical debridement. We believe that this is not the case, because all but two of our patients had previously been treated with surgical debridement in conjunction with four weeks or more of intravenous antibiotics. In addition, two of the five patients, who received more than 14 days of systemic antibiotics, were failures of therapy. We feel that perioperative antibiotics must be used to minimize the risk of infecting the pump pocket and because the soft tissue through which the surgical incision for the debridement was made may not be exposed to the high local level of antibiotic that is in the depths of the wound, and therefore, may become infected.[12]

In these 21 patients, there was no statistically significant correlation between success or failure and: age; number of prior procedures; presence of nonunion; or number and types of organisms. A correlation may become evident when more patients are treated with this method. We did notice three apparent trends: (1) Both patients (cases 3 and 17) who had drained more than 20 years were failures. (2) All patients who had involvement of the upper extremity were successes. (3) The factor that correlated most significantly with failure was our experience. Cases 1, 3, 4, and 5 (all failures of therapy) were four of the first five cases treated with this method at St. Louis University. Case 17 (our other failure of therapy) was the first case treated at Cook County Hospital. Some of these failures can be attributed directly to our inexperience. For example, the pump in case 17 was implanted too closely to his infection (ipsilateral lower quadrant of the abdomen and infected hip). Subsequently, the pump became infected probably by direct spread along the outflow catheters. This necessitated its early removal, despite the fact that the patient seemed to be responding to therapy. Our results have improved as experience is gained and our protocol has been modified. There have been two major modifications in our protocol: (1) In the first seven patients, we found that wound cultures obtained in the clinic by taking swabs of the drainage were not reliable in identifying all the pathogenic organisms. Two of these patients (cases 1 and 3) did not respond to therapy and grew organisms that were not sensitive to amikacin. These organisms grew from material obtained during debridement and pump insertion. In the subsequent 14 patients, we changed our protocol and performed an adequate surgical biopsy at least two weeks prior to debridement and pump insertion. (2) The second and most important modification is that after the first seven patients, pump removal was based upon the clinical course and erythrocyte sedimentation rate. We continued therapy until the wound healed, and the erythrocyte sedimentation rate dropped below 20 mm/h. The first seven patients had their pumps removed at six weeks. The subsequent 14 patients had a longer duration of therapy.

Improvements which must be made are: increasing the number and types of antibiotics that can be used in the pump; and developing a catheter that will disperse the antibiotic over a greater area and occupy the dead space produced by the debridement. With these improvements, it may be possible to achieve an even higher rate of success, and work is proceeding in both of these areas.

Our preliminary results indicate that local delivery of antibiotics via an implantable pump, when used as an adjunct to thorough surgical debridement, has potential for decreasing the disability associated with the treatment of osteomyelitis and increasing the incidence of eradication of infection.

---

# References


1. Buchholz HW, Gartman HD. (1972). Infecktions-prophylaxe and Operative Behandlung der Scheichenden Tiefen Infektion bei der Totalen Endoprosthese. *Chirug* 43:446.
2. Burri C. (1975). *Post-Traumatic Osteomyelitis*, Bern Stuttgart, Vienna, Hans Huber Publishers Bern.
3. Carlsson AS, Josefsson GJ, Lindberg L. (1978). Revision with gentamicin-impregnated cement for deep infections in total hip arthroplasties. *J Bone Joint Surg* 60A:1059.
4. Cierny G, Mader J. (1983). The surgical treatment of adult osteomyelitis. In: Evarts CM, ed, *Surgery of the Musculoskeletal System*, (4) 10:15−35, New York, Churchill-Livingstone.
5. Compere EL. (1962). Treatment of osteomyelitis and infected wounds by closed irrigation with detergent-antibiotic solution. *Acta Orthop Scand* 32:324.
6. Mackey D, Carlet A, Debeaumont D. (1982). Antibiotic loaded plaster of Paris pellets: An invitro study of a possible method of local antibiotic therapy in bone infections. *Clin Orthop* 167:263.
7. Organ CH. (1978). The utilization of massive doses of antimicrobial agents with isolation perfusion in the treatment of chronic osteomyelitis. *Clin Orthop* 76:185.
8. Perry CR, Rice S, Ritterbusch JK, Burdge RE. (1985). Local administration of antibiotics with an implantable osmotic pump. *Clin Orthop* 182:284−290.
9. Perry CR, Ellington LL, Becker A, Vossen MK, Burdge RE, Greenberg RN. (1986). Antibiotic stability in an implantable pump. Accepted by *J Orthopaedic Res*, March.
10. Petty W. (1978). The effect of methylmethacrylate on bacterial phagocytosis and killing by human polymorphonuclear leukocytes. *J Bone Joint Surg* 60A:752.
11. Vecsei V, Barquet A. (1981). Treatment of chronic osteomyelitis by necretomy and gentamicin-PMMA beads. *Clin Orthop* 159:201−207.
12. Wahlig H, Dingeldein E, Buchholz HW, Buchholz M, Bachman F. (1984). Pharmacokinetic study of gentamicin-loaded cement in total hip replacements. *J Bone Joint Surg* 66B:175−179.
13. Weiland AJ, Moore JR, Daniel RK. (1984). The efficacy of free tissue transfer in the treatment of osteomyelitis. *J Bone Joint Surg* 66A:181−193.

# Chapter 26

# Is GnRH-Infusion a Treatment of Polycystic Ovarian Disease (PCOD)


J. Schoemaker
C.W. Burger
C.B. Lambalk


## The Stein−Leventhal Syndrome

In 1935 Stein and Leventhal[1] described a syndrome that was clinically characterized by infertility, menstrual disturbances, and obesity. They discovered that the ovaries of these patients usually were bilaterally enlarged, showing multiple subcortical cysts, a thickened cortex with subscapsular fibrosis, and numerous atretic follicles, of which the theca interna often was thickened and showed luteinization. Luteinization of stroma cells was often found. Closer observation of the clinical syndrome showed that the above-mentioned menstrual disturbances usually consisted of either oligomenorrhea or amenorrhea, sometimes even primary amenorrhea. If oligomenorrhea exists, it is usually of an anovulatory character. However, spontaneous ovulation may occur. Obesity and hirsutism, a symptom added later on to the syndrome, are not obligatory, but the latter often exists. Other virilizing symptoms,


From: Ensminger WD, Selam JL (eds): *Infusion Systems in Medicine*. Mount Kisco, NY, Futura Publishing Co., Inc.,©1987.

such as a deepening of the voice and/or hypertrophy of the clitoris, are rare. In the beginning, the syndrome was referred to as the Stein–Leventhal syndrome; later on it acquired the name "polycystic ovarian disease" or PCOD.

Endocrinologically the syndrome is characterized by a normal FSH level, a moderately elevated LH level, a mild increase in estrogen levels, particularly estrone, and usually, increased levels of androgens such as testosterone, androstenedione, and sometimes dehydroepiandrosterone. Although the pathogenesis of the syndrome is not clear, these abnormal hormonal values seem to be caused by a disturbed feedback of estrogens and possibly androgens, at the hypothalamic and/or pituitary levels. Particularly the increased levels of LH and androgens, in close connection with the clinical picture of oligoamenorrhea, have currently become the most important diagnostic criteria. It has appeared now that many a woman fits into these diagnostic criteria without showing the overt pathological changes in their ovaries, as described by Stein and Leventhal. Since these pathological changes are no longer a prerequisite for the diagnosis, we tend to speak of the PCOD-like syndrome rather than about PCOD.

## Conventional Therapy

Treatment of infertility, and more specifically induction of ovulation, can usually be achieved with clomiphene citrate. Most of these patients are sensitive to this drug. A small number of patients appears to be or gradually becomes resistant to clomiphene. Before clomiphene treatment had become a regular therapy, patients were treated by so-called wedge resections of their ovaries. Stein and Leventhal had already noticed that many women, after removal of a wedge-shaped piece of tissue from their ovaries, became regular ovulators. However, recurrences of the syndrome after one or two years were common. Therefore, this therapy should be reserved for the time at which a woman wants to become pregnant.

If clomiphene treatment failed, the next step, since the early 1960s, has been to induce ovulation with exogenously-administered gonadotropins. This therapy, however, carries the risk of the development of multiple pregnancies and/or the hyperstimulation syndrome. The latter is a particularly serious complication, with massively enlarged ovaries, which are at risk for bleeding and torsion. Ascites and pleural effusion may develop, followed by hypo-volemia with related complications such as venous and arterial thrombosis and emboli. A few deaths from this syndrome have been described in the literature. PCOD-like patients are particularly prone to develop this complication. Other methods of ovulation in-duction in women with clomiphene-resistant PCOD would there-fore be welcomed.

## Treatment with Gn-RH Infusion

On the basis of the findings of Knobil et al., extensively re-viewed in the 1980 volume of *Recent Progress in Hormone Res-earch*,[2] Leyendecker in 1978,[3] started a new therapy for induction of ovulation in women with hypogonadotropic forms of amenor-rhea, by means of pulsatile administration of the hypothalamic peptide GnRH. This therapy is based on the fact that continuous administration of GnRH, SC or IV, causes desensitization of the pi-tuitary. Only when GnRH is administered in small doses every 60 to 120 min. a sustained, albeit intermittent, release of LH and FSH can be achieved.

Pulsatile administration of GnRH is accomplished by portable computerized infusion pumps, of which a number of different types are available on the market now. GnRH may be administered subcutaneously as well as intravenously, the latter giving slightly better results. The GnRH dose may vary between 2 and 20 μg per pulse. Continued pulsatile administration of GnRH leads to induc-tion of ovulation in most women with a hypogonadotropic amenor-rhea of suprapituitary origin. Ovulation rate is as high as 95–98%, and 80% of the women have achieved pregnancy after five months of treatment. For an extensive update of these data, the reader is referred to reference 4.

The overwhelming success of GnRH treatment in hypogonado-tropic women prompted a number of investigators to try whether this treatment would be beneficial to women with PCOD as well. Recent data on larger series were presented at the pulsatile GnRH symposium in Noordwijk, The Netherlands, in September 1985.[4] Berg et al.[5] were able to obtain an ovulatory cycle in 21 out of 26 hyperandrogenic patients and in 41 out of 74 cycles. Only six preg-nancies were achieved. Birckhauser and Huber[6] completed 20 induction cycles in 13 patients. Twelve of these 20 cycles appeared to be ovulatory and four pregnancies were obtained, of which two ended in an early abortion. Bringer et al.[7] performed a crossover randomized study in nine PCOD patients who were resistant to clomiphene treatment, comparing pulsatile GnRH and HMG/hCG treatment. They showed that, although the number of ovulatory cycles achieved with HMG/hCG therapy was higher than that achieved with GnRH, the pregnancy rate was the same under the two treatment regimes. Finally, Adams et al.[8] reported the achievement of 27 ovulatory cycles in 67 cycle attempts in 22 PCOD patients. Eight of 22 patients conceived, but six of those miscarried.

Our own first two successful patients were published in the *Acta Endocrinologica*,[9] showing two and four consecutive ovulatory menstrual cycles and a first pregnancy. Unfortunately, this patient miscarried. The endocrinology of the two cycles of the first patient is shown in Figure 1. From this it can be seen that after the beginning of stimulation, LH levels started to decline and gradually normalized. Even before reaching a completely normal LH/FSH ratio, a rise in LH was seen again, culminating in a normal LH peak. After ovulation, during the luteal phase of the first cycle, LH further decreased, until by the end of the first cycle, a normal LH/FSH ratio was achieved. The second cycle showed endocrinologic values that were hardly distinguishable from a similarly-induced cycle in a woman with amenorrhea of hypothalamic origin.

## Rational Basis for Gn—RH Infusion Treatment of PCOD

As the exogenous application of a strict pulsatile GnRH regime apparently was able to normalize the major endocrine abnormality in the PCO-like syndrome, i.e., the elevated LH levels in the presence of normal FSH levels, we asked ourselves whether an abnormal endogenous GnRH stimulation could probably be responsible for the disturbance of regular follicle growth and ovulation in this

**Figure 1:** The endocrinology of two consecutive cycles induced by means of pulsatile iv GnRH-infusion in a patient with clomiphene-resistant PCOD : Days of menses. In the LH and FSH graphs, the lower end of each bar represents the basal values just prior to a GnRH dose at 9 AM. The upper end of each bar represents the peak value in response to this GnRH dose at 9 AM (reprinted from Reference 10 with kind permission of the editor).

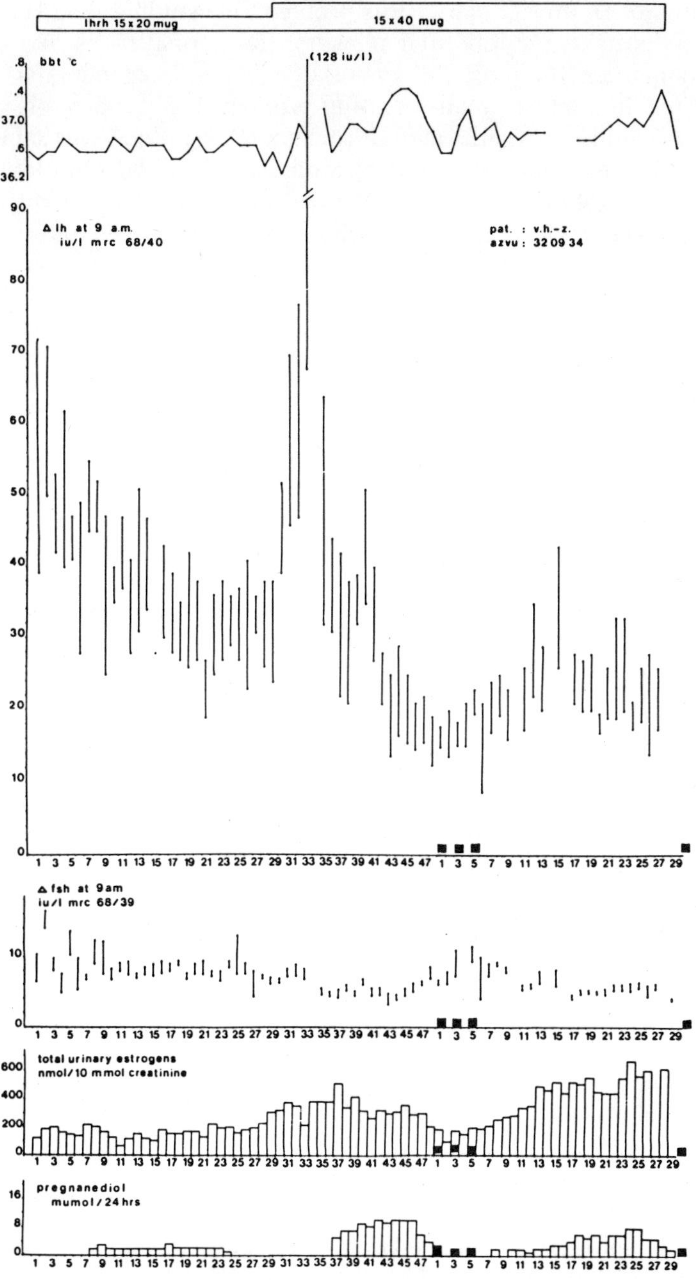
lhrh 15 x 20 mug
15 x 40 mug
bbt °c
(128 iu/l)
.8
.4
37.0
.6
36.2
90
Δ lh at 9 a.m.
iu/l mrc 68/40
pat. : v.h.–z.
azvu : 32 09 34
80
70
60
50
40
30
20
10
0
Δ fsh at 9 am
iu/l mrc 68/39
10
0
total urinary estrogens
nmol/10 mmol creatinine
600
400
200
0
pregnanediol
mumol/24 hrs
16
8
0

syndrome. To further clarify this problem, we studied the LH secretion patterns in the follicular phase of the normal menstrual cycle in comparison to those in anovulatory periods of patients with PCOD.[10] In nine normally cycling women and 11 patients with PCOD, a study was performed during six hours. Blood was sampled every 10 min., and LH was determined in all blood samples. Figures 2 and 3 show examples of these secretion patterns. A variation in LH level was called a pulse when a peak level was found to be elevated at least 20% over the preceding lowest value (nadir). Pulse amplitude was defined as the difference between a peak level and the level of the preceding nadir. As it is assumed that the LH pulse pattern represents the responses to a similar GnRH pulse pattern and as the GnRH pulses are assumed to coincide with the LH nadirs, we chose the interval between the LH nadirs as a measure of the frequency of GnRH pulses.

The results showed that in PCOD, the nadir interval is significantly shorter, with a median of 50 minutes, than during the follicular phase of the menstrual cycle, with a median of 60 minutes. The amplitude of the pulses was significantly larger in PCOD patients (5.75 IU/L) compared to women in the follicular phase (3.0 IU/L).

The increase in amplitude in PCOD patients could be explained by an increased output of GnRH per pulse from the hypothalamus but, by the same token, might also be the result of increased responsiveness of the pituitary due to prolonged estrogen exposure of the gonadotropic cells. The alteration in frequency, however, seems to indicate a hypothalamic alteration of the pulse generator frequency. Therefore, it is concluded that indeed there is a disturbance of LH, and probably of GnRH secretion in PCOD.

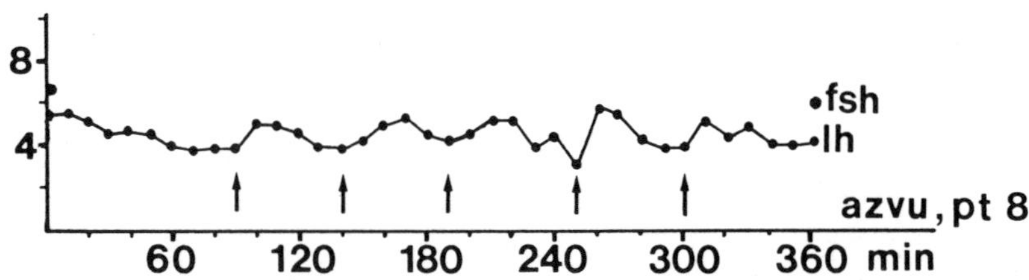


**Figure 2:** LH-secretion pattern in a regularly menstruating woman during the follicular phase of the menstrual cycle. Arrows indicate nadirs.

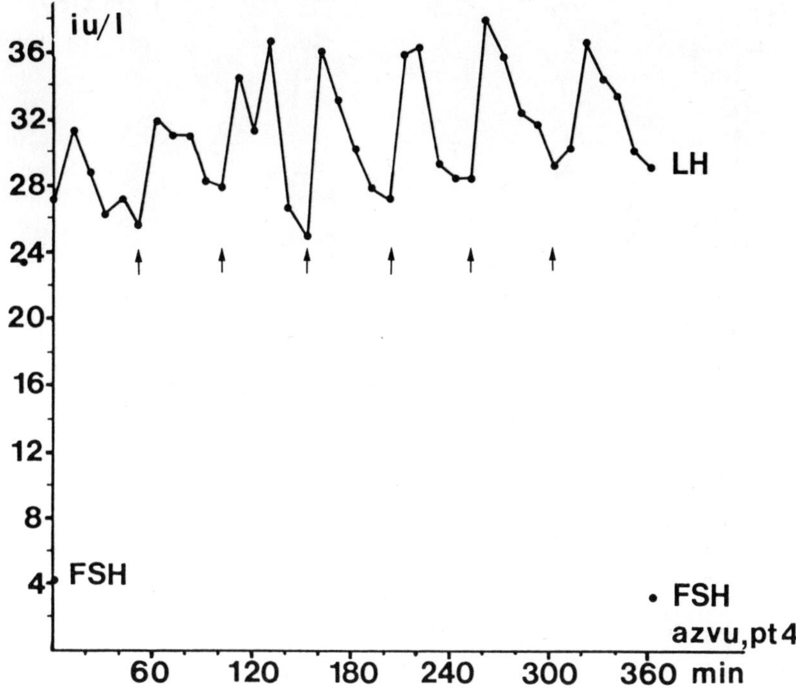


**Figure 3:** LH-secretion pattern in a patient with PCOD. Arrows indicate na-dirs. Note increased level and amplitude as well as the slightly decreased nadir interval in comparison with Figure 2.

The next question to address was: How is it possible that, once exogenous pulsatile administration has been initiated, the pituitary starts to follow the exogenous pulsatile regimen rather than the disturbed endogenous one? Could it be that exogenous GnRH suppressed endogenous GnRH secretion, or was this caused by a different mechanism, possibly at the pituitary level?

In order to investigate this, we chose to mimick the situation in the PCOD patient by stimulating six completely hypogonadotropic women with pulses of 2 and 20 μg of GnRH in a fixed order.[11] The two μg pulses mimicked the endogenous ones, and the 20 μg pulses the exogenous ones. At time zero an IV needle was placed and a baseline blood sample was taken. Two μg pulses were given at t30, t150, t240, and t270, and 20 μg pulses at t90 and t210 (Fig.

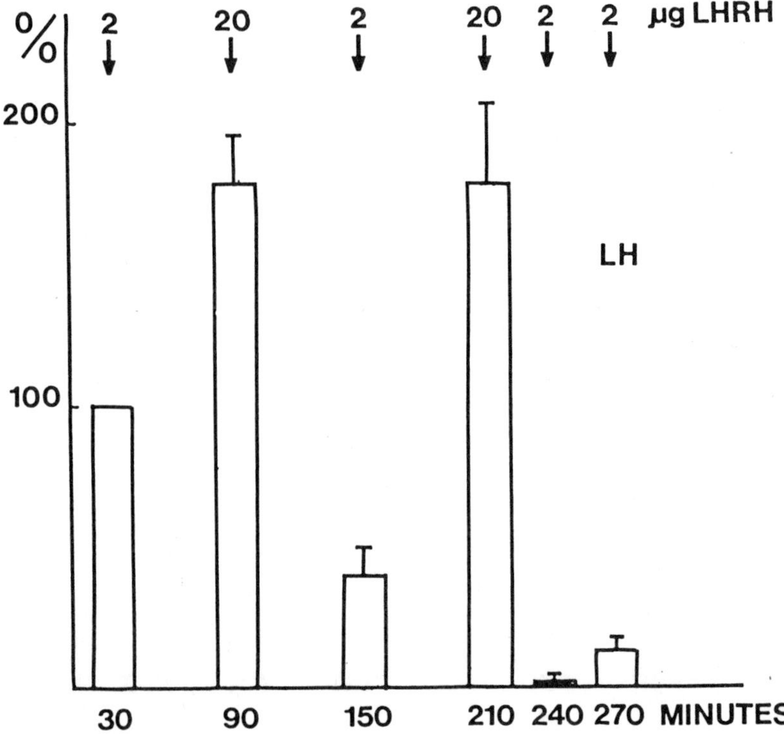


**Figure 4:** Pituitary responses in LH-secretion to subsequent challenges of 2 and 20 µg of GnRH in six hypogonadotropic females with amenorrhea of suprapituitary origin. t150 t240 and t270 are significantly different from t30. t240 and t270 are significantly different from t150; t210 is not different from t90.

4). Blood was sampled every 10 minutes from t0 until t300 for LH determination.

Results show that the response of the pituitary to a 2 µg bolus of GnRH (t150) given one hour after a 20 µg bolus (t90) is significantly smaller than the response to 2 µg at t30. This effect is expressed even more clearly when such a 2 µg bolus (t240) is given 30 min. after a 20 µg bolus (t210).

Although the mean response to the 20 µg bolus of t210 is lower than that of the 20 µg bolus of t90, this difference is not statistically significant. These and more unquoted data show that each pulse of GnRH not only induces a release of LH but induces a short-term refractoriness of the gonadotropic cells of the anterior pituitary too. This refractoriness, at least in the rat, is dose and time dependent.[12]

This short-term refractoriness explains why the pituitary follows the relatively high exogenous pulses and ignores the smaller endogenous ones. The latter usually come when the pituitary is in part refractory, due to the preceding larger endogenous GnRH pulses.

Having found a rational basis now for the pulsatile GnRH treatment in PCOD patients, we continued to treat clomiphene-resistant PCOD-patients in this manner under close monitoring.

A study was performed in 11 patients with clomiphene-resistant PCOD. A patient was considered to suffer from PCOD when her clinical picture of oligo- or amenorrhea was found together with elevated LH levels in the presence of normal FSH values. Usually, the level of at least one androgen was elevated. Patients were treated IV with GnRH in a pulsatile manner with pulse doses varying from 5 to 40 μg and pulse intervals from 60 to 120 min. Patients were monitored by basal body temperature, daily measurement of urinary estrogen excretion, and, after ovulation, total urinary pregnanediol excretion. LH and FSH levels were measured daily in all subjects during the first two months of treatment before the 9 AM pulse of GnRH was administered and 30, 60, and 90 or 120 min. thereafter. Out of 85 cycles in 11 patients, 74 in nine patients were ovulatory. Three patients became pregnant five times. One of the patients, who conceived three times, aborted twice before she carried the third pregnancy to term. One other patient had an early abortion, and a third had an uneventful pregnancy.

In the ovulatory cycles, the cycle length varied from 17 to 60 days with a median length of 33 days. Four patients became quite regular; others, although improving on their regularity, remained irregular ovulators. The development of regularity in the cycle pattern was neither pulse-dose nor pulse-interval dependent. The iregularity, as might be expected, was caused by a wide spread in the time span from the beginning of either stimulation or a menstrual period until the beginning of organized follicular growth, as expressed by an exponential increase in total urinary estrogen output. Eleven cycles in six patients were anovulatory. Two patients did not ovulate once during treatment periods, which lasted for as long as 52 and even 284 days.

It thus appears that under pulsatile GnRH therapy, we still find the whole spectrum of cycle anomalies as we find in untreated PCO patients. Although some become regular ovulators, some develop either ovulatory or anovulatory oligomenorrhea or remain amenorrheic. Therefore, it appears that patients with oligoamenorrhea can be made more regular by means of pulsatile GnRH therapy, but this does not necessarily lead to a completely regular menstrual pattern. Moreover, it tells us that the abnormality in the LH secretion pattern, and by inference of the GnRH secretion pattern, may be a result of the underlying defect, which causes this clinical syndrome, rather than that it is the cause of it.

## Conclusion

We conclude from our studies that induction of ovulation with pulsatile GnRH therapy is certainly possible. Ovulation rate is relatively high, but the pregnancy rate is disappointingly low in our hands. This, in general, is confirmed by the results of other investigators. Of the pregnancies achieved, a relatively large number seem to miscarry. Although this high number of abortions is the finding of some individual investigators, this could not be confirmed in a large series collected from several Dutch centers.[13] Bringer showed that there was no difference in the pregnancy rates in GnRH and HMG therapy, but unfortunately he does not provide us with data on the outcome of the pregnancies. On the basis of the outcome of our study and the data from the literature we have, until new and more favorable data become available, we have decided to abandon this therapy in PCOD patients.

## References


1. Stein IF, Leventhal ML. 1935. Amenorrhea associated with bilateral polycystic ovaries. *Am J Obstet Gynecol* 29:181.
2. Knobil E. 1980. The neuroendocrine control of the menstrual cycle. In: Greep RO, ed, *Recent Progress in Hormone Research*. Vol 36, 53–88 Academic Press, New York, London, Toronto, Sydney, San Francisco.
3. Leyendecker G. 1979. The pathophysiology of hypothalamic ovarian failure. *Eur J Obstet Gynecol Reprod Biol* 9:175–186.

4. Coelingh Bennink HJT, Dogterom AA, Lappohn RE, Rolland R, Schoemaker J, eds, 1986. *Pulsatile GnRH 1985*, Proceedings of the 3rd Ferring Symposium, Noordwijk, Sept. 11–13, 1985 Ferring Publication, Haarlem, The Netherlands.

5. Berg FD, Hinrichsen MJ, Mickan H. 1986. Administration of gonadotropin-releasing hormone in hyperandrogenic women with anovulation. In: Coelingh Bennink, et al. 1986. Pulsatile GnRH 1985. Proceedings of the 3rd Ferring Symposium, Noordwijk, Sept. 11–13, 1985, pp 155–160.

6. Birckhauser MH, Huber P. 1986. Pathophysiological aspects and clinical results of ovulation induction by pulsatile intravenous administration of GnRH in polycystic ovary syndrome. In: Coelingh Bennink, et al. 1986. Pulsatile GnRH 1985. Proceedings of the 3rd Ferring Symposium, Noordwijk, Sept. 11–13, 1985, pp 161–170.

7. Bringer J, Hedon B, Gibert F, Mares P, Jaffiol C, Orsetti A, Boutes C, Vialla JL, Mirouze J. 1986. Treatment of anovulation by HMG or GnRH: Contribution of a cross-over randomized study to a rational management of PCO. In: Coelingh Bennink, et al. 1986. Pulsatile GnRH 1985. Proceedings of the 3rd Ferring Symposium, Noordwijk, Sept. 11–13, 1985, pp 171–180.

8. Adams J, Polson DW, Abdulwahid N, Morris DV, Franks S, Mason HD, Tucker M, Price J, Jacobs HS. 1985. Multifollicular ovaries: Clinical and endocrine features and response to pulsatile gonadotropin releasing hormone. *Lancet* 2:1375–1378.

9. Burger CW, van Kessel H, Schoemaker J. 1983. Induction of ovulation by prolonged pulsatile administration of luteinizing hormone releasing hormone (LRH) in patients with clomiphene resistant polycystic ovary-like disease. *Acta Endocrinol* 104:357–364.

10. Burger CW, Korsen T, van Kessel H, van Dop PA, Caron FJM, Schoemaker J. 1985. Pulsatile luteinizing hormone patterns in the follicular phase of the menstrual cycle, polycystic ovarian disease (PCOD) and non-PCOD secondary amenorrhea. *J Clin Endocrinol Metab* 61:1126–1132.

11. Lambalk CB, van Kessel H, van Rees GP, Schoemaker J. 1985. Short-term pituitary refractoriness for pulsatile luteinizing hormone releasing hormone after pulsatile luteinizing hormone releasing hormone. A clinical experiment. *J Endocrinol Invest* (Abstract) suppl. 3, 8:132.

12. Lambalk CB, van Dieten HAMJ, de Koning J, Scheomaker J, van Rees GP. 1986. Short-term pituitary desensitization after pulsatile LH-RH in the ovariectomized rat. An in vivo experiment. *Neuroendocrinol*, in press.

13. Braat DDM, Boghelman D, Coelingh Bennink HJT, Heineman MJ, Lappohn RE, Rolland R, Willemsen WNP, Schoemaker J. 1986. The outcome of pregnancies established in GnRH induced cycles with special reference to the multiple pregnanacies in five Dutch centers. In: Coelingh Bennink, et al. 1986. Pulsatile GnRH 1985. Proceedings of the 3rd Ferring Symposium, Noordwijk, Sept. 11–13, 1985, pp 207–211.

# Chapter 27

# Chronic Intrathecal Administration of Baclofen in Treatment of Severe Spasticity

Yves Lazorthes

Bowery[1,2] established that the main site of action of Baclofen (beta-(b chlorophenyl) γ aminobutyric acid) is medullary at presynaptic level. Baclofen is a specific agonist of GABA-B receptors. Autoradiographic studies of Price and colleagues[10] showed that GABA-B receptors are very abundant in the superficial layers (I–IV) of the posterior columns of the spine. Although Baclofen is the most frequently used antispastic drug in treatment of spasticity, particularly of spinal origin, effective treatment requires high dosage usually in the range of 40–80 mg per day orally. Side effects correlate with the dosage necessary to obtain a therapeutic effect. Metabolic and pharmacological studies[4] performed with the help of Baclofen containing radioactive C14 showed a very low concentration in the central nervous system. Due to the poor permeability of Baclofen through the brain barrier, intrathecal administration appeared to be logical. This route was first tried in animal studies by Kroin et al.[5] who also demonstrated the effectiveness of direct application of the drug. Intrathecal administration of Baclofen in humans was performed and reported for the first time by Penn and Kroin,[8] in two patients with incapacitating spasticity.

From: Ensminger WD, Selam JL (eds): *Infusion Systems in Medicine*. Mount Kisco, NY, Futura Publishing Co., Inc., ©1987.

Our clinical experience started in 1984 and comprises nine patients presenting with severe medullary or supramedullary spasticity treated by intermittent or continuous application of Baclofen by intrathecal route.

## Material and Method

The following selection criteria were used: (1) Severe chronic and incapacitating spasticity resistant to treatment by systemic route. (2) Stabilized causative disease. (3) Consent obtained from the patient and availability of facilities permitting continuation of treatment on an outpatient basis with regular follow-up. (4) Lack of disturbances of CSF circulation. (5) Positive results of selection test consisting of percutaneous intrathecal administration of Baclofen.

Percutaneous intrathecal testing was the most essential criterion [12]; the test was performed after positioning of intrathecal lumbar catheter, which may be placed directly or may be tunnelized subcutaneously. In order to evaluate the tolerance and therapeutic effect of Baclofen, progressively increasing dosages (5 µg, −25 µg, −50 µg, . . .) were administered at least at 24-hour intervals.

The effect was evaluated clinically (muscular testing). Particular attention was devoted to undesirable secondary effects, mainly the suppression of the possible useful muscular hypertonia. This testing which was extended over 3 to 5 days permitted to determine: (1) patient's response to the therapy, and (2) the effective therapeutic dose for 8 hours.

According to this protocol, we have tested 20 patients and were able to select nine for chronic administration. Two of these patients presented with spasticity due to disseminated sclerosis, three with spasticity due to traumatic spinal lesions (two cervical at C5 and C6 and one thoracic at D6); one patient had cerebral palsy; one patient suffered from spasticity, which did not improve after removal of thoracic meningioma; one patient exhibited spastic syndrome due to cervical trauma and brain stem lesion; and one patient presented with spasticity hemiplegia of vascular origin (Table 1). There were six men and three women; their age ranged between 26 and 74 years. All patients were treated previously with Dantrolene Sodium (100 to 400 µg), Baclofen (60 to 100 mg), and Diazepam (20 to 60 mg). Three of those patients were submitted to the tests of prolonged cervical electrical stimulation without any effect.[11,12,14]

**Table 1**
**Patients Selected for Chronic Intrathecal Administration of Baclofen**

| Case | Age/Sex | Etiology | Duration of spasticity (years) | Spasticity (Ashworth) | Painful spasms |
|---|---|---|---|---|---|
| 1 | 30/H | Trauma C5 | 2 | 5 | |
| 2 | 27/H | Cerebral palsy | 27 | 4 | + |
| 3 | 56/F | Multiple sclerosis | 5 | 5 | + |
| 4 | 26/H | Trauma Th 6 | 2 | 4 | + + |
| 5 | 49/F | Multiple sclerosis | 20 | 5 | + |
| 6 | 30/H | Cranial injury | 6 | 5 | + |
| 7 | 70/H | Cerebrovascular | 3 | 5 | + + |
| 8 | 64/F | Postoperative Th 4 | 2 | 4 | + + |
| 9 | 56/H | Trauma C 6 | 3 | 4 | Deaff. |
| 10 | /H | Trauma | | | |
| 11 | 27/H | Trauma TH 4 | 2 | 5 | |
| 12 | 23/H | | 2 | 4 | |
| 13 | 37/F | Multiple sclerosis | 2 | 5 | |

The administration of the drug was effected with the help of an implanted system: cutaneous port (Cordis) was used in six cases and programmable micropump type D.A.S. (Medtronic) was used in three cases. In one patient, the subcutaneous port had to be removed because of meningitis. After recovery, a mechanical pump "SECOR" (Cordis) was used for reimplantation. The tip of the catheter was located at the level of D7−D8 in three cases, at the level of D11 in two, at the level of D12 on one, and at the level of L1 on three occasions.

## Results

Follow-up of nine patients ranged between 6 to 28 months; the mean follow-up was a 13 months; the total time of follow-up for all patients was 116 months (Table 2).

The effective initial dose was variable from patient to patient and ranged between 50 to 500 µg. It took 1 to 2 hours for the first effect to appear, and spasticity was abolished for 8 to 48 hours. During the initial percutaneous testing performed in 20 patients on four occasions, reversible somnolence was observed, and in two patients disturbing hypotonia occurred with loss of useful spasticity in the lower extremities. In the testing period, we compared the

**Table 2**
**Results in Patients with Chronic Administration of Baclofen**

| Case | Port | Implantation SECOR | D.A.S. | Dose/24 h μg Baclofen | Spasticity (Ashworth) | Follow-up |
|------|------|------|------|------|------|------|
| 1 | | | + | 500 | 1 | 28 |
| 2 | + | ⎯⎯⎯⎯⎯⎯⟶ | + | 100 | 2 | 14 |
| 3 | + | ⎯⟶ + | | 100 | 3 | 12 |
| 4 | | | + | 50 | 1 | 6 |
| 5 | + | | | 200 | 1 | 22 |
| 6 | + | | | 50 | 3 | 12 |
| 7 | + | | | 50 | 1 | 8 |
| 8 | + | | | 50 | 1 | 7 |
| 9 | + | | | 100 | 2 | 7 |

efficiency of Baclofen to that of intrathecal morphine at a dosage of 2.5 to 5 mg on six occasions and to that of water-soluble benzodiazepine (midazolam, 3−4 mg) given intrathecally on four occasions. The effect of midazolam and morphine was markedly less and shorter than that of Baclofen.

When administered chronically, Baclofen retains its efficiency on spasticity if it is applied in minimal intrathecal dosages. The mean daily dose in this series of nine patients was 100 μg; but as mentioned above, this varies from one patient to another in the range of 50 to 500 μg. All patients, independently from the system used for implantation, were treated by intermittent bolus injections 1 to 3 per day. Three out of the nine patients were also managed by continuous perfusion with a programmable system of Medtronic. Ashworth scale was used for evaluation of muscular hypertonia (Grade 1—normal muscular tone, . . . , grade 5—maximal hypertonia and segmental rigidity). Before treatment, five patients were classified as grade 5 and four patients as grade 4. Following application of Baclofen, an improvement was noted: five patients were in grade 1, two patients were in grade 2, and two other patients were in grade 3. This improvement was confirmed in six patients by registration of the H. reflex. The ratio H max/M max before treatment amounted to 75 to 95%, whereas after treatment it normalized to 40 to 55% (Fig. 1). Before treatment, all patients exhibited painful muscular spasms, which disappeared after intrathecal administration of Balcofen. A single patient whose pain did not improve had deafferentation pain in the lower extremities.

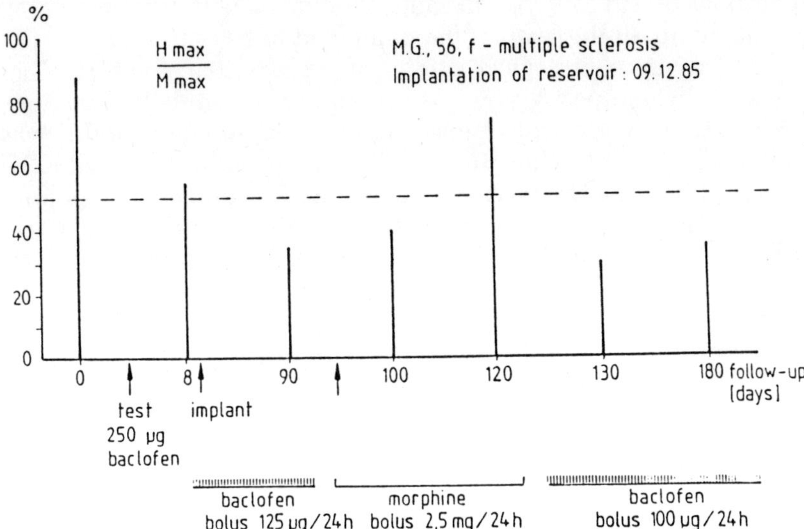


**Figure 1:** H max/M max ratio in the course of treatment with intrathecal Baclofen or morphine (bolus application with the use of an implantable manual release pump).

In two patients, considerable functional gain in their independence in their daily life (moving, feeding, dressing, using the toilet, communication) was very impressive. The first patient, who had post-traumatic paraplegia below D6, regained complete independence and mobility thanks to the preservation of useful spasticity in quadriceps muscles. The second patient with spasticity in flexion due to multiple sclerosis regained complete independence in his daily activities and was able to move without a wheelchair. The remaining seven patients did not obtain a functional gain; however, in two patients, therapy had to be interrupted because of complications.

The complications observed were of mechanical, neurological, and pharmacological types. In one patient, the catheter became disconnected and subcutaneous escape of CSF occurred. In another patient, the catheter became occluded, and in a third patient, the catheter became disconnected at its junction to the port. These complications required small operative corrections. One patient, in whom a programmable pump had been implanted, presented complications due to overdosage, which was linked with malfunctioning of the pump. In this patient the pump had to be removed.

As far as neurological complications are concerned, two patients, in whom port was implanted and in whom daily punctures were necessary, developed local suppuration. In one case this was followed by purulent meningitis. Altogether, the systems had to be removed in three instances (two ports and one implantable pump).

As far as neuropharmacological complications due to application of Baclofen are concerned, in a period of 105 months of treatment in nine patients, in four patients transient somnolence occurred, and in another four cases undesirable muscular hypotonia developed due to overdosage. There were two severe complications in the form of transient coma. In one case, this was accompanied by respiratory depression necessitating reanimation and intensive care with definite interruption of Baclofen administration.

## Discussion

Our experience is similar to that of Penn and Krain[8,9] and confirms the efficacy of intrathecal Baclofen upon spasticity resistant to oral treatment and in a very incapacitating form of spasticity. Baclofen was effective in very low dosages administered directly into the subarachnoid space. All our patients had been unsuccessfully treated with many antispastic drugs, particularly by Baclofen at a daily dose of 80 mg. Therapeutic effect could be achieved by intrathecal administration of the drug at a dose of 100 µg. The ratio of the effective oral/intrathecal dose was therefore 1/1,000. The effective intrathecal threshold was, however, very variable.

It appears, therefore, prudent to be cautious with determination of the initial daily therapeutic dose if the risk of secondary effects such as clouding of vigilance or suppression of muscular tone is to be avoided. Though intrathecal administration of Baclofen is not a particularly invasive procedure and its effect is reversible, the method is not devoid of risks. Factors, which at present limit this type of management of spasticity, are the lack of specific antagonist for Baclofen, unknown pharmacokinetics in the cerebrospinal fluid (half lifetime, distribution), the lack of toxicological data after long-term administration, and lack of studies concerning the stability of Baclofen in ports and implantable pumps. For these reasons, it is necessary to survey patients very closely.

The dose that is effective for 8 hours is usually determined during the period of testing. After implantation, depending on whether the drug is administered by intermittent bolus injection or continuous infusion, the initial dosage for 24 hours is twice the dose that is effective for 8 hours. In the first weeks of chronic administration of the drug, the dose was progressively increased by 10 to 20% until stabilization of the effect required was achieved.

There is an obvious advantage of using an implantable and programmable, flexible system such as D.A.S. (Medronic) over intermittent bolus application. Permanent intrathecal infusion with microdoses of Baclofen assures homogeneous and continuous reduction of spasticity. Constant activation of medullary receptors is superior to discontinuous effects produced by intermittent bolus injections. However, routine use of implantable systems is still very limited. The reasons are the high costs and lack of uniform systems. D.A.S. intrathecal pump for administration of Baclofen is at present in the initial phase of investigation in the United States and in the process of evaulation by the F.D.A.

In order to fill the gap between the simple implantable ports and sophisticated implantable micropumps, which are still in the phase of evaluation, we started to use the SECOR system of Cordis. Implantable reservoir has a volume of 12 mL, and boluses of 0.1 mL can be delivered by mechanical external activation. Once the daily therapeutic dose is established, the appropriate concentration of solution is chosen and multiple boluses can be administered over 24 hours. Thus, for example, if a patient requires 100 µg of Baclofen per day, the solution has a concentration of 200 µg/mL and 5 boluses are given over a period of 24 hours.

Intrathecal administration of Baclofen seems to be superior to other neurosurgical techniques, such as selective posteriod thoracolumbar or cervical radicotomy and more effective than conservative techniques such as neurostimulation of posterior columns or cerebellar cortex.[6,12] Three of our patients treated successfully with intrathecal Baclofen have had successful trial of cervical medullary stimulation.

Finally, in the selection of patients for chronic administration of Baclofen, we have had the opportunity to compare the effect with that of morphine and midazolam. Morphine acts through activation of mu receptors of the posterior columns (substantia gelatinosa). The effect of morphine is dose-dependant, stereospecific, segmental, reversable by administration of naloxone, and selective upon nociception and polysynaptic reflexes. There is no modification of motoricity and monosynaptic reflexes. Willer and Russell[15] demonstrated the mechanism of reaction of morphine in voluntary paraplegic patients. Intravenous morphine (0.2 to 0.3 mg/kg) caused prolonged depression of nocicpetive reflexes without modification of monosynaptic reflexes. The author found a significant reduction of spasticity of medullary origin among his patients. Intrathecal morphine is widely used in the treatment of chronic pain. It has also been used successfully by other authors[3,13] for a reduction of spasticity in paraplegic patients. The effect was obtained with the intrathecal administration of 1 mg of morphine, resulting in a reduction of spasticity within 24 hours. Erickson et al.[3] implanted a constant infusion pump (Infusaid) in eight patients, of whom six were guadriplegic after spinal trauma, and obtained durable, good results with a follow-up period of 1 to 17 months. Administered dosages were 2 and 4 mg per 24 hours respectively. In our patients, we have used a dose of 2.5 and 5 mg per 24 hours respectively, and we were able to register, clinically, a global diminution of spasticity. In two patients, however, within 2 to 3 months, progressive lessening of effect was observed and due to the tolerance, we were obliged to replace morphine by Baclofen.

Midazolam is a water-soluble benzodiazepine which can be administered by intrathecal route; it is physically and chemically stable and contains no additional substances. Müller[7] used midazolam epidurally following his experimental studies in animals. He reported that boluses of 3 to 4 mg produced a therapeutic effect on spasticity of two to four hours' duration; the biological half-time of midazolam is approximately two hours. Increase of dosage did not produce any additional therapeutic effect and caused somnolence. Continuous administration to obtain a therapeutic effect requires a release of 1 to 1.5 mg/hour, and this can cause progressive somnolence. In our experience, we obtained similar results, and were able to confirm the efficiency of midazolam on spasticity; however, the effect was always less pronounced than that of Baclofen and also morphine. Out of the three substances, Baclofen appeared to be the most effective, but its intrathecal administration requires a precise dosage and regular and close surveillance because of the lack of the appropriate antagonist.

In summary, we can conclude that intrathecal administration of Baclofen via the lumbar route is very effective in the control of incapacitating spasticity. The main advantages are reversibility and selectivity of the procedure, for it can normalize the muscular tone without causing modification of the residual motoricity. Furthermore, the procedure is not invasive. The difficulties of the method are connected with the individual variability of the effect, and it is necessary to determine precisely the dose according to the individual patient. Continuous microperfusion is superior to the intermittent bolus administration. The development of this method focused on the biotechnological and neuropharmacological aspects. In the first instance, it is necessary to develop programmable implantable pumps with a sufficient volume reserve, security, and an acceptable price. On the other hand, it is necessary to understand better the intrathecal pharmacokinetics of Baclofen and to find a specific antagonist, giving this method the potential of acquiring a major role in the treatment of spasticity.

## References


1. Bowery NG, Hill DR, Hudson AL. (1980). Baclofen decreases neurotransmitter release at a novel GABA receptor. *Nature* 283:92−94.
2. Bowery NG. (1982). Baclofen: 10 years on. *TIPS* pp 400−403.
3. Erickson DL, Blacklock JB, Michaelson M, Sperling KB, Lo JN. (1985). Control of spasticity by implantable continuous flow morphine pump. *Neurosurgery* 16:215−217.
4. Knutsson E, Lindblom U, Martensson A. (1974). Plasma and cerebrospinal fluid levels of Baclofen (Lioresal) at optimal therapeutic responses in spastic pareses. *J Neurol Sci* 23:473−484.
5. Kroin JS, Penn RD, Beissenger RL. (1984). Reduced spinal reflexes following intrathecal baclofen in the rabbit. *Exp Brain Res* 54:191−194.
6. Lazorthes Y. (1984). Chronic cerebellar cortex stimulation for grades spastic cerebal palsy patients. In: Davis R, Bloedel JR (eds): *Cerebellar Stimulation for Spasticity and Seizures.* CRC Press, pp 217−220.
7. Müller H. (1984). Spinal benzodiazepines for treatment of spasticity. Presented at Symposium on Implantable Pumps, Isle of Palms, South Carolina, September 19−22.
8. Penn RD, Kroin JS. (1984). Intrathecal baclofen alleviates spinal cord spasticity. *Lancet* 1:1078.
9. Penn RD, Kroin JS. (1985). Continuous intrathecal baclofen for severe spasticity. *Lancet* 11:125−127.
10. Price GW, Wilkin GP, Turnbull MJ, Bowery NG. (1984). Are baclofen sensitive GABA-B receptors present on primary afferent terminals of the spinal cord? *Nature* 307:71−74.

11. Sedan R, Lazorthes Y. (1978). La neurostimulation électrique théra-
    peutique. *Neurochirurgie* (suppl 1) 24:1—125.
12. Siegfried J, Lazorthes Y. (1985). La neurochirurgie fonctionnelle de
    l'infirmité motrice d'origine cérébrale. *Neurochirurgie* (suppl 1) 31:
    1—118.
13. Struppler A. (1983). Epidural morphine in spasticity (case report).
    Congress endorphines, neurohormones and transmitters. Garmisch-
    Partenkirchen (FRG), 20th June.
14. Waltz JM, Reynolds LO, Riklan M. (1981). Multi-lead spinal cord
    stimulation for control of motor disorders. *Appl Neurophysiol* 44:
    244—257.
15. Willer JL, Russel B. (1980). Evidence for direct spinal mechanisms in
    morphine induced inhibition of nociceptive reflexes in humans. *Brain
    Res* 187:212—215.

# Conclusion

The editors believe that the chapters in this volume present a good picture of the wide variety of investigative efforts going on internationally in the design and application of drug delivery systems. Examination of these efforts makes it clear that expansion of the market for drug delivery systems hinges on at least several factors: additional appropriate drugs and better sensor technology. Drug analog development and formulation of more potent, more soluble, and more stable agents would make implantable pumps applicable to situations where long-term therapy and precise drug levels are necessary. For example, an immunosuppressive agent as effective as cyclosporine but suitable for an implanted pump with a monthly refill schedule would have wide utility. Similarly, anti-inflammatory agents in arthritis having appropriate pharmaceutical properties might be used with implanted pumps for better effect. An agent equivalent to azidothymidine but pharmaceutically compatible with an implanted pump would lead to a large expansion of pump use in AIDS research and therapy. Unfortunately, to date little effort in the design of such agents has been expended by the pharmaceutical industry. Better sensor technology would provide an opportunity for true physiologic control. Reliable, implantable, long-term sensors/transducers would have obvious application in endocrinology and cardiology.

Opposing forces to advancement in drug delivery technology include the economic constraints of societies aiming to diminish medical costs and of device companies faced with long-term research investment with high risk for no guaranteed return. In certain areas, such as in endocrinology, molecular biology approaches may lead to transplantation of genes curing deficiency diseases, obviating the need (market) for advanced drug delivery systems.

It should prove interesting to participate in and observe the biotechnical revolution we are entering. Hopefully, the Cardiostim meeting and these volumes coming out of the drug delivery sessions of the Cardiostim meeting will provide a window on the state of the art of infusion technology and applications.

---

*From:* Ensminger WD, Selam JL (eds): *Infusion Systems in Medicine.* Mount Kisco, NY, Futura Publishing Co., Inc.,©1987.

# INDEX